4th Edition
CRASH COURSE

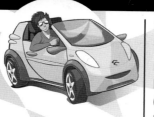

SERIES EDITOR:

Dan Horton-Szar

BSc(Hons) MBBS(Hons) MRCGP
Northgate Medical Practice
Canterbury
Kent, UK

FACULTY ADVISORS:

Naheed Khan

MA PhD FRCP
Consultant Neurologist
Kings College Hospital
London, UK

Katia Cikurel

BSc(Hons) MBBS MD FRCP
Consultant Neurologist
Kings College Hospital
London, UK

Neurology

Mahinda Yogarajah

BSc MBBS MRCP
Specialist Registrar in Neurology
St George's Hospital
London, UK

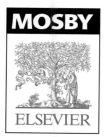

MOSBY

ELSEVIER

Edinburgh London New York Oxford Philadelphia St Louis Sydney Toronto 2015

Senior Content Strategist: Jeremy Bowes
Senior Content Development Specialist: Veronika Watkins / Clive Hewat
Project Manager: Andrew Riley
Design: Christian Bilbow

First edition 1999

Second edition 2006

Third edition 2009

Fourth edition 2013

Updated Fourth edition 2015

ISBN: 978-0-7234-3866-3

British Library Cataloguing in Publication Data
A catalogue record for this book is available from the British Library

Library of Congress Cataloging in Publication Data
A catalog record for this book is available from the Library of Congress

Notices
Knowledge and best practice in this field are constantly changing. As new research and experience broaden our understanding, changes in research methods, professional practices, or medical treatment may become necessary.

Practitioners and researchers must always rely on their own experience and knowledge in evaluating and using any information, methods, compounds, or experiments described herein. In using such information or methods they should be mindful of their own safety and the safety of others, including parties for whom they have a professional responsibility.

With respect to any drug or pharmaceutical products identified, readers are advised to check the most current information provided (i) on procedures featured or (ii) by the manufacturer of each product to be administered, to verify the recommended dose or formula, the method and duration of administration, and contraindications. It is the responsibility of practitioners, relying on their own experience and knowledge of their patients, to make diagnoses, to determine dosages and the best treatment for each individual patient, and to take all appropriate safety precautions.

To the fullest extent of the law, neither the Publisher nor the authors, contributors, or editors, assume any liability for any injury and/or damage to persons or property as a matter of products liability, negligence or otherwise, or from any use or operation of any methods, products, instructions, or ideas contained in the material herein.

your source for books,
journals and multimedia
in the health sciences

www.elsevierhealth.com

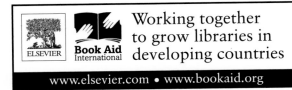

Working together
to grow libraries in
developing countries

www.elsevier.com • www.bookaid.org

The
Publisher's
policy is to use
**paper manufactured
from sustainable forests**

Printed in China

Last digit is the print line: 10 9 8 7 6 5 4 3 2 1

Neurology

First edition authors:

Anish Bahra

Katia Cikurel

Second and third edition author:

Christopher Turner

The *Crash Course* series first published in 1997 and now, 16 years on, we are still going strong. Medicine never stands still, and the work of keeping this series relevant for today's students is an ongoing process. These new editions build on the success of the previous titles and incorporate new and revised material, to keep the series up-to-date with current guidelines for best practice, and recent developments in medical research and pharmacology.

We always listen to feedback from our readers, through focus groups and student reviews of the *Crash Course* titles. For the new editions we have completely re-written our self-assessment material to keep up with today's 'single-best answer' and 'extended matching question' formats. The artwork and layout of the titles has also been largely re-worked to make it easier on the eye during long sessions of revision.

Despite fully revising the books with each edition, we hold fast to the principles on which we first developed the series. *Crash Course* will always bring you all the information you need to revise in compact, manageable volumes that integrate basic medical science and clinical practice. The books still maintain the balance between clarity and conciseness, and provide sufficient depth for those aiming at distinction. The authors are medical students and junior doctors who have recent experience of the exams you are now facing, and the accuracy of the material is checked by a team of faculty advisors from across the UK.

Dr Dan Horton-Szar

Neurological symptoms account for a high proportion of consultations in general practice, 20% of acute medical admissions and many complications of trauma, critical illness, anaesthesia, and surgery. Diagnosis is primarily clinical, based on a careful history and physical examination. Subsequent investigations can only supplement and never replace the process of clinical assessment. For this reason, all medical students and doctors need to acquire and maintain some basic skills in neurology. This book aims to provide a logical and simple approach to understanding the fundamental concepts that underlie most common neurological diseases. In this fourth edition the content has been entirely reorganized and updated to reflect the exciting advances in the diagnosis and management of neurological conditions. The first part of the book deals with the history, examination and investigations relevant to neurology. The second part of the book deals with the analysis and differential diagnosis of common presenting symptoms such as headache, dizziness, speech disturbance and limb weakness. In the final part of the book, the clinical features, investigation and management of specific neurological disorders are discussed in more detail. Where appropriate, NICE and national guidelines are incoporated into the text. Illustrations and diagrams have been revised to emphasize the most important concepts, and comprehension and communication boxes have been rationalized, to focus the reader on essential topics and difficult clinical scenarios. Finally, the self-assessment section at the end of the book has been completely rewritten, and now contains a mixture of single best answer and extended-matching questions. We are confident that this fourth edition of *Crash Course Neurology* will provide not only a solid foundation for medical students preparing for exams and postgraduates working towards MRCP, but also an excellent reference book for those working in hospital medicine and general practice.

Mahinda Yogarajah, Katia Cikurel and Naheed Khan

Acknowledgements

Thanks go to Katia Cikurel and Naheed Khan who were a patient source of guidance, and feedback.

Thanks also to Dr M Mirfenderesky for help with the chapter on infections of the nervous system and to Dr Naheed Khan who re-wrote the Movement Disorders and amended the Parkinson's Disease chapters.

Mahinda Yogarajah

Dedication

To Appa and Amma who made all things possible.

To M, for putting up with me.

Mahinda Yogarajah

Contents

Series editor foreword v

Preface vii

Acknowledgements ix

Dedication xi

Part I: History, Examination and Common Investigations 1

1. Taking a history 3
Structure of the history 3

2. The neurological examination 7
Mental state and higher cerebral functions . . 7
Speech 8
Gait 10
Cranial nerves 10
The motor system 18
The sensory system 23
General examination 24

3. Further investigations 25
Routine investigations 25
Neurophysiological investigations 25
Imaging of the nervous system 29

Part II: The Patient Presents With 31

4. Disorders of higher cerebral function . . . 33
Frontal lobe 33
Parietal lobe 35
Temporal lobe 36
Dysphasia 37
Occipital lobe 37

5. Disturbances of consciousness 39
Transient loss of consciousness 39
Driving and episodes of disturbances of consciousness 42
Coma 42
Brainstem death 47

6. Headache 49
History 51
Examination 52

7. Disorders of smell and taste 53
Differential diagnosis 53
Examination 54
Investigations 55

8. Visual impairment 57
The anatomical path of light stimulation . . 57
Blood supply to the visual pathway 58
Clinical features to aid localization of a lesion 59
Differential diagnosis of visual loss 60
Optic atrophy 62

9. Disorders of the pupils and eye movements 63
Pupillary reflexes 63
Differential diagnosis of pupil disorders . . 64
Disorders of eye movements 66

10. Facial sensory loss and weakness 75
The trigeminal nerve 75
Differential diagnosis of facial sensory loss . 75
Facial nerve 78

11. Deafness, tinnitus, dizziness and vertigo . . 81
Deafness and tinnitus 81
The auditory system 81
Differential diagnosis of deafness 81
Differential diagnosis of tinnitus 83
The vestibular system 84
Differential diagnosis of dizziness and vertigo 84
Investigations for vertigo 86

12. Dysarthria, dysphonia and dysphagia . . . 89
Definitions 89
Dysarthria 89
Dysphagia 91
Dysphonia 91

Contents

13. **Cerebellar dysfunction** **93**
    Clinical features of cerebellar dysfunction . 93
    Localization of a cerebellar lesion 95

14. **Movement disorders** **97**
    The anatomical basis and classification of
      movement disorders 97
    The hyperkinetic movement disorders:
      tremor and dystonia. 97
    Dystonia 99
    The hyperkinetic movement disorders:
      chorea, tics and myoclonus 101

15. **Limb weakness** **103**
    Neuroanatomy. 103
    Terminology 104
    Upper motor neuron weakness 104
    Upper motor neuron syndromes 105
    Lower motor neuron weakness 107
    Lower motor neuron syndromes 108
    Disorders of the neuromuscular junction . . 110
    Myopathy 110

16. **Limb sensory symptoms** **113**
    Dorsal (posterior) column pathway 113
    Spinothalamic pathway. 113
    Trophic skin changes and ulcers 113
    Sensory syndromes. 114

17. **Disorders of gait.** **119**
    Practical approach to the assessment
      of gait 119
    Differential diagnosis of disorders of gait . . 120

Part III: Diseases and Disorders. . . . **123**

18. **Dementia** **125**
    Definition 125
    Differential diagnoses 125
    Epidemiology 125
    General clinical features 125
    History 126
    Examination 126
    Investigations 126
    Management 127
    Primary neurodegenerative dementias . . . 128

Vasculitis 130
Dementia as a part of other degenerative
  diseases 130
Pseudodementia 130

19. **Epilepsy** **131**
    Definitions. 131
    Classification of seizures 131
    Epidemiology 131
    Aetiology 131
    Clinical features 133
    History and investigations to aid
      diagnosis. 134
    Differential diagnoses 135
    Drug treatment 135
    Status epilepticus. 137
    Neurosurgical treatment of epilepsy 137
    Mortality of epilepsy 137
    Driving and epilepsy 138

20. **Headache and craniofacial pains** **139**
    Tension-type headache. 139
    Migraine 139
    Cluster headache 140
    Other neurological causes of headache
      and craniofacial pain 141
    Non-neurological causes of headache
      and craniofacial pain 142

21. **Parkinson's disease and other
    extrapyramidal disorders** **145**
    Akinetic–rigid syndromes 145
    Neuroleptic-induced movement
      disorders 150
    Restless legs syndrome 151

22. **Cranial nerve lesions.** **153**
    Olfactory nerve (first, I) 153
    Optic nerve (second, II) 153
    Oculomotor (third, III), trochlear (fourth,
      IV) and abducens nerves (sixth, VI) . . . 154
    Trigeminal nerve (fifth, V) 155
    Facial nerve (seventh, VII) 156
    Vestibulocochlear nerve (eighth, VIII) . . . 157
    Lower cranial nerves (glossopharyngeal,
      vagus, accessory and hypoglossal) 158

23. **Diseases affecting the spinal cord (myelopathy)** **159**
  Anatomy 159
  Major pathways within the spinal cord. . . 159
  Causes of spinal cord disease 161

24. **Motor neuron disease** **169**
  Types and clinical features of motor neuron disease 169
  Pathogenesis 170
  Differential diagnosis. 171
  Diagnosis 171
  Treatment. 171

25. **Radiculopathy and plexopathy** **173**
  Anatomy 173
  Radiculopathy (spinal nerve root lesions). . 173
  Plexopathies 175

26. **Disorders of the peripheral nerves** . . . **177**
  Anatomy 177
  Definitions of neuropathies 177
  Symptoms of neuropathy. 178
  Investigation of peripheral neuropathy. . . 179
  Specific neuropathies. 180

27. **Disorders of the neuromuscular junction.** . **189**
  Myasthenia gravis 189
  Lambert–eaton myasthenic syndrome . . . 191
  Other myasthenic syndromes 192
  Botulinum toxin 192

28. **Disorders of skeletal muscle** **193**
  Anatomy 193
  Clinical features of muscle disease (myopathy). 193
  Investigation of muscle disease 194
  Specific diseases 195

29. **Vascular diseases of the nervous system.** . **201**
  Cerebrovascular disease 201
  Intracranial haemorrhage 209
  Cerebrovascular involvement in vasculitis. . 211
  Cerebral venous thrombosis. 211
  Dissection 211
  Vascular disease of the spinal cord 212

30. **Neuro-oncology** **215**
  Types of intracranial tumour 215
  Clinical features of intracranial tumours . . 216
  Investigations 218
  Treatment 219
  Prognosis 219
  Neurological complications of cancer . . . 220

31. **Infections of the nervous system** **223**
  General conditions 223
  Specific organisms and their associated diseases 229

32. **Multiple sclerosis** **237**
  Epidemiology 237
  Pathogenesis 237
  Pathology 237
  Clinical features 237
  Differential diagnosis 239
  Investigations 239
  Diagnosis 240
  Management 240
  Other central demyelinating diseases . . . 241

33. **Systemic disease and the nervous system** **243**
  Endocrine disorders 243
  Haematological disorders 244
  Gastrointestinal disorders 244
  Renal disorders 245
  Vasculitides and connective tissue disorders 245
  Cardiac disorders. 245
  Other multisystem diseases 245

34. **The effects of vitamin deficiencies and toxins on the nervous system** **247**
  Vitamin deficiencies 247
  Toxins. 248

35. **Hereditary conditions affecting the nervous system** **251**
  The neurocutaneous syndromes. 251
  Hereditary ataxias 253
  Inherited neuropathies 253
  Inborn errors of metabolism 253

Contents

Self-Assessment 255

Single best answer questions (SBAs) 257

Extended-matching questions
(EMQs) 267

SBA answers. 273

EMQ answers 283

Objective structured clinical examination
(OSCE) stations 285

Glossary. 289

Index 293

PART I
HISTORY, EXAMINATION AND COMMON INVESTIGATIONS

1. Taking a history..........................3

2. The neurological examination....7

3. Further investigations..............25

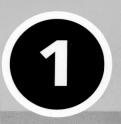

The patient's neurological history often provides more diagnostic information than the examination or investigations and it is therefore important to do it well. Many common conditions, such as headache and epilepsy, are diagnosed solely from the clinical history. It is important to gain the patient's trust and to begin to develop a rapport at the initial contact, so that the patient feels comfortable talking about illnesses that might be embarrassing or stigmatizing:

- Introduce yourself and explain who you are.
- Ask for permission to talk to, and examine the patient.
- Ask the patient's age and occupation.
- Ask whether the patient is right- or left-handed (if you do not ask this at the beginning, you might forget). Handedness is important because the left hemisphere controls language in right-handed patients, and in about 75% of left-handed or ambidextrous patients.

Within the first few minutes of the consultation you should be able to make some inferences about the patient's mood and cognitive state:

- Does the patient respond appropriately (indicating probable preservation of important higher mental functioning)?
- Does he or she appear to be depressed (which can either be part of the patient's neurological condition or might indicate a reaction to it) or behaving inappropriately (as in patients who have frontal lobe dysfunction)?
- Is the patient's speech normal?

STRUCTURE OF THE HISTORY

The presenting complaint

Consider the presenting complaint (PC) from the patient's point of view. Ask:

- What is the main problem?
- What was it that caused you to go to your doctor/come to the hospital?

When presenting the history to others, use the patient's language (e.g. 'This woman complains of seeing double') not the medical terminology (e.g. 'This woman complains of horizontal diplopia').

History of the presenting complaint

Establish the history of the presenting complaint (HPC) by asking:

- When did the patient first notice it?
- Was the onset sudden (over seconds or minutes), subacute (over hours or days), or insidious and gradual (over weeks, months or years)? The time course of onset of symptoms gives an important insight into the underlying pathological process. For example, in a 40-year-old woman with unilateral visual loss, sudden onset over seconds might suggest amaurosis fugax or vascular aetiology; onset over 10–15 minutes followed by a headache might suggest migraine; onset over 1 to 2 days associated with pain on eye movement and resolution over 6 weeks would suggest optic neuritis and an inflammatory aetiology.
- Is the symptom episodic, constant and progressive, or constant with fluctuations in intensity?
- Has it worsened, improved, or stayed the same since?
- What is the character of the symptom (e.g. headache may be throbbing, stabbing or pressure-like) and its distribution (unilateral, bilateral, frontal, occipital, etc.)?
- Is there anything that makes it better (e.g. medicines, sleep, exercise) or worse (e.g. movement, coughing, posture)?
- Are there associated symptoms that may help localize the cause of the symptoms? For example in a patient with bilateral upper motor neuron leg weakness, associated urinary incontinence and a sensory level would localize the cause to the spinal cord.
- Are there associated symptoms that are recognized as part of a particular syndrome? For example in a patient with parkinsonian gait, there may also be an associated tremor, and change in hand writing.
- Has the patient ever had other neurological symptoms in the past? These might be related (e.g. an episode of transient visual loss 5 years previously in a young woman now complaining of difficulty in walking is indicative of possible multiple sclerosis).
- Are there relevant risk factors? For example in a patient presenting with a likely stroke, ask about stroke risk factors such as smoking, diabetes, hypertension, and a history of atrial fibrillation.

Once the HPC has been elucidated, it is useful to ask general questions pertaining to neurological dysfunction including:

- problems with double or blurred vision
- difficulties in speech, swallowing, chewing
- weakness or sensory symptoms in the limbs
- sphincter function (bowels, bladder, sexual function)
- a history of headaches
- a history of dizziness, blackouts or falls
- difficulties with memory or other cognitive functions
- further questions pertaining to the HPC will relate to the differential diagnosis of the main complaint, the most common of which are outlined in Part 2 of the book.

Past medical history

Some clinicians prefer to take the past medical history (PMH) before considering the presenting complaint because there might be important background information. The following may be relevant in neurological cases:

- Birth history and childhood development, e.g. motor and verbal milestones
- Infections and seizures during childhood
- Head injuries
- Hypertension, ischaemic heart disease, rheumatic fever
- Diabetes
- A systemic disorder, e.g. systemic lupus erythematosus.

Drug history

To determine the drug history (DH), find out from the patient:

- is he or she is taking any medicines now, or have any been taken for some time in the past
- are there any known drug allergies.

Prior, and current exposure to drugs can be important in several conditions. For example, movement disorders can occur following phenothiazine exposure, or some peripheral neuropathies can be caused by previous chemotherapeutic agent exposure.

Review of systems

Review of systems (ROS) should include questions relating to symptoms such as:

- Gastrointestinal: appetite, weight loss or gain, swallowing, change in bowel function
- Cardiovascular: chest pain, breathlessness, palpitations, claudication
- Respiratory: cough, breathlessness

- Genitourinary: bladder function, impotence, sexual function
- Musculoskeletal: joint pain, stiffness
- Systemic symptoms: weight loss, appetite decline, lethargy, night sweats.

Family history

Many neurological disorders are familial and have a genetic basis. To determine the family history (FH), find out from patients:

- if there are any 'family illnesses', especially in relatives under the age of 60 years
- if their parents, siblings, and children are alive and well and, if not, what they died from and at what age
- if their parents could possibly be related, i.e. a consanguineous marriage. This is especially important in autosomal recessive conditions when related patients may carry the same defective gene and pass both to their children.

Social history

The social history (SH) is important, because the impact of the neurological problem will vary according to the social circumstances of the individual. The detail necessary in the social history will depend on the neurological problem. For example, in a patient with difficulty walking it will be important to have detailed knowledge of home circumstances (e.g. number of floors, number of stairs, etc.), whereas in someone with headache such knowledge is not necessary. To determine the SH, ask the patient about:

- home circumstances: house or flat, stairs, help from Social Services
- smoking history
- alcohol intake (units/week): is there a past history of heavy alcohol consumption?
- diet (vegetarian or vegan)
- sexual history or orientation: this might be relevant in certain cases.

COMMUNICATION

Sometimes it is critical to acquire a collateral history in patients. For example, in patients who have had episodes of altered awareness or loss of consciousness, a witness account of events will be critical to differentiate between seizures or syncope. Similarly, in patients with cognitive decline it is important to also get a history from family members to aid diagnosis.

COMMUNICATION

The history is the most important part of the neurological assessment, and the time course of the symptoms will often given an insight into the underlying pathological process. The history should be used to construct diagnostic hypotheses that are then tested using the neurological examination. The history should also be used to put the patient's neurological presentation into the context of their past medical history, family history and social circumstances.

Summary

When presenting the history to colleagues (a very important skill), you need to spend several minutes organizing your thoughts and the structure of the history. It is best to start with a general summary such as: 'Miss Randolph is a 40-year-old administrator who complains of numbness in the feet.' The HPC, PMH and ROS should then be described. You do not have to mention all negative points, but it is worth pointing out those that are important (e.g. 'She has no history of diabetes' in a patient who has a peripheral neuropathy).

List the patient's medications and any side-effects or benefits they perceive to be obtained from them.

Describe the FH, if relevant; if it is not, state: 'There is no relevant family history'.

Describe important social points: 'She drinks only moderate amounts of alcohol and has never smoked'.

You will then move on to your examination findings.

The neurological examination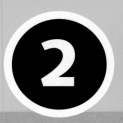

The neurological examination consists of the following elements which should be carried out in sequence:

1. Assessment of mental state and higher cerebral functions
2. Assessment of speech
3. Assessment of gait
4. Testing of the cranial nerves
5. Testing of motor function
6. Testing of sensory function
7. Examination of related structures.

MENTAL STATE AND HIGHER CEREBRAL FUNCTIONS

Consciousness

Consciousness is the state of being aware of self and the environment. A number of ill-defined terms are used to describe different levels of consciousness:

- **Alert:** full wakefulness and immediate and appropriate responsiveness. The patient is orientated in person, time, and place.
- **Confusion:** the inability to think with the usual speed and clarity. There may be lack of attention, disorientation in time and place, and impairment of memory. Delirium is a confusional state characterized by hyperactivity. The patient may be agitated, excited and anxious with visual hallucinations.
- **Obtundation:** the patient is drowsy and indifferent to the environment, but responsive to verbal stimuli.
- **Stupor:** the patient is unconscious, but rousable when stimulated.
- **Coma:** the patient is unaware of self and the environment and is not rousable.

The terms described above are imprecise and often used differently by different clinicians. The level of consciousness is therefore more objectively assessed using the Glasgow Coma Scale (see Ch. 5).

Appearance and behaviour

Assessment of the patient's mental state begins as soon as you meet the patient. The physical appearance can be helpful. Demented patients may look bewildered but unconcerned, or apathetic and withdrawn. Self-neglect is common but may be masked by caring relatives. The patient's response to your questions during the history taking is important in terms of assessing his or her comprehension and whether he or she retains insight into the problem.

Affect

- Does the patient seem depressed?
- Are there any signs of delusions or hallucinations which can be seen in dementia or confusional states?
- Loss of interest, euphoria or social disinhibition may be signs of frontal lobe dysfunction. Emotional behaviour such as aggression and anger may arise from damage to the limbic system.
- Emotional lability, such as uncontrollable laughing or crying, should prompt further examination to look for upper motor neuron signs associated with a pseudobulbar palsy.

Cognitive function

The clarity with which a patient presents their history, and cooperates with the examination may convey a sense of their intellectual capacity. This should be compared with one's own estimate of their pre-morbid ability given their job and educational history. If after taking the history there is no suggestion of a defect of higher cerebral function, then further testing is not required. However, if there is any doubt, more extensive testing with for example, the Mini-mental State Examination, should be carried out. In addition the history should also be corroborated with independent witnesses if possible.

Mini-mental State Examination

The Mini-mental State Examination is a screening test for cognitive function (Fig. 2.1):

- **Orientation** of person, time, and place establishes full awareness of self and the environment. Further testing requires the patient to be alert.
- **Registration and recall** tests immediate and recent memory, respectively. Remote memory may be tested by asking about memories of childhood, work, or marriage. These need corroboration with

Fig. 2.1 Mini-mental State Examination
Orientation
1. What is the year, season, date, month, day? (one point for each correct answer) 2. Where are we? Country, county, town, hospital, floor? (one point for each answer)
Registration
3. Name three objects, taking 1 second to say each. Then ask the patient to name all three. One point for each correct answer. Repeat the question until the patient learns all three, e.g. 'bus', 'rose', 'door'.
Attention and calculation
4. Serial sevens. One point for each correct answer. Stop after five answers. Alternative: spell 'world' backwards
Recall
5. Ask for names of the three objects asked in question 3. One point for each correct answer
Language
6. Point to a pencil and a watch. Ask the patient to name them for you. One point for each correct answer 7. Ask the patient to repeat 'No ifs, ands, or buts'. One point 8. Ask the patient to follow a three-stage command: 'Take the paper in your right hand; fold the paper in half; put the paper on the floor with your left hand'. Three points 9. Ask the patient to read and obey the following: CLOSE YOUR EYES. (Write this in large letters.) One point 10. Ask the patient to write a sentence of his or her own choice. (The sentence must contain a subject and an object and make some sense). Ignore spelling errors when scoring. One point
Constructional/spatial
11. Ask the patient to copy two intersecting pentagons with equal sides. Give one point if all the sides and angles are preserved and if the intersecting sides form a quadrangle Maximum score = 30 points

family or friends to be certain the details are correct. Verbal memory can be tested by asking the patient to remember a sentence or short story and to recall it 15 minutes later. Visual memory can be assessed by asking the patient to memorize three objects on a table and recall them after 15 minutes.

- **Attention and calculation** can be tested by asking the patient to spell a five-letter word backwards and to subtract 7 from 100 and continue to subtract 7 from each answer obtained; if the latter is too complex for the patient's pre-morbid calculation skills, simple arithmetic can be used.
- **Language** examination tests comprehension of speech and written language and includes tests for dysphasia, dyslexia and dysgraphia.
- **Constructional** ability.

The maximum score is 30. Scores of less than 25 suggest the presence of cognitive impairment. Formal psychometric testing should be performed for all patients suspected of having impaired cognition.

SPEECH

The content and articulation of speech should be evident when taking the history. If there is any suggestion

that it is abnormal, further examination is necessary. Speech production is organized at three levels:

1. Phonation
2. Articulation
3. Language production.

Phonation: dysphonia

Phonation is the production of sounds as the air passes through the vocal cords and resonating sound boxes. A disorder of this process reflects either local vocal cord pathology, or an abnormality of the nerve supply via the vagus nerve, and is called dysphonia. The hoarse voice of someone with laryngitis, or the nasal voice of someone with a cold, are common, non-neurological causes of dysphonia.

Assessment

Speech will have already been heard during the history taking. Patients who have dysphonia may present with reduced speech volume and the voice may sound hoarse or husky. Aphonia is the inability to produce sound. Coughing may also be impaired in patients with dysphonia due to vocal cord palsy, because this action requires normal vocal cord function. Coughing should be tested in patients in whom there is a possibility of dysphonia. The patient should also be asked to say a sustained 'eeeee'. If it fatigues and cannot be sustained, consider myasthenia gravis.

Articulation: dysarthria

Voice production requires the coordination of breathing, vocal cords, larynx, palate, tongue and lips. A disorder of this process is called dysarthria, and can reflect problems at any one or more parts of this system. Lesions of the basal ganglia or cerebellum tend to disturb the rhythm of speech. In contrast, lesions of the cranial nerves critical to voice production produce disturbance of certain parts of speech but the rhythm is normal.

Assessment

Articulation is assessed from the patient's spontaneous speech during history taking and also, if necessary, by asking a series of additional questions such as the patient's name and address, what he or she had for breakfast and what he or she has been doing recently. Ask the patient to repeat a series of phrases: 'baby hippopotamus' or 'British Constitution' tests labial (lip) sounds, 'yellow lorry' or 'West Register street' tests lingual (tongue) sounds. More complicated phrases such as 'Peter Piper picked a peck of pickled pepper' can be used to test cerebellar function, which is necessary to coordinate the muscles of speech articulation. The characteristics of the speech can be gained from these phrases and localization of the site of the lesion may be possible based on the type of dysarthria and confirmed by additional signs on formal neurological examination (see Ch. 12).

Although dysarthria can be caused by neurological disorders affecting the muscles of the soft palate, lips, tongue and larynx, a non-neurological cause (such as an inflammatory or infective process affecting the mucosal surfaces) might be responsible and should be sought in the first instance. Ill-fitting or absent dentures can also cause the patient to sound dysarthric.

Dysarthria may result from a lesion of the:

- **upper motor neuron** (pseudobulbar palsy): spasticity of the tongue, palate and mouth produces a slow, high-pitched and forced and often described as 'hot potato' speech' because the patient talks as if they have a hot potato in their mouth
- **lower motor neuron** (bulbar palsy): paralysis of the soft palate causes slurred and indistinct speech, with nasal intonation due to the nasal escape of air; labial (lip) and lingual (tongue) sounds are affected
- **basal ganglia**: slow, low-pitched and monotonous (akinetic-rigid syndromes); loud, harsh and with variable intonation (chorea and myoclonus); loud, slow and indistinct consonants (athetoid)
- **cerebellum**: incoordination of the muscular action necessary for speech causes slow and slurred, scanning (equal emphasis on each syllable) or 'staccato' quality if there is also involvement of the corticobulbar tracts
- **muscle and neuromuscular junction**: similar to those of a bulbar palsy. In myasthenia gravis, there might be a deterioration in the quality of speech (fatigability) during prolonged speech or over the course of the day.

Language production: dysphasia

Language production is the organization of phonemes into words and sentences. It is controlled by the speech centres in the dominant hemisphere (Broca's and Wernicke's areas). A disorder of this process is called dysphasia.

Assessment

To assess language production:

- establish the patient's handedness: dysphasia is a feature of dominant-hemisphere dysfunction. The left hemisphere is dominant in over 95% of right-handed and about 75% of left-handed individuals
- listen to the patient's spontaneous speech, assessing its fluency and content
- assess the patient's comprehension by observing his or her response to simple commands, e.g. 'Open your mouth', 'Look up to the ceiling'. Then try more complicated 2- or 3-stage commands, e.g. 'With your right index finger touch your nose and then your left ear'
- assess the patient's ability to name familiar objects: use your wristwatch (face, hands, strap, buckle). Start with easy objects, before moving onto objects that are used less frequently. Ask the patient to name all the animals he/she can think of (normal >18 in 1 minute), or all the words beginning with a particular letter (normal >12 in 1 minute for letter 's')
- assess the patient's ability to repeat sentences, e.g. 'No ifs, ands, or buts'
- assess the patient's ability to read and write.

An **expressive dysphasia** arises from a lesion of **Broca's** area in the dominant frontal lobe (see Ch. 4). The speech is non-fluent and hesitant, but comprehension mostly intact. The speech may be 'telegraphic' with loss of the conjunctions and articles. Repetition is better than spontaneous speech. The patient has difficulty finding the correct words and often produces an incorrect word. Writing is often also poor. Patients retain insight into their language disturbance, which can therefore frustrate them.

A **receptive dysphasia** arises from a lesion of **Wernicke's** area in the posterior superior temporal lobe and probably also the adjacent parietal lobe (see Ch. 4). The speech is fluent but the words are partly incorrect, and related to the intended word (paraphrasia), or newly created (neologisms). The patient often has poor comprehension of the spoken word and has poor handwriting. The language is therefore mostly unintelligible (as it cannot be internally checked), but the patient is often unaware of the problem. Writing is abnormal, and often there is difficulty understanding the written word (dyslexia).

Conduction dysphasia occurs when there is damage to the tract, called the arcuate fasciculus, that joins Wernicke's and Broca's regions. It causes a syndrome similar to receptive aphasia with fluent speech, abnormal and new words, and loss of repetition but preservation of comprehension.

Nominal dysphasia is the inability to name objects. It can occur following recovery from other types of dysphasia and occasionally as part of a dementia.

Global and mixed dysphasia is often seen in clinical practice where both receptive and expressive defects coexist or only some of the features are seen from each.

The clinical features of the different types of dysphasia are summarized in Figure 2.2.

GAIT

Normal gait requires input from the motor, somatosensory, visual, cerebellar and vestibular systems. Assessing the gait carefully can therefore provide the examiner with a lot of information about each of these systems, which can be examined in detail later in the examination. The assessment and abnormalities of gait are described in Chapter 17.

CRANIAL NERVES

The brainstem is a phylogenetically ancient organ that subserves control of basic functions such as breathing, cardiovascular function, consciousness and thermoregulation. It also acts as a pathway for tracts between the cerebrum and the spinal cord controlling movement and sensation. Finally, it is involved in movement and sensation of the head and neck. Examination of the brainstem provides important prognostic information in the unconscious patient and irreversible damage to the brainstem is the criterion for the legal definition of death.

Olfactory nerve (first, I)

To test the olfactory nerve, first ask the patient about any recent change in the sense of smell or taste. A characteristic-smelling object (e.g. peppermint, clove oil) is held under each nostril in turn while the other is occluded and the patient keeps the eyes closed. An individual who has intact olfaction can not only detect the smell but also discriminate and name it. The recommended special testing bottles are rarely available when needed and most clinicians perform preliminary assessment with nearby objects such as fruit, a coffee jar or cigarette packet. Avoid using irritating odours such as ammonia or camphor because these can non-specifically activate fifth nerve receptors in the nasal mucosa.

Unilateral loss of smell is usually asymptomatic. Bilateral loss of smell may be associated with an altered sensation of taste (dysgeusia or ageusia).

When examining patients who have anosmia, it is important to look carefully for frontal lobe signs and evidence of optic nerve or chiasmal damage, as these structures are anatomically close to the pathways that subserve smell.

The most common cause of impaired smell is pathology in the nasal passages or sinuses.

Fig. 2.2 Classification of dysphasia					
Type	**Lesion**	**Speech fluency**	**Speech content**	**Comprehension**	**Repetition**
Expressive	Broca's area	Non-fluent	Impaired	Normal	Variable
Nominal	Angular gyrus	Fluent	Impaired	Normal	Normal
Receptive	Wernicke's area	Fluent	Impaired	Impaired	Impaired
Conductive	Arcuate fasciculus	Fluent	Impaired	Normal	Impaired
Global	Frontal, parietal and temporal lobe	Non-fluent	Impaired	Impaired	Impaired

Optic nerve (second, II)

Visual acuity

Visual acuity (VA) is tested using a Snellen chart in a well-lit room. Seat or stand the patient 6 m from the chart. Small, hand-held Snellen charts can be read at a distance of 2 m (Fig. 2.3).

Correct the patient's refractive error with glasses or a pinhole. Ask the patient to cover each eye in turn with his or her palm, and find which line of print the patient can read comfortably. VA is expressed as the distance between the chart and the patient and the number of the smallest visible line on the chart. The numbers associated with each line on the chart correspond to the distance (in metres) at which a normal patient should be able to read that line of letters. So 6/6 is normal and 6/24 means that from 6 metres away the patient can only read letters that a normal individual can read from 24 m (Fig. 2.3). If the patient is unable to read characters of line 60 (VA less than 6/60), assess his or her ability to count your fingers at 1 m (VA:CF), see your hand movements (VA:HM), or perceive a torch light (VA:PL). If unable to perceive light (VA:NPL), then the patient is blind. The visual acuity is a measure of the integrity of central macular vision.

Colour vision

Colour vision is tested using Ishihara plates in a day-lit room. Test each eye separately. If at least 15 out of 17 plates are read correctly, colour vision can be regarded as normal. This test is designed principally to detect congenital colour vision defects, but is sensitive in detecting mild degrees of optic nerve dysfunction when the red colours are often lost first.

Visual fields

Sit about 1 m from the patient with your eyes at the same horizontal level. Start by testing for visual inattention (see Ch. 4). Ask the patient to look into your eyes; hold your hands halfway between you and the patient. Stimulate the patient's visual fields by moving each hand separately and then both hands together, and ask the patient to indicate which of your hands has moved each time.

In patients with a non-dominant parietal lobe lesion, a visual stimulus presented in isolation to the contralateral field is perceived, but it may be missed when a comparable stimulus is presented simultaneously to the ipsilateral field.

Visual fields are then examined by confrontation, during which you compare your own visual fields with the patient's on the assumption that yours are normal. The patient's visual field will match yours only if your head positions are exactly comparable and if your hand is exactly halfway between you and the patient. Visual fields in poorly cooperative patients are assessed by the response to visual threat (sudden, unexpected hand movement into the patient's visual field).

Peripheral fields

Examine each eye in turn. To test the patient's right visual field, ask the patient to cover his or her left eye with his or her left palm and to look into your left eye throughout the examination. Initially ask the patient if any part of your face is missing or distorted. Then cover your right eye with your right hand, and test the patient's peripheral field by bringing the moving fingers of your left hand into the upper and then the lower quadrants of the patient's temporal fields. Ask the patient to inform you as soon as he or she sees your

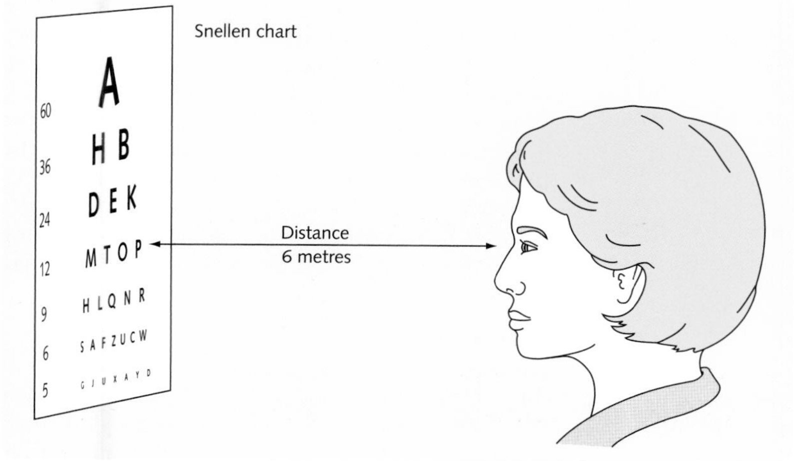

Fig. 2.3 Visual acuity. The patient is able to read line number 24 but not line number 12; visual acuity is therefore 6/24. If the patient could read only three out of the four letters on line number 24 then the visual acuity would be 6/24–1.

Snellen chart

A
H B
D E K
M T O P
H L Q N R
S A F Z U C W
G I U X A Y D

Distance
6 metres

fingers. Now cover your right eye with your left hand and examine the patient's nasal fields with your right hand, using the same method. The peripheral fields can be tested more sensitively by using a white hat pin instead of fingers, and asking the patient to say when they first perceive the pin. A red hat pin is more sensitive to defects of central vision and can be used to map the blind spot. Lesions of different parts of the visual pathway produce characteristic field defects (see Ch. 8).

Blind spot

Routine testing is unnecessary, but enlargement of the blind spot may be an important finding in patients with raised intracranial pressure. The blind spot is tested using a red hatpin. Ask the patient to cover his or her left eye, and move the pin from the central into the temporal field, along the horizontal meridian, having explained to the patient that the pin will disappear briefly and then reappear again, and that he or she should indicate when this happens. Once you have found the patient's blind spot, you can map its shape and compare its size with yours.

Central field

The central field is tested by moving a red hatpin along the central visual field (fixation area) in the horizontal meridian. Ask the patient to indicate if the pin disappears (absolute central scotoma) or if the colour appears diminished (relative scotoma). A central scotoma may extend temporally from the fixation area into the blind spot (centrocaecal scotoma).

Perimetry

Peripheral visual fields are sensitive to a moving target and formally tested with Goldmann perimetry. The patient fixates on a central point and a point of light moves centrally from the periphery. The patient indicates the position of the point of light each time and this is plotted on a chart. Repetitive testing from different directions accurately records the visual fields. Central fields can be tested using this method, but with a less intense light source. Humphrey fields use a static light source. A record of the threshold of the light source with increasing intensity provides information about the central visual field.

Fundoscopy

Ask the patient to fixate on a distant target in dimmed light. Using a direct ophthalmoscope, examine the patient's right eye using your right eye, and the patient's left eye using your left eye.

Adjust the ophthalmoscope lens until the retinal vessels are in focus, and trace them back to the optic disc. Assess the cupping, colour and contour of the optic disc, and the clarity of its margins. The temporal disc margins are normally slightly paler than the nasal margins. The physiological cup varies in size but does not extend to the disc margins. The retinal vessels should then be assessed. The arteries are narrower than the veins and more red in colour. The vessels should not be obscured as they cross the disc margins. Look for retinal vein pulsation, which is present in about 80% of normal individuals and is an index of normal intracranial pressure. This is seen best at the disc margins where the veins cross over the arteries. Note the width of the blood vessels and look for arteriovenous nipping at the crossover points.

Assess the rest of the retina, noting any evidence of discoloration, haemorrhages, or white patches of exudate. Ask the patient to look at the light of the ophthalmoscope, which brings the macula into view. Classify fundoscopic abnormalities into those affecting the optic disc, the retinal vessels or the retina (Fig. 2.4).

Oculomotor (third, III), trochlear (fourth, IV), and abducens (sixth, VI) nerves

Eyelids

Ptosis is drooping of the upper eyelid and the drooping is usually partial. A full ptosis (complete closure of the eyelid) is usually due to a third nerve palsy. Examination of pupil responses and eye movements provide essential information about the cause of the ptosis (Fig. 2.5).

Pupils

Size and shape

Assess the size and shape of the pupils. They should be circular and symmetrical (see Ch. 9). A discrepancy between the size of the pupils is called anisocoria. The most common cause of an irregular pupil is secondary to disease or trauma directly to the anterior chamber of the eye (e.g. anterior uveitis or postsurgical). The Argyll Robertson pupil is associated with tertiary syphilis and consists of irregular pupils that have an accommodation reflex but an absent light reflex. This abnormality occurs more often in examinations than in everyday practice.

Light response

Light responses should be assessed using a bright torchlight. Ask the patient to fixate on a distant target, then shine the light into each eye in turn, bringing the torch beam quickly onto the pupil from the lateral side.

Fig. 2.4   Common fundoscopic abnormalities

Structure	Abnormality	Pathology
Optic disc	Papilloedema – the optic disc is 'swollen' with blurring of the disc margin and engorgement of the retinal veins; there may be flame-shaped haemorrhages near the disc	Raised intracranial pressure (space-occupying lesions, e.g. tumours, particularly of the posterior fossa, hydrocephalus subsequent to meningitis or subarachnoid haemorrhage), venous obstruction (e.g. cavernous sinus thrombosis), malignant hypertension, idiopathic intracranial hypertension
	Optic atrophy – the disc is paler than usual, particularly on the temporal side, with fewer small vessels crossing its margins	Any cause of chronic optic nerve disease – central retinal artery occlusion, optic neuritis (multiple sclerosis, ischaemia), chronic glaucoma, B_{12} deficiency, toxins (e.g. methyl alcohol, tobacco), hereditary (e.g. Leber's optic atrophy), lesion of the optic chiasm and or tract
Retinal arteries	Silver-wiring, increased tortuosity, arteriovenous nipping	Hypertension
	Gross narrowing with retinal pallor and reddened fovea	Central retinal artery occlusion
	Cholesterol or platelet emboli	Cerebrovascular disease
	New vessel formation (on the surface of the optic disc or retina): new vessels develop subsequent to widespread retinal ischaemia; they do not affect vision, but are fragile and may bleed	Diabetes, central or branch retinal vein occlusion
Retinal veins	Venous engorgement	Papilloedema (see above), central retinal vein occlusion
Retina	Haemorrhages	Superficial flame-shaped and deep dot-shaped (hypertension, diabetes); subhyaloid between the retina and the vitreous (subarachnoid haemorrhage)
	Exudates	'Soft cotton-wool spots' (retinal infarcts) and hard exudates (lipid accumulation within the retina from leaking blood vessels in hypertension and diabetes)
	Pigmentation	Retinitis pigmentosa (e.g. Refsum's disease, Kearns–Sayre syndrome), choroidoretinitis (e.g. toxoplasmosis, sarcoidosis, syphilis), post-laser treatment (diabetes)

Observe the direct (ipsilateral) and the consensual (contralateral) responses.

Assess the presence of an afferent pupillary defect by swinging the light from one eye to the other, dwelling 3 seconds on each (see Ch. 9).

Accommodation

The accommodation reflex consists of two components. The first involves convergence of the eyes, which requires simultaneous adduction of both eyes. The second involves bilateral simultaneous constriction of the pupils. This reflex is required for actions such as reading a book or walking downstairs. To test this reflex, ask the patient to look into the distance and then bring an object to within 10 cm of the patient's eyes and ask him or her to fixate on the object. Both components of the reflex should be observed on near fixation.

Eye movements

Inspect the eyes and note the position of the eyelids and the presence of any strabismus (misalignment of the visual axes). Strabismus is non-paralytic or paralytic (see Ch. 9). There are two main types of eye movement:

- Pursuit eye movements are used to follow an object smoothly.
- Saccadic ('jump') eye movements are used to look from one object to a distant object without focusing on objects in between.

Fig. 2.5 Assessment of ptosis

Cause	Additional clinical features	Pupil responses	Eye movements
Congenital	Hereditary; unilateral or bilateral	Normal	Normal
Neurogenic			
3rd nerve palsy (see Ch. 9)	Complete ptosis	Dilated pupil, absent response to light and accommodation	Eye looks 'down and out' ophthalmoplegia with diplopia in all positions of gaze
Horner's syndrome	Partial ptosis, apparent enophthalmos; ipsilateral anhidrosis	Constricted pupil, impaired response to light and accommodation	Normal
Myogenic			
Senile	This is due to degenerative changes in the levator superioris muscle of the upper eyelid	Normal; senile pupil – constricted with impaired dilatation in the dark	Normal
Myasthenia gravis	Fatigable and therefore variable ptosis	Normal	Variable diplopia and ophthalmoplegia
Myopathy	Associated bulbar/limb weakness	Normal	Abnormal if extraocular muscles involved

Conjugate eye movements occur when the visual axes stay correctly aligned during either pursuit or saccadic movements. If the visual axes are misaligned, the patient experiences diplopia. Sometimes, the brain tries to correct a partial failure of gaze with a saccadic movement. The cycle of failure to sustain gaze and correction by saccadic movement is called nystagmus.

Pursuit eye movements

To test pursuit eye movements, ask the patient to focus on an object, such as a finger or pen, held approximately 50 cm in front of the patient's nose. Any strabismus, ptosis, or nystagmus in the 'primary position' should be noted. The patient should be asked to follow the object as it describes the shape of an 'H' in front of the patient and to inform the examiner of any double vision. In the presence of diplopia, identify the direction of the maximum separation of images and the two muscles responsible for moving the eyes in this direction (see Ch. 9). Cover each eye in turn and observe when the outer image disappears. The outer image is always produced by the pathological eye, irrespective of where the double vision occurs. The presence of nystagmus should also be noted, whether it is horizontal or vertical, and in which direction it is maximal. The smoothness and speed of pursuit eye movements should also be noted.

Saccadic eye movements

To test saccadic eye movements, hold a finger approximately 50 cm in front of the patient's nose and a fist approximately 50 cm lateral to the finger. Ask the patient to move his or her gaze rapidly back and forth between the fist and finger. This is repeated in all four directions keeping a finger in front of the patient and moving the fist to the appropriate direction. Assess the velocity and the accuracy of these movements. The presence of slow or absent adduction in the horizontal plane is consistent with an internuclear ophthalmoplegia: (see Ch. 9). There may also be horizontal gaze-evoked nystagmus in the abducting eye.

If pursuit or saccadic eye movements are absent, the oculocephalic reflex (doll's eye movements) will differentiate between supranuclear and nuclear gaze palsy. The oculocephalic reflex is tested by asking the patient to fixate on your eyes while you rotate his or her head in the horizontal and the vertical planes. The reflex in supranuclear lesions is intact, allowing the patient's eyes to remain fixated on the examiner's eyes. This reflex is intact because the afferent (information from neck muscle and vestibular apparatus) and efferent (nerves and muscles controlling eye movements) loop is intact. If there is a nuclear or more peripheral lesion (i.e. pathology in the brainstem, nerves, or muscles) then the reflex loop is broken and doll's eye movements are absent.

Fig. 2.6 Causes of nystagmus

Type	Description	Pathology
Pendular	Oscillations of equal velocity	Longstanding impaired macular vision (since early childhood), e.g. albinism, congenital cataracts, congenital nystagmus; lesions in upper brainstem, e.g. MS
Jerky	Fast phase towards the side of the lesion	Unilateral cerebellar lesions
	Fast phase to the opposite side of the lesion	Unilateral vestibular lesions or VIIIn lesions
	Direction of nystagmus varies with the direction of gaze	Brainstem pathology
	Upbeat nystagmus Downbeat nystagmus	Lesions at or around the superior colliculi (midbrain) Lesions at or around the foramen magnum
Rotatory	Specific to one head position, and fatigues with repeated testing	Unilateral labyrinthine pathology
Mixed	Jerky and rotatory	Brainstem pathology

HINTS AND TIPS

Normal pursuit movements depend on intact posterior cortical areas and cerebellum. Normal saccadic eye movements depend on intact basal ganglia, cerebellum, anterior cortical areas and the superior colliculi of the midbrain.

Ocular nerve palsies

Clinical signs and causes of ocular nerve palsies are discussed in Chapter 9.

Nystagmus

Nystagmus is an involuntary, rhythmic oscillation of the eyes caused by lesions affecting the vestibular apparatus, the vestibulocochlear (eighth) nerve, brainstem centres involved in controlling gaze or the cerebellum. Nystagmus is usually asymptomatic but patients sometimes describe an unpleasant experience of alternating movements of their visual fields, which is called oscillopsia.

In normal individuals a few beats of nystagmus can often be observed at the extremes of gaze. This is not pathological or sustained. It may also occur during voluntary rapid oscillation of the eyes. These physiological movements are called nystagmoid jerks.

Nystagmus should be looked for in the primary position of gaze (i.e. when the patient is looking straight ahead) and also during the testing of eye movements. Nystagmus can be jerky (the oscillation has a fast and a slow phase) or pendular (the oscillation occurs with equal velocity in all directions). The nystagmus may be horizontal, vertical, rotatory or a mixture of these. The amplitude of the nystagmus and its persistence should be noted. The direction of jerky nystagmus is defined by the direction of the fast phase by convention. Causes of nystagmus are shown in Figure 2.6.

Trigeminal (fifth, V) nerve

The motor part of the trigeminal nerve is highly robust and is not often affected by the many pathologies that involve the surrounding structures. However, the sensory aspect of the fifth nerve is often affected by local pathologies and loss of the corneal reflex is often one of the first clinical signs of a lesion at the cerebellopontine angle.

Motor

Inspect for wasting of the temporalis muscles, which produces hollowing above the zygoma. Ask the patient to clench his or her teeth and palpate the masseters for contraction and relaxation. Note any loss of bulk. Assess the pterygoid muscles by resisting the patient's attempts to open the mouth. In unilateral trigeminal lesions, the lower jaw deviates to the paralytic side as the mouth is opened.

Jaw jerk

Jaw jerk is a brainstem stretch reflex. Ask the patient to open the mouth slightly. Rest your index finger on the apex of the jaw and tap it lightly with the patella hammer. The normal response is closure of the mouth, which is caused by reflex contraction of the pterygoid muscles. An absent reflex is not significant but the reflex becomes pathologically brisk with upper motor neuron lesions (i.e. bilateral damage to the upper motor neurons (UMNs) to the motor fifth nucleus in the pons).

Sensory

Sensory testing is performed using the techniques described below. Test light touch, pin-prick, and temperature over the forehead, the medial aspects of the cheeks, and the chin. These correspond to the ophthalmic, maxillary and mandibular branches of the trigeminal nerve, respectively (see Ch. 10). It should be noted that the angle of the jaw is not innervated by the trigeminal nerve. A partial loss can be detected by comparing the response to the same stimulus on different areas of the face. The clinical pattern of sensory loss depends on the anatomical site of the lesion (Fig. 2.7).

The corneal reflex is elicited by lightly touching the cornea (not the conjunctiva) with a wisp of cotton wool. Synchronous blinking of both eyes should occur. An afferent defect (fifth cranial nerve lesion) results in depression or absence of the direct and consensual blinking reflex. An efferent defect (seventh cranial nerve lesion) results in an impairment or absence of the reflex on the side of the facial weakness.

Facial (seventh, VII) nerve

Motor

Inspect the patient's face, looking for asymmetry of the nasolabial folds and the position of the two angles of the mouth. Assess the movements of the upper part of the face by asking the patient to:

- elevate his or her eyebrows
- close his or her eyes tightly and resist your attempt to open them. Look for Bell's phenomenon – this is a reflex upward deviation of the eyes in response to attempted but failed forced closure of the eyelids.

Movements of the lower part of the face are assessed by asking the patient to:

- blow out the cheeks with air
- purse the lips tightly and resist your attempt to open them
- show the teeth
- whistle
- smile (observe any facial asymmetry).

If you detect any weakness or asymmetry, decide if the weakness is confined to the lower part of the face (upper motor neuron lesion) or both the upper and the lower parts of the face (lower motor neuron lesion). Do not miss bilateral facial weakness. In this case, the face appears to sag, with lack of facial expression even though it is symmetrical.

Hyperacusis (oversensitivity to noise) is suggestive of a lesion affecting the nerve to the stapedius, which comes off the facial nerve in the facial canal within the petrous bone.

Sensory

Taste (visceral afferent)

Examine taste by applying a solution of salt, sweet (sugar), sour (vinegar) or bitter (lemon) to the anterior two-thirds of the tongue and comparing the response on the two sides. The mouth should be rinsed with water between testing. Lesions of the chorda tympani will cause loss of taste.

A few somatic afferent fibres from the seventh nerve subserve parts of the outer pinna. In Ramsay Hunt syndrome, there may be vesicles in this position with unilateral facial weakness associated with reactivation of herpes zoster in the geniculate ganglion.

Fig. 2.7 Clinical syndromes of the trigeminal nerve	
Site of lesion	**Pattern of sensory loss**
Supranuclear	Contralateral discriminative sensory loss in lesions of the primary somatosensory cortex
Upper pons	Ipsilateral loss of light touch with preserved pain and temperature sensation (spinal tract of trigeminal nerve)
Lower pons, medulla, upper cervical cord (lesion above C2)	Contralateral loss of pain and temperature sensation in an 'onion-skin' distribution; preserved light touch
Cerebellopontine angle	Ipsilateral loss of all modalities
Cavernous sinus	Ipsilateral loss of all modalities in the V_1 and occasionally V_2 distribution
Trigeminal root, ganglion, and peripheral branches of the nerve	Loss of all sensory modalities in the V_{1-3} distributions; there will be a more selective distribution of loss with lesions of the peripheral nerve

Vestibulocochlear nerve (eighth, VIII)

Hearing

Clinical bedside assessment of hearing is not sensitive and can detect only gross hearing loss. Audiometry is usually required for detailed assessment.

Assess each ear separately while masking the hearing in the other ear by occluding the external meatus with your index finger. Test patients' hearing sensitivity by whispering numbers into their ears and asking them to repeat these.

Determine if the hearing loss is conductive or sensorineural by performing Rinne and Weber's tests (see Ch. 11).

Vestibular function

There are no satisfactory bedside tests for vestibular function. Examination of the patient's gait and eye movements for nystagmus may be helpful. The findings in a patient who has vestibular dysfunction are summarized in Chapter 11. The use of caloric testing and the Hallpike manoeuvre for patients presenting with positional vertigo is discussed in Chapter 11. A patient suspected of having vestibular dysfunction will sometimes require formal vestibular testing.

Glossopharyngeal (ninth, IX) and vagus (tenth, X) nerves

Motor

The motor component of the vagus nerve supplies the muscles of the palate, pharynx and larynx via the recurrent laryngeal nerve. Check the patient's speech quality and volume for hoarseness and quietness as well as strength of cough to assess for dysphonia. Nasal intonation of speech arises from palatal weakness and causes a bulbar dysarthria.

Palatal movement can be assessed by:

- asking the patient to say 'ah' (voluntary activity)
- touching the posterior pharyngeal wall with the end of an orange stick on both sides (the 'gag' reflex).

Assess the afferent pathway of the 'gag' reflex (ninth cranial nerve) by asking the patient whether sensation is comparable on both sides. Assess the efferent pathway (tenth cranial nerve) by observing the normal response of a symmetrical rise of the soft palate and movement of the pharyngeal muscles; characteristically, a 'gagging' sound is made.

Supranuclear (upper motor neuron) innervation of the palatal and pharyngeal muscles is bilateral. Unilateral lesions will therefore not cause significant and prolonged dysfunction of swallowing and speech. In patients who have bilateral upper motor neuron lesions, the palate cannot be elevated voluntarily, but moves normally when testing the 'gag' reflex. This is part of a syndrome called a 'pseudobulbar palsy' and is associated with a brisk jaw jerk, spastic tongue and speech, and emotional lability.

If the voluntary and reflex movements are bilaterally impaired, then the patient may have a bilateral bulbar palsy (i.e. damage to the lower motor neurons [LMNs] or their nuclei in the brainstem on both sides). If the palate does not elevate on one side, the lesion almost always involves the lower motor neuron because the palate has bilateral UMN innervation. Therefore, in unilateral lower motor neuron lesions, the palate lies slightly lower on the affected side and deviates towards the unaffected side.

Minor and inconsistent deviations of the uvula should be ignored.

Sensory

The posterior pharyngeal wall and tonsillar region is innervated by the glossopharyngeal (ninth cranial) nerve and sensation is tested by a wooden probe as described above. The ninth nerve also subserves sensation and taste to the posterior third of the tongue but taste is difficult to test in this location.

Accessory (eleventh, XI) nerve

The spinal part of the accessory nerve is a purely motor nerve that arises from the upper five segments of the cervical cord. It supplies the trapezius and sternocleidomastoid muscles and wasting or weakness of these muscles should be noted on inspection.

The strength of the sternocleidomastoid muscles is assessed by asking the patient to turn his or her head to each side against the resistance of the examiner's hand. Turning of the head to the left involves contraction of the right sternocleidomastoid and vice versa. In a patient with a hemispheric stroke, it is the sternocleidomastoid muscle ipsilateral to the hemisphere that is affected. Therefore, there is weakness in head-turning towards the side of the hemiparesis.

Assess the strength of the trapezius muscles by asking the patient to shrug his or her shoulders upwards against resistance and note the bulk of the muscles on palpation.

Hypoglossal (twelfth, XII) nerve

The hypoglossal nerve is a purely motor nerve that supplies the muscles of the tongue. Inspect the tongue as it lies in the floor of the mouth for evidence of wasting

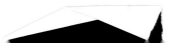

Fig. 2.8 Clinical patterns of tongue weakness

Lower motor neuron lesions	Unilateral	Atrophy and fasciculations ipsilateral to the side of the lesion and deviation of the protruded tongue towards the affected side
	Bilateral	Bilateral atrophy and fasciculations (see bulbar palsy)
Upper motor neuron lesions	Unilateral	Slight deviation of the tongue away from the side of the lesion but usually asymptomatic
	Bilateral	Tongue has limited protrusion and appears contracted (see pseudobulbar palsy)

(which may be unilateral or bilateral), fasciculations (wriggling movements at the tongue surface) or other involuntary movements. Then ask the patient to protrude the tongue. Abnormalities caused by upper and lower motor neuron lesions are summarized in Figure 2.8.

THE MOTOR SYSTEM

The examination should start by simply observing the patient. Important information may be obtained through observing the patient during history taking. Is the patient not moving one side of the body? Was the patient unstable when sitting in the chair? The formal examination should be started by assessing the nature of the patient's gait and should then proceed to bedside examination of the motor system.

Inspection

- **Posture:** look for the characteristic posturing of a patient with a hemiparesis (see Ch. 17). Ask the patient to hold out both arms in front of the body with eyes closed. If the patient has an UMN lesion, he or she may demonstrate a drift of the arm downwards from the horizontal into a pronated and eventually flexed position. This is called 'pronator drift'. The fingers of the outstretched arm may move spontaneously, as if the patient was playing the piano. This is called 'pseudoathetosis' and is caused by loss of joint-position sense. In cerebellar disease, if the outstretched arms are rapidly displaced, they may oscillate about the horizontal rather than quickly returning to the initial position. This is called 'rebound'.
- **Muscle wasting:** look for the degree and distribution of muscle wasting. This is usually characteristic of LMN disorders, i.e. anterior horn cell, spinal nerve, plexus, or peripheral nerve disorders as well as myopathies.
- **Fasciculations:** these are seen as brief, localized twitches or flickers of movement within the muscle

at rest and are also a feature of lower motor neuron disorders. Each muscle should be carefully studied for up to several minutes if there is a strong suspicion of an LMN disorder.
- **Involuntary movements,** e.g. a resting tremor may be evident in patients who have Parkinson's disease (see Ch. 14).
- **Atrophic skin changes** such as smooth, hairless, purple oedematous skin may be a sign of associated sensory nerve damage in an LMN disorder or from disuse in a UMN disorder.
- **Any scars** should be noted, particularly over the lateral aspect of the foot from a sural nerve biopsy or over the vastus lateralis or triceps from a muscle biopsy. Some patients may have scars from orthopaedic surgery such as arthrodesis at the ankle in foot drop.
- **Walking sticks, ankle–foot orthoses, and other orthotic devices** can often give an early clue as to the patient's main functional difficulty.

Tone

Tone refers to the activity of the stretch reflexes as assessed by the degree of resistance that occurs on stretching a muscle at different velocities.

Some patients have difficulty relaxing during an examination, which can artificially increase stiffness in their limbs. Relaxation can be achieved by asking the patient to loosen up the limbs so that they are limp.

Arm

Pyramidal hypertonia: spasticity

Take the patient's arm and flex and extend the elbow. Spasticity may be especially observed during extension. Then hold the patient's hand, with the elbow flexed, and rapidly pronate and supinate the forearm. If tone is increased, you may feel a 'supinator' or 'spastic catch', which is an interruption of the smooth movement on supination by increased tone of a spastic type. Alternatively, there may be increased tone on extending the elbow, which suddenly gives way to low tone. This is sometimes referred to as the 'clasp-knife' effect. These signs are suggestive of a UMN lesion.

Extrapyramidal rigidity

If there is increased tone throughout movement of a limb, this is called 'lead-pipe' rigidity. When the patient has a tremor, which may be subclinical, and lead-pipe rigidity, they may have 'cog-wheel' rigidity. These two types of rigidity are typical of idiopathic Parkinson's disease but can occur in many other extrapyramidal syndromes. All extrapyramidal types of increased tone can be enhanced by asking the patient to move the other arm up and down. If this brings out increased tone, then the rigidity is said to occur 'with synkinesis'. Extrapyramidal rigidity is best looked for by rotating the wrist in both directions.

Legs

- Rock each leg from side to side on the bed, holding it at the knee. Normally, the foot lags behind the leg. If tone is increased, the foot and leg move stiffly together. If tone is decreased, the foot moves limply from side to side with each movement.
- Passively flex and extend the knee at varying speeds, supporting both the upper leg and the foot.
- With the patient's legs extended on the couch, place your hand under the patient's knee and quickly lift the knee about 15 cm. The foot will normally stay on the bed as the knee is flexed. If tone is increased, the foot may jump up with the lower leg and if tone is decreased the limb will feel lax and slightly heavier than normal.

'Clonus' describes the rhythmic unidirectional contractions evoked by a sudden passive stretch of a muscle. This is elicited most easily at the ankle. A few beats may be normal but 'sustained clonus' is characteristic of an upper motor neuron lesion.

Power

Power is tested in each of the main muscle groups by the examiner stabilizing the limb proximal to the joint movement that is being tested. Power in each muscle is given a grade as defined by the Medical Research Council (MRC) scale (Fig. 2.9).

The scheme in Figure 2.10 shows testing of the main muscle groups of the arms. The scheme in Figure 2.11 shows testing of the main muscle groups of the legs.

Figure 2.12 summarizes the typical pattern of physical signs arising from lesions in different parts of the motor system.

Fig. 2.9	The MRC scale for assessment of muscle power
Grade	**Response**
0	No movement
1	Flicker of muscle when patient tries to move
2	Moves, but not against gravity
3	Moves against gravity but not against resistance
4	Moves against resistance but not to full strength
5	Full strength (you cannot overcome the movement)

HINTS AND TIPS

Increased tone may be due to an upper motor neuron or extrapyramidal disorder. Spasticity occurs in patients who have increased tone due to an upper motor neuron lesion – look for a supinator catch, clasp-knife phenomenon and clonus, brisk reflexes, and extensor plantar responses. In patients who have increased tone due to an extrapyramidal disorder, there is characteristic 'lead-pipe' rigidity or 'cog-wheel' rigidity if there is a superimposed tremor. The reflexes are usually normal and plantar responses flexor.

Reflexes

Tendon reflexes are most easily determined by briskly stretching the tendon. To perform this, the tendon hammer is held near the end of the shaft and the heavy end is swung onto the tendon directly or onto a finger placed over the tendon (biceps and supinator jerks). The tendon reflexes shown in Figure 2.13 A and B should be examined. The tendon reflexes may be increased ('brisk'), decreased or absent. If they are absent, this should be confirmed by reinforcement (Fig. 2.13C). Abdominal reflexes can be tested as shown in Figure 2.13D. The abdominal reflexes are lost in an upper motor neuron lesion, but may also be lost after abdominal injury or in an obsese patient. The plantar response is elicited by scratching the sole as demonstrated in Figure 2.13E.

Tendon reflexes are conventionally annotated as shown in Figure 2.14.

Coordination

The ability of a patient to perform smooth and accurate movements is dependent on power, intact joint-position sense and coordination. Weakness and loss of joint-position sense may give rise to apparent

Fig. 2.10 Testing muscle groups of the upper limb. The orange arrow indicates the direction of movement of the patient, and the black arrow the direction of resistance by the examiner. Each muscle group should be given a grade as defined by the MRC scale (see Fig. 2.9).

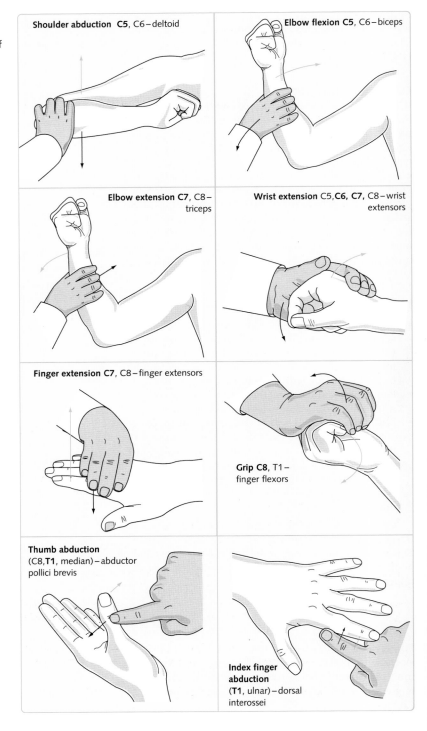

Shoulder abduction **C5**, C6 – deltoid

Elbow flexion **C5**, C6 – biceps

Elbow extension **C7**, C8 – triceps

Wrist extension C5, **C6**, **C7**, C8 – wrist extensors

Finger extension **C7**, C8 – finger extensors

Grip **C8**, T1 – finger flexors

Thumb abduction (C8, **T1**, median) – abductor pollicis brevis

Index finger abduction (**T1**, ulnar) – dorsal interossei

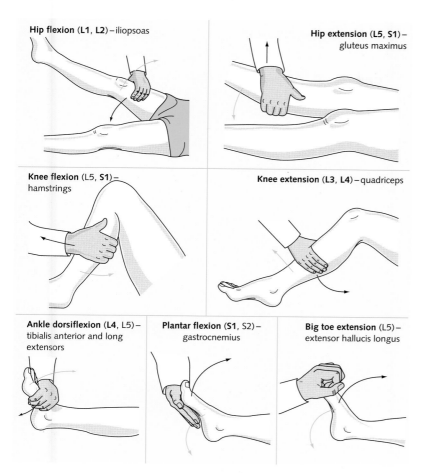

Fig. 2.11 Testing muscle groups of the lower limb. The orange arrow indicates the direction of movement of the patient, and the black arrow the direction of movement of the examiner. Each muscle group should be given a grade as defined by the MRC scale (see Fig. 2.9).

Hip flexion (**L1, L2**) – iliopsoas

Hip extension (**L5, S1**) – gluteus maximus

Knee flexion (**L5, S1**) – hamstrings

Knee extension (**L3, L4**) – quadriceps

Ankle dorsiflexion (**L4**, L5) – tibialis anterior and long extensors

Plantar flexion (**S1, S2**) – gastrocnemius

Big toe extension (**L5**) – extensor hallucis longus

Fig. 2.12   Clinical features of patients presenting with limb weakness

Site of lesion	Wasting	Tone	Pattern of weakness	Reflexes	Plantar response
Upper motor neuron	None	Increased	'Pyramidal' pattern weakness	Increased	Extensor
Lower motor neuron	Present	Decreased	Individual or groups of muscles	Decreased/ absent	Flexor or absent
Neuromuscular junction	Uncommon	Usually normal, may be decreased	Bilateral and predominantly of the proximal limb girdle (fatigable)	Usually normal	Flexor
Muscle	From mild to severe	Decreased in proportion to wasting	Bilateral and predominantly of the proximal limb girdle	Decreased in proportion to wasting	Flexor

Note: Not every patient will have all the features of their syndrome.

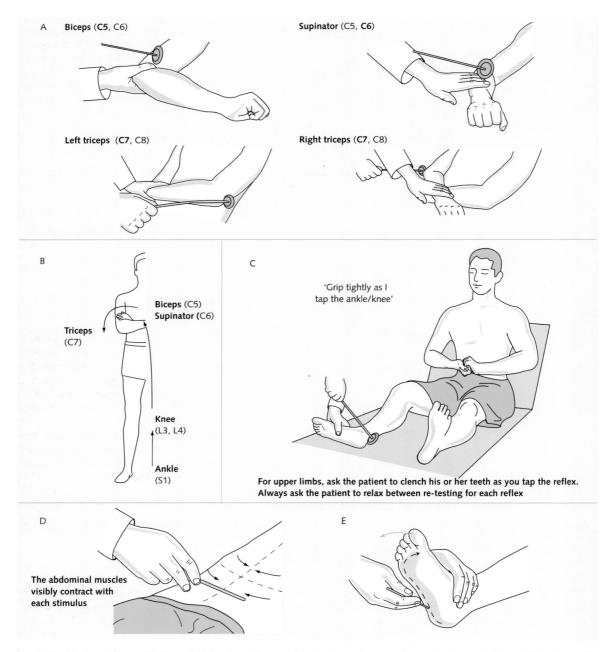

Fig. 2.13 Eliciting reflexes. (A) Upper limb tendon reflexes. (B) A simple way to remember root values of reflexes. (C) Testing ankle jerk reinforcement. (D) Abdominal reflexes: test in the four quadrants shown. (E) Plantar reflex. The normal response is a downgoing hallux. In an upper motor neuron lesion, the hallux dorsiflexes and the other toes fan out (the Babinski response).

Fig. 2.14 Annotation of tendon reflexes

Reduced	+
Normal	++
Very brisk (with associated clonus)	+++
Absent	0
Present with reinforcement only	±

clumsiness, which may be misinterpreted as incoordination. Cerebellar dysfunction can only be accurately detected if weakness and/or joint-position sense loss is mild or there is severe incoordination.

Gait

A wide-based, sometimes lurching gait is seen in cerebellar disease. Unsteadiness is made more obvious if the patient is asked to walk 'heel to toe'.

Arms

Cerebellar dysfunction can be assessed as follows:

- **The finger–nose test:** the examiner places a finger 50 cm in front of the patient's nose and asks the patient to move his or her index finger between the nose and the examiner's finger; both index fingers are tested. In patients who have a cerebellar lesion, on approaching the examiner's finger, the patient's arm may coarsely oscillate. This is called an intention tremor. The inability to perform smooth, accurate, and targeted movements is called dysmetria. If the patient overshoots the intended target, this is called 'past pointing'.
- **Dysdiadochokinesis:** this is the inability to carry out rapid, alternating movements with regularity. It can be tested by asking the patient to alternately pronate and supinate his or her arm and correspondingly tap the palm and then dorsum of his or her hand on the examiner's palm. In cerebellar disease, the movements are irregular in amplitude and speed.
- **The 'rebound phenomenon':** if the wrists are gently tapped when the patient's arms are outstretched, then the arms should rapidly come to the resting horizontal position. In patients with cerebellar disease, the arms oscillate about the horizontal before coming to rest. This is called the rebound phenomenon.

Legs

Cerebellar dysfunction can be assessed as follows:

The heel–shin test

Ask the patient to place one heel on the other knee and slowly slide the heel down the shin, then lift the heel off the shin and repeat the test. This test should be performed on each side in turn.

The tapping test

The rapid tapping of the foot is impaired in cerebellar disease. This test should be performed on each side in turn.

The combination of these abnormalities in a patient is called cerebellar ataxia and may be associated with other signs of cerebellar disease such as horizontal jerky nystagmus and slurring dysarthria (see Ch. 13).

THE SENSORY SYSTEM

Patients use various terms to describe sensory disturbance, including numbness, tingling, 'pins and needles', and burning. Medical terms include paraesthesia (tingling), dysaesthesia (unpleasant awareness of touch or pressure), hyperaesthesia (exaggeration of any sensation), and hyperalgesia (exaggerated perception of painful stimuli).

To test the sensory modalities, ask the patient to close his or her eyes and, for all modalities except joint-position sense, apply the test to a reference point such as the skin over the sternum and ask the patient if he or she can feel the sensation normally. Subsequently, test each sensory modality distally to proximally in each limb and ask the patient if it feels the same as the reference point on the chest.

Sensory testing

It is not recommended to spend too much time doing sensory testing because you will exhaust the patient and yourself. It is best to tailor your examination to the patient's complaint. In coming to the sensory examination in the neurological evaluation, one should have a hypothesis as to the pattern of sensory loss that is expected. The sensory examination can be tailored towards that pattern. Patterns of sensory impairment are discussed in more detail in Chapter 16.

Sensory modalities

Pain

A safety pin or specialized disposable device (e.g. 'neurotip'), and not a hypodermic needle, should be used to test pain sensation. The patient will either feel nothing, a blunt sensation (which is abnormal), or a sharp pain (which is normal). If an abnormal area is found, then its margins should be further defined by moving from the area of reduced sensation to the normal area.

Temperature

A cold object such as the flat surface of a non-vibrating tuning fork can be used to test perception of cold temperature.

Light touch

A wisp of cotton wool is used to test light touch with brief static stimuli. Remember that 'tickle' is carried by spinothalamic fibres.

Joint-position sense

Move the distal interphalangeal (DIP) joint of the index finger/big toe up and down while stabilizing the digit with your other hand. Ask the patient to indicate the direction in which the digit is being moved. If perception of joint position is abnormal, then test more proximal joints until the test is normal (e.g. DIP, wrist, elbow, shoulder).

Vibration

A 128-Hz tuning fork should be used to test vibration sense. Start the tuning fork vibrating and place it on the DIP joint of the finger/big toe and ask if the patient can feel it vibrating. If the patient cannot feel these vibrations, move the tuning fork proximally (e.g. lateral malleoli, tibial tuberosity, iliac crest, sternum). The tuning fork should always be touching bony elements under the skin. Vibration sense is often lost early in peripheral polyneuropathies.

Two-point discrimination

Test two-point discrimination with specific compasses. The pulp of the index finger (normal: 2–3 mm) and hallux (normal: 5 mm) are normally tested and the patient asked whether they feel one or two points.

GENERAL EXAMINATION

The conclusion of the neurological examination should include a more general examination of the other, relevant, body systems. In particular, where it is important, autonomic function should also be assessed. The easiest method of assessment is measurement of the blood pressure as the patient lies supine and again after standing for a couple of minutes. Orthostatic hypotension, defined as a fall in systolic blood pressure of >20 mmHg and >10 mmHg diastolic blood pressure, can be associated with autonomic dysfunction.

Further investigations 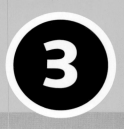 3

ROUTINE INVESTIGATIONS

You should be aware of simple tests of neurological relevance. In this section, four areas of investigation are presented:

- Haematology (Fig. 3.1)
- Biochemistry (Fig. 3.2)
- Immunology (Fig. 3.3)
- Microbiology (Fig. 3.4)
- Cerebrospinal fluid findings (see Ch. 31)

For each test, normal ranges are given, with neurological differential diagnoses for high and low values.

NEUROPHYSIOLOGICAL INVESTIGATIONS

Electroencephalography

Electroencephalography (EEG) measures electrical potentials generated by the neurons lying underneath an electrode on the scalp, and compares these with recordings from either a reference electrode or a neighbouring electrode. The normal trace is symmetrical, and therefore asymmetries, as well as specific abnormalities, may indicate an underlying disorder.

Before accurate brain imaging was possible, EEG was used to detect focal lesions. These are now more commonly picked up with computed tomography (CT) or magnetic resonance imaging (MRI), but EEG remains useful for detecting underlying abnormalities of cerebral function, and especially for:

- epilepsy (see below)
- diagnosis of encephalitis (especially herpes simplex infection)
- coma
- aid to diagnosis of Creutzfeldt–Jakob disease
- diagnosis of subacute sclerosing panencephalitis.

The main role of EEG is in the assessment of epilepsy. It can help in the following ways:

- Support of the diagnosis: (although this is made primarily on the clinical history and the EEG may be normal in patients who have clearly had seizures) an increased yield of abnormalities may be obtained if recording is made under conditions of sleep

deprivation, with hyperventilation, and with photic stimulation
- Classification of seizure type, which may optimize therapy
- Assessment for surgical intervention
- Diagnosis of non-epileptic seizures (especially with simultaneous video recording: 'video telemetry').

'Invasive EEG monitoring' refers to prolonged recording from electrodes inserted directly into the brain, undertaken preoperatively, before surgery to remove an epileptic focus.

Different normal rhythms are characteristically found over different regions of the brain (Fig. 3.5). Other than these rhythmic activities, other abnormal activity may be generated in certain conditions (Figs 3.6 and 3.7).

Electromyography and nerve conduction studies

Electromyography (EMG) and nerve conduction studies (NCS), usually performed together, examine the electrical activity of muscle, neuromuscular junction and lower motor neurons. They are useful in:

- determining the cause of weakness, e.g. neuropathy, myopathy, anterior horn cell disease
- determining the distribution of the abnormality, e.g. generalized or focal
- suggesting the type of myopathy (e.g. dystrophy or myositis) or neuropathy (e.g. axonal or demyelinating and motor, sensory or sensorimotor)
- diagnosing myasthenia gravis
- assessing baseline deficits before surgery, e.g. carpal tunnel syndrome
- objectively assessing the response to medical therapies, especially new treatments currently under trial, e.g. intravenous human immunoglobulin in Guillain–Barré syndrome.

EMG

EMG involves the insertion of a needle electrode into muscle.

Normal muscle at rest is electrically silent (apart from actually during needle insertion, 'insertional activity')

Fig. 3.1 Possible clinical relevance of abnormalities in blood or serum levels of haematological indices. Individual laboratories may have different normal ranges

Test	Normal range	Abnormality	Possible clinical explanation
Full blood count			
Haemoglobin (Hb)	13.5–18.0 g/dL male; 11.5–16.0 g/dL female	Low; anaemia	May cause non-specific neurological symptoms (e.g. dizziness, weakness, faintness); may suggest an underlying chronic illness
		High; polycythaemia	Predisposes to stroke and chorea
Mean cell volume (MCV)	76–96 fL	High; macrocytic	Vitamin B_{12} deficiency (peripheral neuropathy, dementia)
		Low; microcytic	May indicate an underlying chronic illness; associated with idiopathic intracranial hypertension
White cell count (WBC)			
Neutrophils	$2–7.5 \times 10^9$/L	High; neutrophilia Low; neutropenia	Meningitis or other infection Leukaemia or lymphoma (infiltrative disease, space-occupying lesions, peripheral neuropathy) Multiple myeloma (neuropathy, vertebral collapse, hyperviscosity syndrome)
Lymphocytes	$1.5–3.5 \times 10^9$/L	High; lymphocytosis Low; lymphopenia	Viral infection (transverse myelitis, Guillain–Barré syndrome) Leukaemia or lymphoma, as above
Eosinophils	$0.04–0.44 \times 10^9$/L	High; eosinophilia	Hypereosinophilic syndrome (rare)
Platelet count	$150–400 \times 10^9$/L	High; thrombocythaemia Low; thrombocytopenia	Predisposes to stroke Intracranial bleeding
Erythrocyte sedimentation rate (ESR)	20 mm/h	High	Vasculitis (e.g. PAN, SLE, giant-cell arteritis) may cause cerebral, cranial, and peripheral nerve infarcts, confusion and fits
Coagulation tests			
Activated partial thromboplastin time (APT or PTTK)	35–45 s	High	SLE; antiphospholipid syndrome
Protein C, protein S	Varies with laboratory	Low; deficiency	Inherited predisposition to thrombosis (arterial and venous)
Factor 5 Leiden	Varies with laboratory	Present	Mutation causes a single amino acid substitution in factor 5, which results in activated protein C resistance and predisposition to thrombosis (arterial and venous)
Vitamin B_{12}	>150 ng/L	Low; deficiency	Peripheral neuropathy, myelopathy, confusion/dementia, optic neuropathy, SCDC, ataxia
Folate	4–18 µg/L	Low; deficiency	Peripheral neuropathy, dementia

APT, activated thromboplastin; PAN, polyarteritis nodosa; PTTK, partial thromboplastin time; SCDC, subacute combined degeneration of the cord; SLE, systemic lupus erythematosus.

Fig. 3.2 Possible clinical relevance of abnormalities in blood or serum levels of biochemical indices. Individual laboratories may have different normal ranges

Test	Normal range	Abnormality	Possible clinical explanation
Urea and electrolytes (U and Es)			
Sodium	135–145 mmol/L	High; hypernatraemia low; hyponatraemia	Both may cause weakness, confusion and fits
Potassium	3.5–5.5 mmol/L	High; hyperkalaemia Low; hypokalaemia	Hyper- or hypokalaemic periodic paralysis
Urea	2.5–6.7 mmol/L	High; renal failure	Confusion, peripheral neuropathy
Creatinine	<120 mmol/L	High; renal failure	Confusion, peripheral neuropathy
Glucose (fasting)	4–6 mmol/L	High; diabetes Low; hypoglycaemia	Neuropathy, coma Confusion, coma, focal signs
Calcium	2.2–2.6 mmol/L	Low; hypocalcaemia	Tetany, seizures
Liver function tests (LFTs)			
Bilirubin and liver enzymes	Bilirubin range: 3–17 mmol/L; enzyme levels vary between laboratories	High	Liver disease: confusion, tremor, neuropathy
Creatine kinase (CK)	24–195 U/L	High	Muscle disease: myositis, dystrophy
Thyroid function tests			
Thyroid-stimulating hormone (TSH)	0.5–5.0 mU/L	High T_4 Low TSH; thyrotoxicosis	Tremor, confusion, hyperreflexia
Thyroxine (T_4)	10–24 pmol/L	Low T_4 High TSH; hypothyroidism	Apathy, confusion, hyporeflexia, neuropathy, dementia

Fig. 3.3 Immunology: selected autoantibodies and their associated syndromes (see Chs 30 and 33 for further details)

Test	Associated disorder
Antinuclear factor (ANA)	Systemic lupus erythematosus (SLE): fits, confusion, neuropathy, aseptic meningitis, Sjögren's syndrome: gritty eyes, neuropathies, mixed connective tissue disease (MCTD)
Anti-double-stranded DNA (dsDNA) antibodies	SLE
Rheumatoid factor	Rheumatoid arthritis: cervical spine subluxation, neuropathies, vasculitis
Anti-Ro (SSA), anti-La (SSB) antibodies	Sjögren's syndrome
Antiphospholipid antibodies (e.g. anticardiolipin)	Antiphospholipid syndrome
Anti-ribonucleoprotein (RNP) antibodies	MCTD; myositis, trigeminal nerve palsies
Jo-1 antibodies	Polymyositis and pulmonary fibrosis
Antineutrophil cytoplasmic antibodies (ANCA)	pANCA (peripheral): polyarteritis nodosa cANCA (classical): Wegener's granulomatosis
Anti-acetylcholine receptor (AChR) antibodies	Myasthenia gravis
Anti-GM1 antibodies	Multifocal motor neuropathy, Guillain–Barré syndrome
Anti-GAD antibodies	Stiff-man syndrome
Anti-Hu, -Yo and -Ri antibodies	Paraneoplastic syndromes
Anti-voltage gated potassium channel, NMDA receptor, glycine receptor, GABA receptor antibodies	Autoimmune or paraneoplastic (limbic) encephalitis or encephalomyelitis

Fig. 3.4 Microbiology: investigations that should be carried out if infections are implicated as the cause of neurological disease

Test	Associated disorder
Bacterial microscopy and culture (including blood, CSF, urine, stool, sputum and wounds)	Bacterial infections can cause a wide range of conditions – septicaemia, meningitis, pneumonia, urinary tract infections, cerebral abscess, etc. – or are implicated in their pathogenesis, e.g. Guillain–Barré syndrome (*Campylobacter pylori*)
	Do not forget atypical infections caused by *Listeria, Mycoplasma, Legionella,* etc.; diagnosis of TB requires special stains (Ziehl–Neelsen) and culture media (Lowenstein–Jensen)
Viral serology and culture (blood, CSF)	Viruses can cause a wide range of neurological infections, e.g. meningitis, encephalitis, shingles (herpes zoster)
VDRL (Venereal Disease Research Laboratory) (blood)	Primary syphilis (false positives in pregnancy, systemic lupus erythematosus, malaria)
TPHA (*Treponema pallidum* haemagglutination assay) (blood)	Syphilis, false positives in VDRL and other treponemal infections (yaws, pinta)
Borrelia serology (blood, CSF)	Lyme disease (see Ch. 31)
HIV (blood)	AIDS (see Ch. 31)
HTLV-1 (blood)	Myelopathy

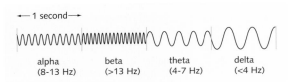

← 1 second →

| alpha | beta | theta | delta |
| (8-13 Hz) | (>13 Hz) | (4-7 Hz) | (<4 Hz) |

Fig. 3.5 Normal electroencephalographic rhythms.

Fig. 3.6 Some abnormal electroencephalographic activities

Activity	Interpretation
Generalized slow-wave activity	Metabolic encephalopathy, drug overdose, encephalitis
Focal slow-wave activity	Underlying structural lesion
Focal or generalized spikes, or spike and slow-wave activity	Epilepsy
Three-per-second (3/s), bilateral, symmetrical spike-and-wave activity (Fig. 3.7)	Typical absence seizures and other 'primary generalized epilepsy' syndromes
Periodic complexes (generalized sharp waves every 0.5–2.0 seconds)	CJD

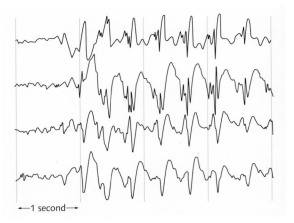

←1 second→

Fig. 3.7 Three-per-second (3/s) spike-and-wave activity, characteristic of typical absence seizure.

activity may be seen at rest. The most common types of spontaneous activity include fibrillation potentials, positive sharp waves and fasciculations.

Fibrillation potentials and positive sharp waves are due to spontaneous contractions of individual muscle fibres, probably due to abnormal rhythmic fluctuations of membrane potential. They cannot be seen clinically through the skin. They are most commonly seen in denervation, but may be found in some muscle diseases, especially inflammatory muscle disease (e.g. polymyositis).

Fasciculation potentials are much larger than fibrillations and represent the contractions of groups of muscle fibres supplied by a motor unit. They occur following denervation. They may be seen as a clinical fasciculation. They are common in motor neuron disease.

unless the needle is placed in the region of a motor end-plate (when miniature end-plate potentials are recorded).

In abnormal muscles, either due to primary muscle disease or to denervation of the muscle, spontaneous

Fig. 3.8 Common abnormalities found with electromyography (EMG) and nerve conduction studies (NCS)

Abnormality	Change in electromyographic trace
Denervation	Increased insertional activity; fibrillations, positive sharp waves, and fasciculations; large amplitude, long duration, polyphasic MUPs
Myopathy	Small, short, polyphasic MUPs
Myasthenia gravis	Abnormal decrement of amplitude of response on repetitive stimulation using nerve conduction tests; increased 'jitter' with single-fibre EMG (indicating variable neuromuscular transmission time)
Abnormality	**Change in nerve conduction**
Axonal neuropathy	Small action potential; normal nerve conduction velocity
Demyelinating neuropathy	Slow nerve conduction velocity; prolonged latency (time to travel from one point to the next); normal or slightly reduced action potential

MUPs, motor unit potentials.

Fasciculations may occur as normal phenomenon, especially after excess caffeine or in thyrotoxicosis. However, in these situations the firing rate is far more rapid than in diseases caused by denervation.

During voluntary movement, individual motor unit potentials (MUPs; the activity of a single anterior horn cell) can be seen on the EMG. Common abnormalities of EMG are shown in Figure 3.8.

Nerve conduction studies

Nerve conduction studies involve stimulating a nerve with an electrical impulse via a surface electrode and recording further along the nerve (sensory studies) or recording the muscle action potential (motor studies).

The amplitude of the response, the latency to the beginning of the response, and the conduction velocity are measured. As a general rule, a reduction in conduction velocity suggests demyelination whereas a reduction in amplitude suggests axonal loss (see Fig. 3.8).

Evoked potentials

Evoked potentials (EPs) use EEG electrodes to record responses centrally to peripheral stimuli:

- Visual EPs (VEPs): these are delayed in patients who have had an episode of optic neuritis (even if this was not clinically symptomatic) and this is therefore a useful test to help confirm a diagnosis of multiple sclerosis

- Brainstem auditory EPs (BSAEPs)
- Somatosensory EPs (SSEPs).

IMAGING OF THE NERVOUS SYSTEM

Plain radiography

Skull radiography

Skull radiography has a limited role in current neurological practice. The main indication is head injury when more sophisticated imaging is not immediately indicated or available. The standard views are:

- lateral
- posteroanterior
- Towne's view (fronto-occipital).

Spinal radiography

The standard views in spinal radiography are:

- lateral
- posteroanterior.

Computed tomography scanning

Using an X-ray source and a series of photon detectors housed in a gantry, CT produces a series of consecutive two-dimensional axial brain digital images that show the X-ray density of the brain tissue.

The densities of different brain tissues vary according to their X-ray absorption properties, ranging from low (black: air, cerebrospinal fluid) to high (white: bone, fresh blood).

The diagnostic yield of CT scanning is increased by injecting iodine-containing contrast agents. These enhance the distinction between the different brain tissues and outline areas of breakdown in the blood–brain barrier (around tumours, infarcts, or abscesses).

Magnetic resonance imaging

The term 'nuclear magnetic resonance' describes the interaction between the hydrogen protons in the different body structures and strong external magnetic fields. As the patient lies in the scanner, the naturally spinning hydrogen protons align with the strong magnetic field of the scanner. When a further external magnetic field (radiofrequency pulse) of a specific frequency is applied at a right angle, the protons 'flip' out of the main external magnetic field.

As the protons 'relax' back to their original position, they emit a radiofrequency signal that can be digitally analysed and displayed as an image. This 'relaxation' time has two components, known as T1 and T2, which determine the MRI parameters of the different brain tissues. MRI is especially useful at looking at small detail of intracranial structures, especially in the posterior fossa and spinal column where the surrounding bone distorts the image on CT.

The paramagnetic agent gadolinium-labelled DTPA (diethylene triamine penta-acetic acid, or pentetic acid) is used as contrast agent. Modification of the field conditions can now produce good-quality images of the cervical or cerebral blood vessels (either arterial or venous). This is called magnetic resonance angiography or venography, respectively.

Despite the better resolution of MRI, CT is faster and cheaper and is often better at examining fresh blood and bony structures.

Myelography

This procedure has now been largely supplanted by spinal MRI. A water-soluble iodine-based medium is injected into the subarachnoid space through a lumbar or a cervical approach. This outlines the spinal canal and nerve root sheaths, allowing the assessment of the spinal canal and the nerve roots. Cord compression caused by extramedullary or intramedullary lesions is identified as a compression or interruption of the column of contrast.

Postmyelographic CT scanning provides more detailed images of the nerve roots within the theca.

Imaging of the spinal cord is now performed largely by MR scanning but myelography can be helpful in specific conditions (nerve root lesions, spinal dural arteriovenous malformation) or in patients unable to undergo MRI because of claustrophobia or a cardiac pacemaker.

Catheter arteriography

Serial cranial radiographs are taken after the injection of an iodine-containing contrast agent into a large artery (aorta, carotid, vertebral) to allow the identification of cerebral vessels. Simultaneous digital subtraction of the surrounding soft tissues and bony structures allows the use of more-dilute contrast and a shorter procedure time, although the spatial resolution of the images will be compromised.

Venous digital subtraction angiography is possible, but the quality of the images obtained is distinctly inferior to those obtained through the arterial route.

The indications for traditional arteriography are:

- diagnosis of extracranial atherosclerotic cerebrovascular disease (stenosis, lumen irregularities, or occlusions), when not shown by Doppler study or MR angiography
- detailed evaluation of aneurysms and arteriovenous malformations
- diagnosis of cerebral vasculitis and other rare angiopathies
- assessment of cerebral vessel anatomy and tumour blood supply before neurosurgery
- interventional angiography: therapeutic embolization of aneurysms and vascular malformations.

Duplex ultrasonography

Duplex ultrasonography offers a combination of real-time and Doppler-flow ultrasound scanning, allowing a non-invasive assessment of extracranial arteries. It is particularly helpful as a screening test for lesions at the carotid bifurcation, which avoids the need for angiography in many patients. The quality of this technique is dependent on the experience and skill of the operator.

PART II
THE PATIENT
PRESENTS WITH. . .

4. Disorders of higher cerebral function 33

5. Disturbances of consciousness 39

6. Headache 49

7. Disorders of smell and taste 53

8. Visual impairment 57

9. Disorders of the pupils and eye movements .. 63

10. Facial sensory loss and weakness 75

11. Deafness, tinnitus, dizziness and vertigo 81

12. Dysarthria, dysphonia and dysphagia 89

13. Cerebellar dysfunction 93

14. Movement disorders 97

15. Limb weakness 103

16. Limb sensory symptoms 113

17. Disorders of gait 119

Disorders of higher cerebral function

4

● **Objectives**

- Understand the major functions of the four lobes of the cerebral neocortex
- Sketch the cortical homunculus
- Describe the main clinical symptoms and signs expected in lesions of each lobe
- Understand the difference between focal and diffuse cortical dysfunction

The term 'cognition' refers to our ability to perform complex intellectual behaviours such as speaking and writing, navigating our way around our environment, and recognizing and communicating with other people.

Focal damage to the cerebral hemispheres usually results from vascular events (infarction or haemorrhage), tumours, trauma or localized inflammatory/ infective lesions (e.g. abscess, tuberculoma). Generalized or multifocal cerebral dysfunction results from degenerative diseases (Alzeimer's disease, dementia with Lewy bodies), multiple infarcts, demyelination or diffuse infections (encephalitis, meningitis). For these reasons it is important to understand the basic functions of the different lobes and anatomical areas of the cerebral hemispheres.

The left and right cerebral hemispheres each contain a frontal, parietal, temporal and occipital lobe (Fig. 4.1). The side of the brain that controls writing and speech is called the 'dominant' hemisphere and the other side is the 'non-dominant' hemisphere.

The left hemisphere is dominant in over 90% of right-handed people and in about 60% of left-handed people.

FRONTAL LOBE

Normal functions

- Primary motor cortex: this is located in the precentral gyrus and is concerned with motor function of the opposite side of the body. The upper motor neuron cell bodies are topographically organized in the primary motor cortex in a 'homunculus' (Fig. 4.2). These neurons project axons in the corticospinal and corticobulbar tracts. The axons travel in the internal capsule to reach the brainstem and spinal cord to synapse with lower motor neuron cell bodies.
- Supplementary motor and premotor cortices: these areas are concerned with coordinating and planning complex movements.

- Frontal eye field: this is involved in making eye movements to the contralateral side.
- Broca's area (dominant hemisphere only): the motor or 'expressive' centre for the production of speech.
- Prefrontal cortex: the anterior and orbital parts of the frontal cortex govern personality, emotional expression, initiative and the ability to plan.
- The cortical micturition centre: this region lies in the paracentral lobule and is involved in the cortical inhibition of voiding of the bladder and bowel.

Blood supply

The blood supply to the frontal lobe is from the anterior cerebral artery (ACA) and middle cerebral artery (MCA). The ACA supplies the medial surface of the primary motor cortex, which controls the leg; the MCA supplies the lateral surface of the primary motor cortex, which controls the face and arm (see Ch. 29).

Symptoms from lesions of the frontal lobe

- Contralateral weakness: this is caused by damage to the precentral gyrus and can cause contralateral mono- or hemiparesis and facial weakness in an upper motor neuron pattern.
- Gait apraxia: this is the inability to walk normally in spite of preservation of normal power, coordination and sensory function, and no extrapyramidal dysfunction. The gait is slow and shuffling but upright and wide based, distinct from the flexed posture and narrow base of the parkinsonian gait (see Ch. 17). It can be caused by damage to the premotor and supplementary motor area.
- Conjugate eye deviation: both eyes look towards the side of the lesion and away from the side of weakness due to damage to the frontal eye field. This is

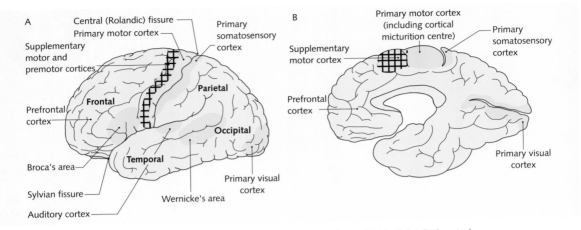

Fig. 4.1 Functional regions of the cerebral cortex. (A) Lateral left hemisphere. (B) Medial right hemisphere.

Fig. 4.2 Topographical distribution of the sensorimotor cortices or 'homunculus'.

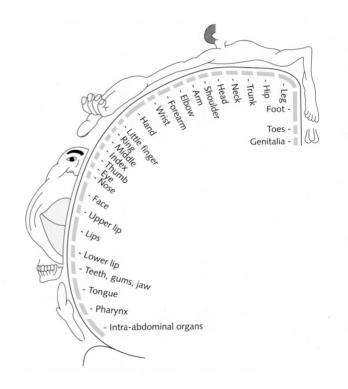

most commonly seen in a large middle cerebral artery stroke and carries a poor prognosis.

- Focal seizures arising from the frontal cortex give rise to clonic movements of the contralateral lower face, arm and leg, and conjugate deviation of the head and eyes towards the convulsing side (i.e. away from the side of the lesion).
- Expressive dysphasia: this is caused by damage to Broca'a areas and comprises non-fluent, hesitant speech with intact comprehension. The patient knows what he or she wants to say but has difficulty finding the correct words, often producing the wrong word. The ability to repeat words is better than spontaneous speech. Handwriting is also often poor.
- Personality and behavioural change: damage to the prefrontal cortex causes altered behaviour, including social disinhibition, loss of initiative and interest, inability to solve problems with loss of abstract thought, and impaired concentration and attention

without intellectual or memory decline. Loss of abstract thought can tested by the patient's interpretation of proverbs, which tends to be concrete or literal in nature e.g. people in glass houses should not throw stones; and by the patient's ability to identify similarities between pairs of objects, e.g. cow and dog, chair and table. These symptoms usually occur with bilateral lesions resulting from head injury, small vessel disease, frontal degenerations (e.g. the frontotemporal dementias) and acute hydrocephalus. Severe bilateral pathology, especially of the orbital surfaces, can result in akinetic mutism, in which the patient appears awake and is able to move the eyes but does not spontaneously move and is incontinent.

- Anosmia: lesions of the inferior or 'orbital' frontal lobes can be accompanied by disturbances of the olfactory pathway and optic nerves as a result of the close proximity of these pathways to the orbital surfaces of the lobes.

- Primitive (grasping, sucking, pouting, rooting and palmomental) reflexes: these reflexes may originate from the parietal cortex and are usually inhibited by the prefrontal cortex, although the exact anatomical substrate is uncertain. They are essential as a baby but are subsequently suppressed as the child grows. The grasp reflex consists of flexion of the thumb and fingers on stroking the skin of the palm. The sucking reflex can be elicited by lightly stroking the lips, which produces a sucking response. The palmomental reflex involves a brief muscular twitch on one side of the chin in response to a scratch by the examiner across the patient's palm on the same side.

- Incontinence of urine and/or faeces: this results from loss of cortical inhibition. There is no desire to micturate. Milder symptoms are frequency and urgency of micturition.

> **COMMUNICATION**
>
> Patients with frontal lobe disease often have poor insight into their cognitive problems. It is vital that a relative is interviewed to obtain a full history.

PARIETAL LOBE

Function

- Primary somatosensory cortex (dominant and non-dominant): this is located in the postcentral gyrus and is concerned with perceiving complex somatosensory stimuli from the contralateral side of the face and body. It receives afferent (incoming) projections via the thalamus from the somatosensory pathways. The fibres are represented topographically, in a homunculus, similar to that of the primary motor cortex.

- Language (dominant hemisphere): pathways within the arcuate fasciculus connecting Broca's area (frontal) with Wernicke's area (posterior temporal) pass through the inferior parietal region.

- Use of numbers, e.g. calculation (dominant hemisphere).

- Integration of somatosensory, visual and auditory information (mainly non-dominant): this allows awareness of the body and its surroundings, appropriate movement of the body and constructional ability.

- Visual pathways (dominant and non-dominant): the upper part of the optic radiation (subserving the lower quadrant of the contralateral visual field) passes deep within the parietal lobe and might be affected in lesions of the deep white matter.

Blood supply

The blood supply to the parietal lobe is from the middle cerebral artery.

Symptoms from lesions of the parietal lobe

- Cortical contralateral sensory loss (dominant and non-dominant): there is an inability to integrate sensory information which manifests as impairment of joint position and two-point discrimination, an inability to recognize objects by form and texture (astereognosis or tactile agnosia – e.g. patient cannot recognize a key or coin in the hand with the eyes closed) or figures drawn on the hand (agraphaesthesia). Cortical damage alone (as opposed to deep hemispheric damage) does not impair the ability to be able to appreciate light touch, pain, temperature or vibration, but that information cannot be used to make sensory judgements.

- Visual disturbances: if the deeper fibres of the parietal lobe are involved, a contralateral homonymous inferior quadrantanopia can arise.

Syndromes of the dominant parietal lobe

- Wernicke's receptive 'fluent' dysphasia: this arises from inferior parietal and superior temporal lesions (Wernicke's area and dorsally). There is impaired comprehension of speech and written language. The speech is fluent but words are replaced with partly correct words and an incorrect word related to the word intended (paraphasia) or newly created meaningless words (neologisms). The speech does not make sense and the patient has poor insight into the problem.

- Gerstmann's syndrome: this consists of the inability to differentiate the right and left sides of the body, inability to distinguish the fingers of the hands (finger agnosia), and impairment of calculation (dyscalculia) and writing (dysgraphia). Difficulty with reading (dyslexia) may also occur; this is a function of the dominant parieto-occipital cortex. Any of these symptoms may also occur in isolation in lesions of the dominant parietal lobe.
- Bilateral ideomotor and ideational apraxia: this is the inability to carry out a sequence of tasks when there is normal comprehension and intact motor and sensory function. Ideomotor apraxia occurs when a patient fails to mimic a meaningful or meaningless hand gesture by the examiner or cannot perform a movement to command such as sticking out their tongue, closing their eyes, whistling, or pretending to brush their hair. Ideational or 'conceptual' apraxia is more profound and is due to disturbances in the temporal sequencing of motor actions, and a failure to understand the use of tools and objects at a basic level, e.g. squeezing toothpaste onto a toothbrush.

Syndromes of the non-dominant parietal lobe

- Contralateral sensory inattention: there is an inability to perceive a contralateral stimulus when two simultaneous sensory stimuli are applied with equal intensity to corresponding sites on opposite sides of the body. However, when the stimulus is applied unilaterally it is perceived. This inattention or neglect when severe can be motor, sensory or visual. For example, a hemiplegic patient may ignore the paralysed side or there may be denial of the hemiplegia (anosognosia). Sensory and visual neglect are discussed in Chapter 16.
- Constructional apraxia (visuospatial dysfunction): there is difficulty in drawing simple objects (e.g. a house) and with construction (e.g. using building blocks). This also occurs to a lesser extent with dominant lesions.
- Dressing apraxia: there is difficulty with putting on clothes
- Topographical disorientation or topographagnosia: the patient cannot find his or her way around normally familiar spaces, e.g. home.

TEMPORAL LOBE

Function

- Wernicke's area (dominant hemisphere): this area, in the posterior part of the superior temporal gyrus, is concerned with comprehension of written and spoken language.

- The auditory and vestibular cortices: the primary auditory cortex receives fibres arranged in order of frequency of tone. The auditory pathways from each ear project to both auditory cortices. The dominant temporal lobe is important for the comprehension of spoken words, and the non-dominant for the appreciation of sounds and music. Vestibular fibres terminate just posterior to the auditory cortex.
- The limbic system: the olfactory and gustatory cortices lie in the medial temporal lobe. The limbic system is important in memory, learning and emotion.
- Visual pathways: the fibres of the lower part of the optic radiation (subserving the upper quadrant of the contralateral visual field) pass deep through the white matter of the temporal lobe.

Blood supply

The blood supply to the temporal lobe is from the posterior cerebral (medial part of the lobe) and middle cerebral (lateral part) arteries.

Symptoms from lesions of the temporal lobe

- Wernicke's receptive dysphasia (temporoparietal region): this is associated with fluent speech but a loss of comprehension of speech.
- Visual disturbances: a lesion involving the deeper fibres within the temporal lobe will cause a contralateral superior homonymous quadrantanopia (most commonly stroke or tumour).
- Memory impairment: this occurs with lesions of the medial temporal lobe involving the hippocampus and parahippocampal gyrus (e.g. neurodegenerative conditions like Alzheimer's disease). Difficulty in learning verbal information occurs in dominant lesions and non-verbal information in non-dominant lesions. Bilateral damage results in marked impairment of retention of new information.
- Emotional disturbances: emotional disturbances from damage to the limbic system can include aggression, rage, apathy, hyperorality and hypersexuality.
- Auditory agnosia: this is the inability to recognize sounds, e.g. ringing of a bell, without seeing or feeling the bell. It occurs in lesions of the non-dominant hemisphere.
- Cortical deafness: this will occur only with bilateral lesions of the primary auditory cortices and is uncommon. The patient might be unaware of the deficit.

HINTS AND TIPS

Hearing is normal in auditory agnosia and Wernicke's receptive dysphasia, but the interpretation of sounds and speech are abnormal.

DYSPHASIA

Dysphasia is a disorder of spoken and written language; it occurs with damage of the frontal, parietal or temporal cortices. Broca's expressive and Wernicke's receptive dysphasias occur with damage of the dominant hemisphere and are discussed above. The cortical areas subserving these functions are linked by the arcuate fasciculus, which runs in the sub-cortical white matter. This enables the comprehension of language with subsequent production of speech. There are other types of dysphasia associated with more isolated focal lesions:

- Conduction dysphasia: occurs with damage to the arcuate fasciculus in the dominant parietal lobe. The speech is fluent but contains 'jargon' and is non-sensical, with paraphrasia and neologisms as in Wernicke's dysphasia. However, comprehension of language is intact, the patient is aware of the problem, and repetition is markedly impaired.
- Global dysphasia: occurs with lesions of both Broca's and Wernicke's areas. There is a combination of non-fluent speech and impaired comprehension of language. This is the most common type of dysphasia and is usually caused by a stroke affecting the left middle cerebral artery territory.
- Nominal dysphasia: is an inability to name objects and arises from a lesion of the dominant parietotemporal cortex. It may occur during recovery from other dysphasias.

OCCIPITAL LOBE

Function

The function of the occipital cortex is the perception of vision and recognition of whatever is visualized.

Blood supply

The blood supply is from the posterior cerebral artery but the occipital poles, subserving macular vision, have additional supply from a branch of the middle cerebral artery.

Frontal lobe

Contralateral mono-/hemiparesis, facial weakness
Broca's dysphasia: Motor, expressive dysphasia (dominant)
Behavioural change: Social disinhibition, loss of abstract thought, apathy, mutism
Primitive reflexes: Grasp and sucking
Apraxic gait
Urinary incontinence
Contralateral horizontal gaze paresis

Parietal lobe

Contralateral discriminatory sensory impairment
Wernicke's dysphasia: Sensory, receptive dysphasia (dominant)
Visual field deficit: Contralateral lower homonymous quadrantanopia
Dominant syndromes: Gerstmann's syndrome, bilateral ideomotor and ideational apraxia
Non-dominant syndromes: Constructional apraxia, dressing apraxia,contralateral sensory inattention

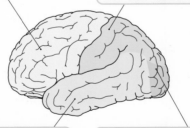

Temporal lobe

Wernicke's dysphasia: Sensory receptive dysphasia (dominant)
Auditory agnosia: Inability to recognize sounds (non-dominant)
Visual field deficit: contralateral upper homonymous quadrantanopia
Learning difficulties: Auditory (dominant) and visual (non-dominant) information
Memory impairment
Emotional disturbances: Aggression, rage, hypersexuality, olfactory and gustatory hallucinations

Occipital lobe

Visual field deficit: Contralateral homonymous hemianopia
lesions of posterior cerebral artery – spare the macula
lesions of the middle cerebral artery/occipital pole – contralateral macular homonymous hemianopic field defect
Visual agnosia: Impaired recognition of faces and objects
Visual illusions: Disturbance of size, shape, colour and number of objects
Visual hallucinations: Unformed and formed

Fig. 4.3 Summary of localization of symptoms arising from focal lesions of the cerebral hemispheres.

Symptoms from lesions of the occipital lobe

- Contralateral homonymous hemianopic field defect: if this arises from a lesion of the posterior cerebral artery, there will be sparing of the macular area leaving central vision intact with loss of peripheral vision.
- Cortical blindness: bilateral occipital lesions render the patient blind, with retention of the pupillary reflexes. The patient might deny the blindness (Anton's syndrome).
- Visual agnosia: lesions of the visual association cortices cause impairment of perception or identification of faces and objects, even though visual acuity and fields are normal. Achromatopsia refers to an inability to distinguish different colours, whereas prosopagnosia refers to an inability to recognise human faces. A patient knows that they are looking at a face but cannot recognise who they are.
- Visual illusions: objects might appear larger (macropsia) or smaller (micropsia); there might be disturbances of shape, colour and number. This is more common with lesions of the non-dominant hemisphere.

A summary of the localization of symptoms arising from focal syndromes is shown in Figure 4.3.

Disturbances of consciousness

- Describe the common causes of transient and persistent loss or change in consciousness
- What are the clinical differences between the presentation of syncope and epilepsy?
- What are the driving regulations after an episode of altered consciousness?
- How would you assess a patient in a coma? What is the Glasgow Coma Scale?
- Define the term non-convulsive status epilepticus

When consciousness is disturbed, patients usually exhibit an alteration in the awareness of their external environment. The ascending reticular activating system is a network of neurons originating in the brainstem that is modulated by external stimuli and projects to both cerebral cortices. The normal conscious state depends on the integrity of both the brainstem reticular activating system and the cerebral hemispheres. This provides an anatomical framework with which to approach impairment of consciousness clinically, which can range from either complete loss of awareness or 'unconsciousness' through varying degrees of impairment. The prodrome features during an event and the duration of impaired consciousness are also important in formulating a differential diagnosis. Impairment of consciousness can be transient or short-lived with a return to normal function between attacks or ongoing, prolonged unconsciousness otherwise called 'coma'.

TRANSIENT LOSS OF CONSCIOUSNESS

Transient loss or disturbance of consciousness is a very common presenting problem. The patient usually has no ongoing symptoms or physical signs when seen, and subsequent investigations are often unhelpful in ascertaining the cause. The diagnosis depends on taking a careful history from the patient, and from any available witness. The most common causes of transient loss of consciousness (LOC) are (Fig. 5.1):

- syncope
- seizures.

    Uncommon causes include:

- hypoglycaemia
- narcolepsy/cataplexy
- hyperventilation

- vertebrobasilar ischaemia
- vertebrobasilar migraine
- psychogenic or 'non-epileptic' attacks.

Syncope

Syncope is the transient loss of consciousness and posture that results from a global reduction in blood flow to the brain. There are five common causes.

1. Vasovagal syncope

Vasovagal syncope, or 'fainting', is caused by a sudden drop in blood pressure resulting from peripheral vasodilatation. There is a subsequent reduction in cardiac output, which is followed by vagal stimulation and therefore bradycardia. Typical precipitating situations are strong emotion, sudden intense pain and prolonged standing in hot oppressive circumstances such as a crowded train.

The patient is usually upright at the onset of syncope. Prodromal symptoms include feeling light-headed, gradual dimming of vision, ringing in the ears, salivation, sweating, nausea and sometimes vomiting. These symptoms can last from several seconds to a few minutes. The attack can be aborted if the patient lies flat but a patient who remains standing will lose consciousness and fall. The patient is usually pale and clammy, the pulse is low volume and slow, and the systolic blood pressure drops to approximately 60 mmHg. If this state persists for a sufficient time to cause cerebral hypoxia, the eyes may roll upward and there may be brief myoclonic movements, which can be mistaken for a seizure. This typically occurs if the patient is kept standing by unwitting onlookers, which prevents a return of blood flow to the brain. Sphincter control is usually maintained and a typical postictal state is not seen, although malaise may persist.

Fig 5.1 Differentiating syncope from seizures

	Syncope	Seizures
Relationship to posture	Usually when standing	Unrelated
Prodrome	Hypotensive symptoms: e.g. light-headed/faint, blurred/dim vision, sounds seem distant, tinnitus, perception of weakness, nausea, hot/cold, sweating	None or symptoms of a simple partial seizure/aura, e.g. déjà vu, epigastric rising sensation, feeling of anxiety and fear, focal sensory symptoms, focal twitching
Skin colour	Pale	Blue or normal
Respiration	Shallow	Stertorous (noisy)
Tone	Floppy (may jerk)	Tonic–clonic in a generalized seizure
Convulsion	Rare	Common
Urinary incontinence	Rare (though can occur)	Common
Tongue biting	Rare	Common
Recovery phase	Rapid Usually no confusion Pallor may persist	Often prolonged Confusion common and prominent
Focal neurological symptoms	No	Occasional
Clues to underlying aetiology	Situational, e.g. having blood taken Cardiac arrhythmia Aortic stenosis Cardiomyopathy Postural hypotension	History of known epileptic seizures Structural lesion in brain, e.g. tumour Severe head injury

2. Situational syncope – micturition and cough syncope

Micturition syncope usually occurs in men who get up during the night to pass urine. It results from a combination of vasodilatation (which occurs with emptying of the bladder), a degree of postural hypotension on standing and bradycardia. The loss of consciousness is sudden with a rapid recovery.

Sustained coughing can elevate the intrathoracic pressure sufficiently to impair the venous return to the heart. Increase of the cerebrospinal fluid pressure, reduction in pCO_2, and resultant vasoconstriction may also be contributory. Unconsciousness may also be associated with the Valsalva manoeuvre (exhalation against a closed glottis) and is seen in syncope following breath-holding attacks in children and strenuous activity (e.g. heavy lifting or laughing). The mechanism here is probably similar to cough syncope.

3. Postural hypotension

In a number of clinical conditions, the upright posture is accompanied by an uncompensated fall in blood pressure and therefore also cerebral blood flow. Postural hypotension can occur in:

- normal individuals, especially adolescents
- debilitating illness with prolonged recumbency
- autonomic neuropathy, e.g. diabetes, Guillain–Barré syndrome, amyloidosis
- hypovolaemia, e.g. loss of blood, diuretic therapy, Addison's disease
- neurodegenerative diseases, e.g. Parkinson's disease, multisystem atrophy
- drugs, e.g. antihypertensives.

4. Syncope due to primary cardiac dysfunction

Syncope of direct cardiac origin is usually abrupt and without prodrome. The upright position is not a prerequisite. Loss of consciousness is brief and classically accompanied by marked pallor with a rapid return of colour as cardiac output is restored (pallor can be prolonged after vasovagal syncope). Brief tonic or clonic movements and urinary incontinence may occur but recovery is usually rapid. The history, examination and further investigations including a 24-hour electrocardiogram (ECG) monitoring and an echocardiogram will further support a cardiac cause. These include:

- cardiac arrhythmias (usually profound bradycardia or pulseless ventricular tachycardia)

- left ventricular outflow obstruction: aortic stenosis, hypertrophic obstructive cardiomyopathy (HOCM)
- right ventricular outflow obstruction: pulmonary stenosis, pulmonary hypertension, pulmonary embolism
- ventricular failure, e.g. acute anterior myocardial infarction, dilated cardiomyopathy.

5. Carotid sinus disease

The carotid sinus responds to stretch by sending signals to the medullary cardiac centre. This produces a reflex bradycardia or drop in blood pressure. If a patient with a hypersensitive sinus, e.g. atheromatous disease, turns their head rapidly when wearing a tight collar, or if the carotid sinuses are massaged, then the patient can become hypotensive and lose consciousness.

Seizures

The most common diagnostic problem is distinguishing a syncopal attack from a seizure. Certain clinical features aid the differentiation of these common problems (Fig. 5.1):

- A seizure can occur in any position. Syncopal attacks tend to occur in the upright position, although this is less so with those of cardiac origin.
- The onset of a seizure is more sudden. There may be preceding aura symptoms but these usually last only seconds, shorter than the characteristic prodrome of syncope. The notable exception is the abrupt onset of syncope secondary to cardiac arrhythmia.
- During syncope patients usually have normal or reduced tone, although may transiently have mild stiffening or brief jerks of the limbs. In a generalized seizure, usually there is a prolonged and marked increase in tone with prominent jerking (tonic–clonic seizure).
- Urinary incontinence often accompanies a generalized seizure, although it can sometimes also occur with syncope.
- Patients may bite their tongue during a generalized seizure, especially the lateral edge. Tongue biting can occur infrequently in syncope, but more commonly affects the tip.
- Following recovery from a seizure, the patient is often confused, drowsy, with a headache and has aching muscles. This is called the 'postictal' state, and may be prolonged for several hours or days. Following a syncopal attack, the patient recovers consciousness and orientation within minutes, though there may be prolonged malaise.
- Injury is more common during a seizure.

> ### COMMUNICATION
>
> It is important to have a witness account of an episode of loss or disturbed consciousness. A correct history is usually vital to make a diagnosis. If the relative or friend who witnessed the event does not come to clinic with the patient, then ideally they should be contacted.

The different types of seizure are dealt with in more detail in Chapter 19.

Hypoglycaemia

Prodromal symptoms of hypoglycaemia include feeling tremulous and sweaty, palpitations and disorientation and may result in loss of consciousness. Seizures can occur as a secondary phenomenon. Causes of hypoglycaemia include overtreatment of diabetes, liver failure and, more rarely, hypopituitarism, Addison's disease and insulinomas. Hypoglycaemia does not occur in a healthy subject who has not eaten.

Narcolepsy/cataplexy

Narcolepsy is a disorder associated with excessive sleepiness and sleep attacks at innapropriate times. It can be associated with cataplexy (attacks of sudden reduction in muscle tone, lasting several seconds to minutes, usually precipitated by excitement or emotion), hypnogogic (on going to sleep) and hypnopompic (on waking) hallucinations. The disorder has a strong genetic component and there may be a family history.

Hyperventilation

Over-breathing results in a reduction of pCO_2, cerebral vasoconstriction, a metabolic alkalosis, and a reduction in ionized calcium. Characteristic features are:

- breathlessness and air hunger with rapid respiration
- light-headedness
- perioral and digital paraesthesia
- carpopedal spasm
- variable submammary or axillary chest pain
- anxiety and fatigue.

The attacks may occur in particular situations due to phobic anxiety, commonly in crowds, or sometimes after physical exertion. Hyperventilation rarely causes complete loss of consciousness.

Vertebrobasilar ischaemia

The brainstem reticular formation is supplied by the vertebrobasilar system and, if this is compromised, loss of consciousness might occur. This may be transient or prolonged depending on aetiology. Symptoms of brainstem origin, such as vertigo and diplopia, are often associated, and cerebrovascular risk factors may be present.

> **HINTS AND TIPS**
>
> Loss of consciousness due to a transient ischaemic attack (TIA) is extremely rare and is usually associated with focal symptoms of brainstem ischaemia. This should therefore be a diagnosis of exclusion.

Non-epileptic attacks

This is a diagnosis which is based on the exclusion of other causes, and features suggestive of non-epileptiform events. Patients should assessed by a specialist before being given this diagnosis.

Investigating transient loss of consciousness

In patients presenting with episodes of transient loss of consciousness, the first step is to establish whether the attacks might have been syncopal or a seizure. The diagnosis is made primarily from the history and an eyewitness account.

If a seizure is suspected, electroencephalography (EEG) may give information about the presence of abnormal activity but it is not a diagnostic test, and, despite the presence of epilepsy, is often normal between seizures. The diagnosis is made primarily from the history, and an eyewitness account of the event is essential. Imaging with computed tomography (CT) or magnetic resonance imaging (MRI) may help to identify structural causes of epilepsy.

If the history and examination are more suggestive of syncope, then a 12-lead, 24-hour ECG monitoring and echocardiogram need to be considered. If the attacks have a postural component, then tilt table testing should also be considered. Twenty-four-hour ECG monitoring may detect arrhythmias if they occur every day. For less frequent attacks, a REVEAL device may need to be inserted to detect infrequent, but clinically important, arrhythmias.

Often, investigations are normal in both conditions and the diagnosis is made by the history alone.

DRIVING AND EPISODES OF DISTURBANCES OF CONSCIOUSNESS

Patients are required to notify the DVLA after a single episode of loss of consciousness or altered awareness, unless the event is a simple vasovagal faint with clear provoking factors, and doctors should inform the patient of this fact. If the aetiology is likely to be cardiovascular and there is an identified cause which has been treated, patients are not allowed to drive for 4 weeks. If the aetiology is likely to be cardiovascular but no cause has been identified, patients are not allowed to drive for 6 months. After a single episode of loss of consciousness or altered awareness with seizure markers (i.e. strong clinical suspicion of seizure but no definite evidence) patients should not drive for 6 months. Finally after a solitary episode of loss of consciousness or altered awareness with no clinical pointers, patients should not drive for 6 months. Driving restrictions are more severe for those with group 2 licenses. Driving implications after epileptic seizures are covered in Chapter 19.

COMA

Coma is a state of impaired consciousness in which the patient is not rousable despite external stimuli. Confusion, delirium, obtundation and stupor are terms describing progressive states between full alertness and coma. However, they are not clearly defined and therefore interobserver interpretation is highly variable. The Glasgow Coma Scale (Fig. 5.2) provides a more objective and reproducible method by which conscious level can be assessed and documented. It is based on eye opening and verbal and motor responses. A patient with a normal conscious state will score 15 out of a total score of 15.

Differential diagnosis of coma

There are a number of conditions that may resemble coma, but are not true coma. The most important is non-convulsive status epilepticus, which is potentially reversible.

Non-convulsive status epilepticus

Non-convulsive status epilepticus should be suspected in patients who do not regain consciousness after convulsive status epilepticus. It can also occur spontaneously and should be suspected in any patient with ongoing confusion/disturbance of consciousness. An EEG usually confirms ongoing non-convulsive epileptic activity.

Akinetic mutism

Akinetic mutism is caused by damage to the prefrontal or premotor areas responsible for intiating movements. Patients have preserved awareness, and can follow with their eyes, but are unable to initiate movements or obey commands.

Fig. 5.2 Glasgow Coma Scale	
Eye opening	
1 None	
2 In response to pain	Patient responds to pressure on fingernail bed – if this does not elicit a response, supraorbital and sternal rub may be used
3 In response to speech	Not to be confused with an awakening of a sleeping person
4 Spontaneous	
Verbal responses	
1 None	
2 Incomprehensible sounds	Moaning but no words
3 Inappropriate words	Random or exclamatory articulated speech, but no conversational exchange
4 Disorientated speech	Patient responds to questions coherently but there is some disorientation and confusion
5 Orientated speech	Patients respond coherently and appropriately to questions such as their name and age, where they are, and what year/month/time it is
Motor responses	
1 None	
2 Extensor response to pain	Decerebrate response (see Fig. 5.5)
3 Flexor response to pain	Decorticate response (see Fig. 5.5)
4 Flexion/withdrawal to pain	Flexion of elbow, supination of forearm, flexion of wrist when supraorbital pressure is applied; pulls part of body away when nail bed pinched
5 Localization of painful stimulus	Purposeful movements towards a painful stimuli, e.g. hand crosses midline and gets above clavicle when supraorbital pressure applied
6 Obeys commands	

Locked-in syndrome

Locked-in syndrome results from an extensive lesion of the ventral pons which interrupts the corticobulbar and corticospinal pathways, with sparing of the reticular pathways and therefore sparing of consciousness. Patients are alert but unable to speak or move their face or limbs. The pathways for eye movement are relatively spared, so patients can communicate with vertical eye movements and blinking. This carries a grave prognosis and requires ventilatory support.

Persistent vegetative state

A persistent vegetative state, which can follow coma, refers to a state in which individuals have lost cognitive neurological function and awareness of the environment but retain non-cognitive function and a preserved sleep–wake cycle. The individual loses the higher cerebral powers of the brain but the functions of the brainstem, such as respiration and circulation, remain relatively intact. Spontaneous movements may occur and the eyes may open in response to external stimuli, but the patient does not speak or obey commands. Patients may occasionally grimace, cry or laugh. This condition usually follows diffuse damage to the cerebral cortex.

Catatonia

A catatonic patient is silent and there is no volitional motor or emotional response to external stimuli. The patient may resist an examiner's attempt to move, for example, a limb, and if the limb is moved, the patient may keep it fixed in this position for some time. This may be seen in catatonic depressive and schizophrenic states.

Causes of persistent disturbance of consciousness

The causes of persistent loss or disturbance of consciousness may be structural or non-structural (Fig. 5.3). Alteration in awareness is caused by damage to the ascending reticular activating system in the brainstem or damage to the cerebral hemispheres. In the latter case the damage is typically bilateral, or if unilateral, is large enough to exert remote effects on the brainstem or other hemisphere.

Fig 5.3 Common causes of persistent loss (coma) or disturbance of consciousness

Symmetrical and non-structural	Symmetric and structural	Asymmetric and structural
Toxins	**Supratentorial**	**Supratentorial**
Alcohol Carbon monoxide Methanol Ethylene glycol Cyanide Mushrooms	Bilateral internal carotid occlusion Bilateral anterior cerebral artery occlusion Sagittal sinus thrombosis Subarachnoid haemorrhage Thalamic haemorrhage Trauma–contusion Hydrocephalus	Unilateral hemispheric mass (tumour, abscess, subarachnoid/subdural/extradural bleed) with herniation Intracerebral bleed Pituitary apoplexy Massive or bilateral supratentorial infarction Multifocal leukoencephalopathy Acute disseminated encephalomyelitis
Drugs	**Infratentorial**	**Infratentorial**
Opiates Sedatives Barbiturates Lithium Anticholinergics Salicylate	Basilar occlusion Midline brainstem tumour Pontine haemorrhage Central pontine myelinolysis	Brainstem infarction Brainstem haemorrhage
Metabolic		
Hypoxia Hypercapnia Hypoglycaemia Hypernatraemia Hypothermia Hypothyroidism Hypopituitarism Adrenal crisis Thiamine deficiency (Wernicke's encephalopathy) Liver failure Renal failure		
Infections		
Bacterial meningitis Viral encephalitis Sepsis Malaria		
Other		
Seizures or postictal state Diffuse ischaemia (e.g. MI, heart failure, arrhythmias) Hypotension Hypertensive encephalopathy		

Clinical approach to the comatose patient

The first step is to ascertain:

- Airway: establish and clear the airway
- Breathing: ensure the patient is adequately ventilated with oxygen
- Circulation: ensure there is cardiac output; otherwise begin external cardiac massage.

If there is respiratory or circulatory failure, this must be corrected and the potential causes investigated. Once a stable cardiorespiratory status has been established, a history should be taken from a relative, friend or eyewitness, and a clinical examination and initial investigations must be performed to ascertain the cause of coma.

Examination of the comatose patient

Examine the patient for:

- signs of head injury
- neck stiffness (if no evidence of cervical spine injury)
- respiratory pattern
- pupil responses
- resting position of the eyes
- ocular movements
- fundoscopic abnormalities
- corneal reflexes
- limb posture and spontaneous movements
- reflexes and plantar responses
- assess the Glasgow Coma Scale.

Signs of head injury

Lacerations and bruising may be present and occur over an underlying fracture. A basal skull fracture may present with a normal skull X-ray. It is important to look for evidence of an anterior fossa fracture such as rhinorrhoea, bilateral periorbital haematoma, and subconjunctival haemorrhage. A fracture of the petrous bone may produce cerebrospinal fluid (CSF) or blood otorrhoea and be associated with Battle's sign (swelling and bruising over the mastoid process).

Neck stiffness

Resistance to passive neck flexion may be present in meningism, which can be seen in meningitis and subarachnoid haemorrhage.

Respiratory pattern

- Cheyne–Stokes respiration: alternate hyper- and hypoventilation; seen in metabolic and iatrogenic (opiate) disturbances, impaired cardiac output, bilateral deep hemisphere lesions (thalamus or internal capsule) and brainstem or medullary dysfunction
- Central neurogenic hyperventilation: lesions of the lower midbrain and upper pons
- Apneustic respiration: pauses of 2–3 seconds occur after inspiration; seen in pontine lesions.

Pupil responses

- Pin-point pupils: pontine lesions, opiates, parasympathomimetics
- Bilateral fixed mid-position: midbrain lesion, severe sedative drug overdose or hypothermia

- Bilateral fixed and dilated pupil: significant brainstem damage or overdose of anticholinergics or sympathomimetics
- Unilateral fixed and dilated (associated with ipsilateral third nerve palsy): supratentorial mass with uncal herniation, posterior communicating artery aneurysm, or primary brainstem lesion
- Enlarged, slowly reactive pupils: metabolic or toxic.

Resting position of the eyes

- Conjugate lateral deviation: large cerebral lesions produce eye deviation towards a lesion (contralateral to limb paralysis), whereas seizures produce eye deviation away from the lesion
- Lateral and downward deviation: usually due to an ipsilateral third cranial nerve palsy (often associated with a fixed and dilated pupil)
- Inward deviation: usually due to an ipsilateral sixth cranial nerve lesion
- Conjugate depression of eyes: midbrain lesion or compression.

Ocular movements

- Oculocephalic reflex (Fig. 5.4): seen in patients with an intact brainstem. On rotating the head to the left

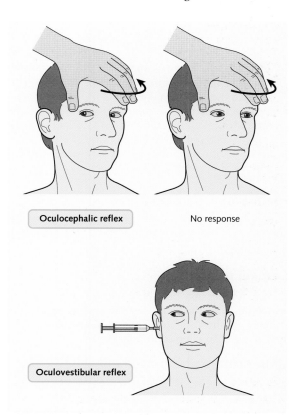

Fig. 5.4 Oculocephalic and oculovestibular reflexes.

Fig. 5.5 Decerebrate and decorticate posturing.

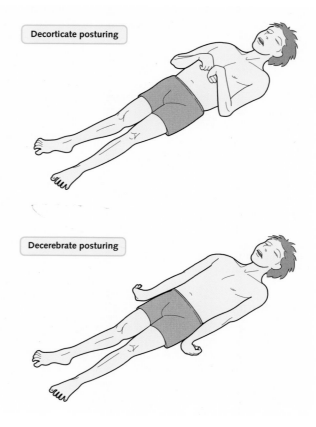

and right, the eyes will maintain their position by conjugate movement in the opposite direction. This is called the 'doll's eye' reflex
- Oculovestibular reflex: pouring cold water into the ear, or 'caloric stimulation', causes deviation of the eyes towards the side irrigated (Fig. 5.4)
- Lesions of the midbrain or pons may result in absent reflexes or dysconjugate movements of the eyes.

Fundoscopic abnormalities

Look for papilloedema suggestive of raised intracranial pressure, and subhyaloid haemorrhage associated with subarachnoid haemorrhage.

Corneal reflexes

Corneal reflexes may be suppressed (no blink with corneal stimulation) in large, contralateral acute cerebral lesions and intrinsic brainstem lesions. Ensure the patient is not wearing contact lenses.

Limb posture and movement

- Look for asymmetry of muscle tone, movement and reflexes, which may indicate a lesion in the contralateral cerebral hemisphere or within the brainstem

- Decerebrate posturing: extension at the elbow, pronation and flexion at the wrist, extension at knee and ankle, plantar flexed feet (Fig. 5.5). Classically associated with lesions at the level of the upper brainstem, but can occur in association with massive hemispheric lesions, or in setting of metabolic coma
- Decorticate posturing: arms flexed at the elbow and wrist, legs extended at the knee and ankle (Fig. 5.5). Classically associated with lesions at or above level of the diencephalon.

Investigations in the comatose patient

Immediate investigations include:
- temperature (hypothermia)
- blood glucose
- electrolytes, calcium, urea and creatinine
- full blood count and coagulation screen
- arterial blood gases
- blood culture and toxicology
- ECG and chest X-ray.

Neurological investigations in selected cases include:
- brain imaging (CT or MRI)

- lumbar puncture for CSF examination
- EEG
- cerebral angiography.

Prognosis of coma

In patients where a drug overdose or a reversible metabolic cause has caused coma and there has not been a prolonged period of unsupported cardiorespiratory failure, then the prognosis can be excellent with appropriate critical care. Other causes have a poorer prognosis. In patients with a Glasgow Coma Scale score of 3 for more than 6 hours there is a mortality of over 50% and, of the remainder, only a small minority will return to independent existence.

HINTS AND TIPS

Two common causes of coma are head injury and post-anoxic brain injury following cardiopulmonary resuscitation.

BRAINSTEM DEATH

Guidelines have been drawn up to diagnose brainstem death. Certain preconditions need to exist before testing can take place:

- The patient requires ventilatory support in the absence of depressant drugs.
- There is a known cause for the coma, capable of resulting in brainstem death.
- The patient's core temperature and any metabolic abnormality or effects of drugs must be normalized.
- The effects of any neuromuscular drugs must have worn off.

Specific clinical features on examination indicate brainstem death:

- Mid-position, fully dilated, fixed and non-reactive pupils
- Absent corneal reflexes
- Absent oculocephalic and oculovestibular reflex
- Absent gag reflex – no cough in response to pharyngeal or tracheal stimulation or suction
- No grimace in response to facial pain (from firm supraorbital pressure)
- Absent ventilatory reflexes – no spontaneous respiration even when pCO_2 rises to >6.5kPa

It should be noted that the tendon reflexes might be intact because these occur at spinal level. There might also be limb posturing to painful stimuli in some cases. The examination should be repeated within 24 hours by a second experienced clinician to confirm that irreversible brainstem death has occurred. Electroencephalography is not a diagnostic investigation. It might show slight residual activity in some brain-dead subjects and, exceptionally, might be flat in reversible coma resulting from hypothermia, drug intoxication or recent cardiac arrest.

● **Objectives**

- Describe the structures that are pain-sensitive in the head and neck
- What are the main clinical presentations of headache and what are the common causes?
- Which features in the history and examination would suggest a secondary cause for headache?

Headaches can be classified as either primary or secondary in nature. The most common primary headache syndrome is migraine. True tension headache and cluster headaches are uncommon. The diagnosis in these cases is made entirely from the history because there are no physical signs. Headache can also be secondary to other disorders affecting the head and neck, and it is sometimes the predominant symptom of serious intracranial disease such as a brain tumour, infections of the brain parenchyma or meninges or a subarachnoid haemorrhage. The most common cause of secondary headache is systemic infection.

Pain in the head and neck may be referred from the ears, eyes, nasal passages, teeth, sinuses, facial bones and cervical spine (Fig. 6.1). It is conveyed predominantly by the trigeminal nerve (fifth cranial nerve), and also by the seventh, ninth and tenth cranial nerves, and the upper three cervical roots. Structures of the anterior and middle cranial fossa generally refer pain to the anterior two-thirds of the head through the branches of the trigeminal nerve and structures of the posterior fossa refer pain to the back of the head and neck via the upper cervical roots. The brain parenchyma itself does not evoke pain, but pain arises from structures encasing it such as the meninges, and the blood vessels within the brain.

The approach to assessing a patient with headache should be based on the temporal pattern of symptoms, especially the mode of onset and subsequent course. This may be:

- recurrent and episodic with acute or subacute onset
- chronic and daily with fluctuations in severity over months or years
- new daily persistent headache
- subacute onset and progressive over days to weeks
- acute onset and progressive over hours.

Recurrent episodic headache

Recurrent episodic headache is usually benign and is very rarely due to sinister pathology. The most common causes are migraine, tension-type headaches and the trigeminal autonomic cephalgias, specifically, cluster headaches. These causes and their clinical features are listed in Figure 6.2. Other forms of trigeminal autonomic cephalgia such as paroxysmal hemicrania and short-lasting unilateral neuralgiform headache attacks with conjunctival injection and tearing (SUNCT) are much rarer and are not discussed in this book.

Chronic daily headache

Chronic daily headache is a descriptive term that is characterized by headaches occurring ≥ 15 days per month. The most common cause is chronic migraine, which is complicated by medication overuse headache (Fig. 6.3). Medication overuse headache is the term used when a primary headache develops or worsens when painkillers are taken too frequently (>8 to 10 days per month), and is typically preceded by an episodic headache disorder.

New daily persistent headache

New daily persistent headache is another descriptive term used to describe patients who present with a history of headache on most, if not all, days from the start of their initial presentation. The most common causes are the primary headache syndromes of migraine and tension-type headaches. However, this descriptive term also serves to highlight a group of secondary headaches which are potentially treatable. These include subarachnoid haemorrhage, low/high CSF pressure headaches, chronic meningitis and post-traumatic (including head injury and post-infection) headache. This type of presentation of headache should therefore prompt a thorough investigation to rule out secondary causes.

Fig. 6.1 The pain-sensitive structures in the head and neck, and disorders that may give rise to secondary headache.

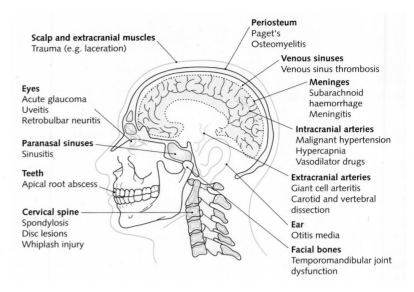

Scalp and extracranial muscles
Trauma (e.g. laceration)

Eyes
Acute glaucoma
Uveitis
Retrobulbar neuritis

Paranasal sinuses
Sinusitis

Teeth
Apical root abscess

Cervical spine
Spondylosis
Disc lesions
Whiplash injury

Periosteum
Paget's
Osteomyelitis

Venous sinuses
Venous sinus thrombosis

Meninges
Subarachnoid
haemorrhage
Meningitis

Intracranial arteries
Malignant hypertension
Hypercapnia
Vasodilator drugs

Extracranial arteries
Giant cell arteritis
Carotid and vertebral
dissection

Ear
Otitis media

Facial bones
Temporomandibular joint
dysfunction

Fig. 6.2 Common causes of recurrent episodic headache

Cause	Clinical features
Migraine	Unilateral subacute onset throbbing headache exacerbated by movement and typically lasting 4 to 72 hours Accompanied by nausea, vomiting, vertigo, photo-, phono- and osmophobia ± aura symptoms (visual, sensory, motor, or speech) May be triggered by bright light, strong smells, loud sounds, sleep deprivation/excess, exercise, tiredness, hunger/dehydration, fatigue, exercise, menstruation
Cluster headache	Severe unilateral retro/peri-orbital ± temporal pain of acute onset reaching crescendo within minutes Associated autonomic features: conjunctival injection/lacrimation, ptosis, miosis, nasal congestion/rhinorrhoea, facial flushing/ sweating/pallor Associated restlessness/agitation Attacks last 15–180 minutes, can occur up to 8 times per day and may have circadian periodicity Triggered by alcohol
Tension-type headache	Tight band around the head or a pressure-like sensation; usually mild-to-moderate severity and waxes and wanes lasting variable amount of time; otherwise completely featureless
Benign coital, exertional, cough and hypnic headache	Headaches precipitated by exertion, coughing, straining, sexual activity and sleep; may be benign, but this diagnosis is one of exclusion

Fig. 6.3 Common causes of chronic daily headache

Cause	Clinical features
Chronic migraine ± analgesic overuse	Daily, mild, bilateral, usually featureless headache with superimposed episodes of characteristic migraine headaches
Tension-type headache ± analgesic overuse	A tight band around the head and otherwise featureless headache; mild-to-moderate intensity
Chronic cluster headache	Defined as cluster headaches occurring ≥ 1 year without remissions or remission lasting < 1 month
Secondary headaches	Post-traumatic headaches (head injury, iatrogenic, post-infectious), inflammatory (giant cell arteritis, sarcoidosis, Behcet's disease), chronic CNS infections, substance abuse

Subacute-onset and progressive headache

The category of subacute-onset headache includes most of the serious secondary causes of headache. Worrying features include acute/subacute onset, increasing severity of headache, persistent associated neurological symptoms or signs, a deterioration of conscious level, seizures, associated fever or local tenderness, such as of the temporal artery (Fig. 6.4).

Fig. 6.4 Common causes of subacute-onset headache

Cause	Clinical features
Intracranial tumour	Features associated with raised intracranial pressure – headache exacerbated by coughing, sneezing, bending over or straining; blurring of vision on bending over; papilloedema; associated nausea and vomiting May be associated focal neurological symptoms and signs including seizures
Idiopathic intracranial hypertension	Most common in young, overweight women Features associated with raised intracranial pressure (as above) CT or MRI/MRV is normal
Meningitis/encephalitis	Fever, neck stiffness, +ve Kernig's sign, inflammatory (infective) CSF
Venous sinus thrombosis	Nausea, vomiting, drowsiness, seizures, focal signs; usually female gender, pregnancy and puerperium are risk factors
Subdural haematoma	History of head injury (falls in elderly and alcoholics), fluctuating level of consciousness, confusion, focal neurological signs
Intracranial abscess	Direct extension from local disease (e.g. frontal sinusitis) or metastatic spread (e.g. lung abscess), fever, systemically unwell, focal neurological signs
Giant-cell arteritis	Patients usually over 50 years of age Visual disturbance–acute monocular loss of vision – signs include papillitis with normal blind spot Associated polymyalgia rheumatica Elevated ESR and CRP Tender thickened superficial temporal artery $\pm$ absent pulsation
Acute hydrocephalus	Nausea, vomiting, diplopia (6th nerve palsy–false localizing sign) $\pm$ fluctuating conscious level, papilloedema, ataxia of gait, diagnosis confirmed on CT head scan
Acute glaucoma	Pain typically frontal, orbital or ocular, accompanied by persisting visual impairment, fixed oval pupil and conjunctival injection This is an ophthalmological emergency
Post-traumatic headache	Post-traumatic headache syndromes include several subtypes, the most common being migrainous headaches
Low CSF volume/ pressure headache	Orthostatic headache occurs following lumbar puncture or a spontaneous or traumatic chronic leakage of CSF – headache better with recumbency

Acute-onset headache

The instantaneous onset should always raise the suspicion of a subarachnoid haemorrhage, the dissection of an artery such as the carotid or basilar artery or a haemorrhagic stroke. There are also benign causes such as recurrent coital or exertional headache and a thunderclap presentation of migraine, as listed in Figure 6.5.

A good history is essential to differentiate the type of headache. Determine:

- age at onset
- presence or absence of an aura and prodrome
- mode of onset: acute, subacute, chronic, or recurrent and episodic
- subsequent course: episodic, progressive or chronic
- site: unilateral or bilateral; frontal, temporal or occipital; radiation to neck, arm or shoulder
- character of pain: constant, throbbing, stabbing, dull ache, pressure-like or a tight band
- frequency and duration: constant or intermittent with pain lasting seconds, hours or days
- accompanying features: neck stiffness, autonomic symptoms and aura-like symptoms (visual, motor, sensory or speech).
- exacerbating factors: movement, light, noise, smell, coughing, sneezing or bending
- precipitating factors: alcohol (cluster headache, migraine), menstruation (migraine), stress (all headache types), postural change (high or low

Fig. 6.5 Common causes of acute-onset headache

Cause	Clinical features
Subarachnoid haemorrhage	Explosive and instantaneous 'thunderclap' headache Neck stiffness, photophobia CT head scan – subarachnoid blood (within 48 hours) CSF – xanthochromia (12 hours to 1 week) CT or formal angiography may show aneurysm ± seizures and focal neurological signs if there has been intracerebral extension of blood
Haemorrhagic stroke	Note history of hypertension, smoking, diabetes, anticoagulation Focal neurological signs depending on site of bleed
Arterial dissection	This presents with head and neck pain; can be spontaneous or secondary to rapid deceleration or high/low-velocity rotation of the head and neck
Migraine	Migraine can present with an explosive 'thunderclap' headache; the diagnosis of a migrainous aetiology is one of exclusion
Coital/exertional headache	Can occur with an explosive onset before or during orgasm. At initial presentation this is a diagnosis of exclusion.

CSF volume headache) or head injury (subdural haemorrhage or post-traumatic migraine).

- particular time of onset: mornings (raised intracranial pressure, sleep apnoea syndrome) or awoken at night (cluster headache).
- past history of headache and response to any previous treatment
- family history: migraine or intracranial haemorrhage
- general health: systemic ill health, existing medical conditions, overweight (sleep apnoea), stress, low mood and depression
- Drug history: analgesic overuse, the oral contraceptive pill, recreational drugs, anticoagulants, vasodilators, e.g. nitrates, nifedipine.

EXAMINATION

When examining a patient with headache, look for:

- level of consciousness including GCS
- focal neurological signs including papilloedema
- signs of local disease of the ears, eyes or sinuses; restriction of neck movements and pain; temporomandibular joint dysfunction; thickening of the superficial temporal arteries and an absence of pulsation; tenderness of the scalp and neck muscles
- signs of systemic disease, and, if overweight, measure the body mass index (sleep apnoea)
- abnormal blood pressure.

COMMUNICATION

The clinical examination is often entirely normal in patients with headache. The history is therefore vital, especially with regard to migrainous symptoms and overuse of analgesics, particularly paracetamol and opiate based analgesics.

HINTS AND TIPS

Features that should alert the clinician to the presence of a secondary headache and prompt further investigation are:

- recent-onset headaches in middle or old age with no previous history of headache
- associated features: new focal neurological symptoms and signs, papilloedema, seizures, personality change, fever or systemic illness
- known systemic illnesses that predispose to secondary headaches (e.g. immunosuppression such as HIV, cancer)
- subacute or acute onset (especially if maximal intensity reached within seconds to minutes) or progressive course
- recent change in established pattern or character of headache
- headaches associated with manoeuvres that increase or decrease intracranial pressure (e.g. orthostatic headaches, Valsalva-induced headaches)
- head pain radiating to the neck or between shoulders (meningeal irritation due to infection or subarachnoid blood)
- increasing severity despite treatment.

Disorders of smell and taste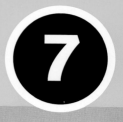

- Understand the basic anatomy of the olfactory system
- Describe the common causes of disturbances of smell
- Be aware of the serious pathologies which may rarely present with loss of smell

Alteration of the sense of smell is not a common presenting symptom, and impairment of olfaction as a physical sign is not often important in making a neurological diagnosis. Consequently, smell is not always tested during a routine clinical examination. However, anosmia, or the loss of sense of smell, is a significant problem after some head injuries and, rarely, it can be the only physical sign of a serious structural lesion involving the frontal lobes.

Odours enter the nose and sinuses where they stimulate olfactory receptors on cells of the nasal mucosa. These cells are bipolar neurons that have peripheral and central processes. The peripheral processes contain many cilia, which carry the olfactory receptors. The unmyelinated central processes enter into the cranial cavity through the cribriform plate of the ethmoid bone to synapse with dendrites of the mitral cells in the olfactory bulb. Axons from mitral cells, in the olfactory bulb, form the olfactory tract, and run in the olfactory groove of the cribriform plate beneath the frontal lobes and above the optic nerve and chiasm. Some of these axons synapse within the anterior perforated substance but most continue into the brain and ultimately terminate in the primary olfactory cortex (in the anterior aspect of the parahippocampal gyrus and the uncus of the temporal lobe) and nuclei of the amygdaloid complex (Fig. 7.1).

DIFFERENTIAL DIAGNOSIS

Anosmia and hyposmia

Anosmia is loss of the sense of smell. Hyposmia is impairment of the sense of smell. Anosmia or hyposmia may be due to:

- inability of odours to reach the olfactory receptors (hypertrophy or oedema of the nasal mucosa)
- destruction of the receptor cells and their central connections
- central lesions including neurodegeneration.

The anosmia or hyposmia may be temporary or permanent. The patient will not notice unilaterally impaired olfaction. Olfaction tends to naturally deteriorate with age.

The following causes should be considered:

- Upper respiratory tract infection: chronic rhinitis, sinusitis (allergic, vasomotor, or infective)
- Heavy smoking causing metaplastic changes in the nasal epithelium
- Viral infections, e.g. influenza, herpes simplex (may cause permanent destruction of the receptor cells)
- Drugs, e.g. antibiotics, antihistamines, penicillamine
- Local trauma to the olfactory epithelium
- Head injury: unmyelinated fibres from the receptor cells are damaged along their vulnerable course through the cribriform plate, particularly if there is an associated fracture. If the dura is torn there may be cerebrospinal fluid rhinorrhoea; this can be differentiated from mucous secretion by its higher glucose concentration. This is the most common neurological cause of anosmia
- Tumours: meningioma of the dura in the olfactory groove may extend posteriorly to involve the optic nerve. Rarely, frontal lobe gliomas and pituitary tumours
- Aneurysm of the anterior cerebral or anterior communicating artery
- Raised intracranial pressure: olfaction may be impaired without evidence of damage to the olfactory structures
- Frontal lobe abscess
- Degenerative disorders such as Alzheimer's disease and Parkinson's disease are often associated with anosmia.

Ageusia and dysgeusia

Ageusia is the perception of loss of taste. Dysgeusia is the perception of an impaired sense of taste.

Many patients with bilateral anosmia complain of loss or impairment of taste. This is because the

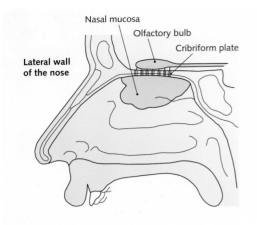
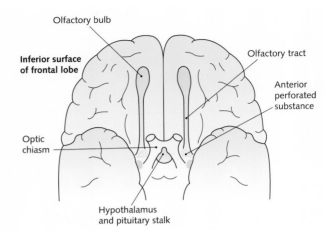

Fig. 7.1 The anatomical relations of the olfactory nerve.

appreciation of food and drink is by olfaction rather than by elemental taste. Taste itself is normal if tested formally in anosmic subjects.

Hyperosmia

Hyperosmia is an abnormally increased sensitivity to odours and may be seen in the following conditions:

- Anxious patients may complain of hypersensitivity to various odours
- Migraine attacks with and without aura may be accompanied by hypersensitivity to light, sound and smell (osmophobia).

Olfactory hallucinations

- Complex partial seizures of temporal lobe origin can give rise to brief olfactory hallucinations, which are part of the aura.
- Olfactory hallucinations may occur following alcohol withdrawal.
- Olfactory hallucinations and delusions of unpleasant nature can be due to a psychotic illness, e.g. depression or schizophrenia.
- Hallucinations and delusions may also occur in patients with some forms of dementia.
- A persistent unpleasant smell may occur from local disease of the nasopharynx such as purulent sinusitis.

HINTS AND TIPS

Disorders of smell:

- Anosmia/hyposmia is the loss/impairment of smell. The patient will notice this if the impairment is bilateral but not if it is unilateral. It is most often caused by disease of the nasopharynx and alterations of the nasal epithelium in smokers but head injury is the most common neurological cause.
- Ageusia/dysgeusia is an apparent alteration in taste perception in individuals with bilateral anosmia.
- Hyperosmia is a hypersensitivity to odours and is usually seen in anxious patients or migraine.
- Olfactory hallucinations may occur with temporal lobe seizures, following alcohol withdrawal, as a manifestation of psychosis or in patients with some dementias.

EXAMINATION

A stimulus for smell (e.g. peppermint, clove oil) is held under each nostril in turn while the other is occluded and the patient keeps the eyes closed. An individual with intact olfaction will be able to detect the smell and name it. The recommended special testing bottles are rarely available when needed and most clinicians perform preliminary assessment with nearby objects such as fruit, a coffee jar or cigarette packet. When examining patients with anosmia, it is important to look carefully for frontal lobe signs and evidence of optic nerve or chiasmal damage.

Pathology in the nasal passages or sinuses is a more common cause of anosmia than any neurological condition.

INVESTIGATIONS

Unexplained anosmia may require referral for more expert ear, nose and throat (ENT) examination if there is no suspicion of a neurological cause or obvious ENT cause.

If the patient has any evidence in the history or examination of frontal lobe or visual field defects in combination with anosmia, then it is appropriate to image the brain with computed tomography or magnetic resonance imaging to look for a structural lesion such as a tumour or abscess. Established post-traumatic anosmia requires no investigation unless there are also features to suggest a cerebrospinal fluid fistula or intracranial infection. The prognosis for a return of smell in post-traumatic patients is often poor, but late recovery can occur.

COMMUNICATION

In any patient complaining of loss of smell, it is important to take an accurate history for use of recreational drugs such as alcohol (head trauma) and smoking (olfactory epithelial metaplasia) as these are the commonest causes. Visual fields and frontal release signs should be accurately assessed as dysfunction in these systems may be the only other abnormal physical signs. If no obvious cause can be found, then CT or MRI of the brain and sinuses is warranted. It should be noted that the sinuses are not formally assessed on a routine CT scan of the brain and appropriate views need to be requested specifically.

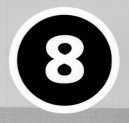

Objectives

- Understand the anatomical pathway from light stimulation of the retina to visual cortex
- Be able to sketch the common visual field defects associated with abnormalities in the visual pathway
- Describe the main causes of acute transient and persistent visual loss

Disturbance of vision is often due to ocular disease and is largely dealt with by the ophthalmologist. Visual impairment presenting to the neurologist usually involves a lesion in the visual pathway from the retina to the occipital cortex.

THE ANATOMICAL PATH OF LIGHT STIMULATION

1. Retina to optic nerve

- The visual fields and retina have an inverted and reversed relationship such that light from (Fig. 8.1):
  - the upper visual field falls on the inferior retina
  - the lower visual field falls on the superior retina
  - the nasal visual field falls on the ipsilateral temporal retina and contralateral nasal retina
  - the temporal visual field falls on the ipsilateral nasal retina and contralateral temporal retina.
- The retina consists of three distinct neuronal levels: photoreceptors, bipolar and ganglion cells.
- There are two types of photosensitive cells: 'rods' and 'cones'.
- Rods are responsible for night vision and detection of peripheral movement and are in greatest density in the periphery of the retina. They do not detect colour.
- Cones are responsible for daytime and colour vision and are concentrated at the macula.
- The macula is a region of the retina specialized for perception of detailed images and colour.
- The rods and cones convert light into electrical impulses and transmit these to bipolar cells, which in turn pass the signal to the ganglion cells.
- The ganglion cells have unmyelinated axons so that their fibres do not interfere with the path of light reaching the rods and cones.

- The unmyelinated axons converge at the optic disc and at that point become myelinated as they form the second cranial or 'optic' nerve.

The physiological blind spot corresponds to the optic disc, which has no overlying photoreceptors, and is located approximately 15° temporally in each eye.

2. Optic nerve to optic chiasm

- Fibres from the temporal half of each retina run in the temporal half of the optic nerve and those from the nasal half of the retina, in the nasal half of the nerve. The macular fibres run centrally.
- The optic nerve then passes through the orbit and exits at the optic foramen to the undersurface of the frontal lobe to join the other optic nerve forming the optic chiasm.

3. Optic chiasm to lateral geniculate nucleus

- The optic chiasm lies anterior to the pituitary stalk, superior to the pituitary and inferior to the hypothalamus (see Fig. 8.2).
- Optic nerve fibres carrying impulses from the nasal part of the retina lie medially and cross in the chiasm whilst those subserving the temporal retina lie most laterally and continue unchanged.
- Fibres in the inferior part of the chiasm carry information regarding the upper visual field and upper part from the lower visual field.
- The ipsilateral temporal fibres and the contralateral nasal fibres join to form the optic tract. This travels to the midbrain and the posterior thalamus where it synapses within the lateral geniculate nucleus (LGN).
- A few fibres leave the tract before the LGN and pass directly to the tectal area at the back of the upper midbrain and mediate the light and accommodation reflexes.

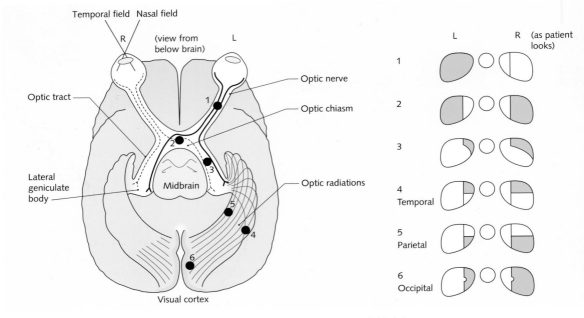

Fig. 8.1   Lesions of different parts of the visual pathway produce characteristic field defects.

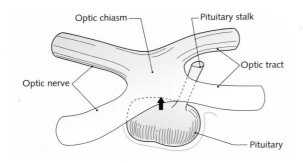

Fig. 8.2   Relation of the optic chiasm to its surrounding structures and in particular to the pituitary fossa, with which it is closely associated. The arrow indicates upward pressure on the inferior part of the chiasm by a pituitary tumour.

4. Lateral geniculate nucleus to occipital cortex

- The axons from the cell bodies in the LGN form the optic radiation, which passes in the posterior part of the internal capsule. Within the optic radiation, those that subserve the upper part of the visual field travel around the temporal portion, and those subserving the lower visual field pass around the parietal portion, of the lateral ventricle (see Fig. 8.1).

- Both paths terminate in the calcarine or primary visual (calcarine) cortex on the medial surface of the occipital cortex.

BLOOD SUPPLY TO THE VISUAL PATHWAY

Figure 8.3 is a schematic diagram of the blood supply to all elements of the visual pathway. The ophthalmic artery is the first branch of the internal carotid artery and gives rise to the central retinal and posterior ciliary arteries, which supply the retina and orbital portion of the optic nerve. The intracranial portion of the optic nerve and optic chiasm is supplied by the internal carotid, anterior cerebral and anterior communicating arteries. The optic tract is supplied mainly by the anterior choroidal artery, which is a branch of the internal carotid. The lateral geniculate nucleus is supplied by the anterior and posterior choroidal arteries. The optic radiations are supplied by the middle and posterior cerebral arteries. The posterior cerebral artery supplies the visual cortex.

Visual field defects

Lesions at different sites of the optic pathway give specific visual field defects, as shown in Figure 8.1.

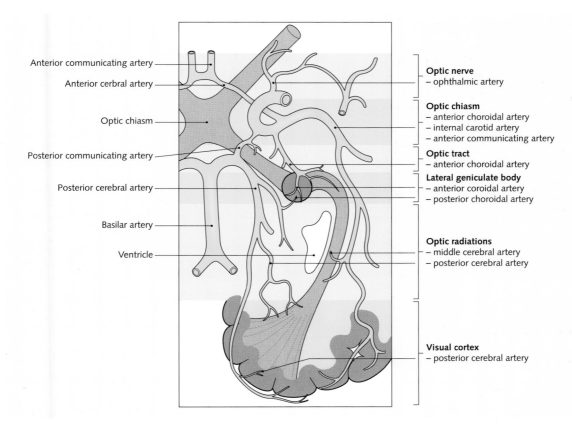

Fig. 8.3 Blood supply to the visual pathway

Descriptive terms for field defects

The terms used to describe visual field deficits can confuse students initially. There are several basic principles:

- 'Monocular' deficits occur anterior to the optic chiasm in the retina or optic nerve.
- 'Binocular' deficits occur posterior to the optic chiasm.
- 'Hemianopia' means affecting half the vision in one or both sides.
- 'Quadrantanopia' means affecting a quarter of the visual field in one or both eyes.
- 'Homonymous' means affecting the same part of the visual field in both eyes.
- 'Incongruous' means the affected part of the visual field is in the same region in both eyes (i.e. homonymous) but it is asymmetrically affected, e.g. lesions of the optic tract.
- If you have difficulty understanding a visual field defect then try and follow the anatomical path it takes from the retina to the lesion.

CLINICAL FEATURES TO AID LOCALIZATION OF A LESION

Retinal lesion

Macular lesions produce central or paracentral defects, whereas most degenerative retinopathies, such as retinitis pigmentosa, produce progressive constriction of the peripheral fields.

Optic nerve lesion (see 1, Fig. 8.1)

The patient complains of impaired vision in one eye. If the cause is inflammatory, then there may be pain with movement of the eye. On examination, there is reduced visual acuity, reduction of colour vision, a central scotoma and afferent pupillary defect may be present. If the lesion is long-standing, the vision may be completely lost in the affected eye and the optic disc becomes pale; this is the appearance of optic atrophy. There are many causes of an optic neuropathy as shown in Figure 8.4.

Fig. 8.4 Causes of optic neuropathy

Mechanism	Examples
Inflammatory (optic neuritis)	Demyelination associated with multiple sclerosis – most common but others include: - acute disseminated encephalomyelitis (ADEM) - sarcoidosis - systemic autoimmune disease (e.g. SLE, Wegener's granulomatosis) - infection (e.g. toxoplasmosis, cat scratch fever, syphilis, Lyme disease)
Vascular	Ischaemic optic neuropathy – can be associated with vasculitis (e.g. giant cell arteritis) or associated with small vessel disease due to age, hypertension or diabetes
Space-occupying lesions	Compressive optic neuropathy due to optic nerve or orbital neoplasm (e.g. meningioma or glioma)
Toxins/drugs	Alcohol overuse, methanol, tobacco, amiodarone, ethambutol, post-radiotherapy
Nutritional deficiencies	Vitamins B_{12} and B_1, folate
Genetic	Leber's hereditary optic neuropathy – presents with subacute painless, sequential optic neuropathy over weeks to months
Raised intracranial pressure	Long-standing papilloedema can cause optic neuropathy
Trauma	

HINTS AND TIPS

A central scotomatous deficit may be caused by:
• retinal disease involving the macula
• lesions of the optic nerve causing an optic neuropathy.

Optic chiasm lesion (see 2, Fig. 8.1)

A chiasmal lesion causes a bitemporal hemianopia due to involvement of the decussating fibres. Pressure from a lesion below the chiasm (e.g. pituitary tumour) will involve the inferior nasal fibres first, resulting in a bitemporal superior quadrantanopia. Compression from a lesion above the chiasm (e.g. hypothalamic craniopharyngioma) will cause a bitemporal inferior quadrantanopia. The patient often either complains of loss of vision in one eye,

or may repeatedly bump into furniture in either visual field field.

The anatomical relations of the optic chiasm are shown in Figure 8.3. Double vision is uncommon but can occur if the lesion extends to involve the oculomotor nerves in the cavernous sinus.

Lesions of the optic chiasm include:

• tumours, e.g. pituitary adenoma, meningioma, craniopharyngioma or metastatic deposits
• cerebral aneurysm
• granulomatous disease of the pituitary or meninges such as tuberculosis, sarcoidosis.

Optic radiation and optic tract lesions (see 3, 4, 5, Fig. 8.1)

Lesions of the optic tract or radiation cause a contralateral homonymous hemianopia or quadrantanopia. The more congruent the hemianopia or quadrantanopia, the more posterior the lesion. Those confined to the parietal fibres give rise to an inferior quadrantanopia and those confined to the temporal lobe fibres give rise to a superior quadrantanopia. The patient often attributes the problem only to the eye on the hemianopic side. Lesions of the optic tract and optic radiation include:

• stroke (infarction or haemorrhage) in the territory of the middle cerebral artery
• tumours
• trauma.

Isolated optic tract lesions are uncommon and are usually caused by posterior extension of a pituitary tumour. They cause an incongruous hemianopia.

Occipital cortex lesions (see 6, Fig. 8.1)

Unilateral lesions of the posterior cerebral artery, e.g. embolism from the vertebrobasilar arterial tree, cause a contralateral homonymous hemianopia sparing the fibres that originate from the macula. This is because of the dual blood supply (posterior and middle cerebral artery) of the pole of the visual cortex which subserves macular function.

DIFFERENTIAL DIAGNOSIS OF VISUAL LOSS

When a patient presents with visual impairment it is important to establish:

• if it is monocular or binocular
• the mode of onset (abrupt or gradual)
• subsequent course
• whether it is transient or permanent
• if it is associated with symptoms such as pain.

The patient's characteristics and associated symptoms are also important: for example, a hypertensive diabetic male is more likely to have painless anterior ischaemic optic neuropathy compared to a young female, who is more likely to have a painful optic neuritis.

Monocular or binocular visual impairment

Monocular visual loss results from lesions anterior to the chiasm (lens, retina or optic nerve), whereas binocular visual loss results from either bilateral anterior lesions or chiasmal, or retrochiasmal lesions.

Acute transient visual impairment

- Amaurosis fugax
- Migraine with aura
- Papilloedema.

Amaurosis fugax

This is a transient ischaemic event. The patient complains of sudden, painless unilateral altitudinal visual loss, often described as a shutter coming down from the superior to inferior part of the visual field. This lasts several seconds or minutes, followed by complete recovery.

The most common cause is atheroma of the ipsilateral carotid artery, causing embolism into the central retinal artery and its distal branches. The patient may have risk factors for vascular disease.

Migraine with aura

The visual symptoms, or 'aura', that precede migraine headache can consist of unformed flashes of white or, less commonly, coloured lights (photopsia) or formations of dazzling zig-zag lines (fortification spectra or teichopsia). This visual aura can move across the visual field over several minutes leaving scotomatous defects that are bilateral and may be homonymous. The aura

generally precedes the headache and lasts less than 60 minutes, although it can occur with the migraine.

The aura can occur without the headache and is known as 'migraine equivalent'. Positive phenomena, such as tingling in a hand or the face as well as visual loss, can occur. The key features are a history of migraine or migraine equivalent, symptoms developing gradually over minutes, unlike a transient ischaemic attack, which usually comes on over seconds. The visual symptoms in migraine often move slowly across the visual field.

Papilloedema

Papilloedema is swelling of the optic disc due to raised intracranial pressure. It is almost invariably bilateral. The optic nerve is covered with meninges and therefore surrounded by subarachnoid fluid. The surrounding dura mater eventually fuses with the periosteum of the orbit, and the pia and arachnoid mater with the sclera. Raised intracranial pressure in the optic nerve sheath impedes venous drainage and restricts axoplasmic flow in the nerve. Patients with moderate papilloedema may have no visual symptoms. In severe cases, fleeting bilateral loss of vision, lasting a few seconds, can occur and are referred to as 'visual obscurations'. On examination, visual acuity is normal but the blind spot is enlarged, with restriction of the peripheral field of vision. The disc is swollen, pink and has blurred or absent disc margins. There is engorgement of the retinal veins, and, if severe, flame-shaped haemorrhages may be visible on or adjacent to the disc. If the condition becomes chronic, optic atrophy and visual failure ultimately occur.

Acute persistent visual impairment

Most causes of optic neuropathy (Fig. 8.4) can cause persistent visual impairment. However, the most common causes of acute persistent visual impairment to be aware of are:

- optic neuritis
- retinal or optic nerve ischaemia
- arterial thromboembolism of the middle or posterior cerebral artery.

Optic neuritis

Optic neuritis is inflammation of the optic nerve. Acute anterior optic nerve involvement causes visible swelling of the optic nerve head or 'papillitis'. This can have a similar appearance to papilloedema. If the optic nerve is inflamed in the posterior part of the optic nerve, known as retrobulbar neuritis, then the optic disc will initially appear normal. Loss of central vision may be mild or severe. Eye movements, particularly elevation are painful. A central scotoma, defective colour vision and an afferent pupillary defect are often elicited. Following recovery, temporal pallor of the optic disc is common. The most common cause is demyelination either confined to the optic nerve or in multiple sclerosis.

HINTS AND TIPS

The swollen optic disc seen in acute papillitis and papilloedema can appear clinically very similar. However, papillitis is typically unilateral and associated with visual symptoms (impaired acuity and colour vision, central scotoma, afferent pupillary defect). Papilloedema is typically bilateral and patients have preserved vision and an enlarged blind spot.

Retinal or optic nerve ischaemia

Sudden monocular visual loss results from embolism into the central retinal artery (retinal ischaemia) or occlusion of small posterior ciliary arteries by local small vessel disease or inflammation such as giant cell arteritis (optic nerve ischaemia). The visual loss is typically painless.

Arterial thromboembolism of the middle or posterior cerebral artery

Arterial thromboembolic events are usually of sudden onset, although the patient may be asymptomatic. The characteristic findings described are of a homonymous hemianopia (occipital cortex) or quadrantanopia (optic radiation). The history and examination should focus on cerebrovascular risk factors, e.g. ischaemic heart disease, diabetes, hyperlipidaemia, hypertension and atrial fibrillation.

OPTIC ATROPHY

This results from damage to the nerve fibres in the visual pathway at any point between and including the ganglion cells of the retina and the lateral geniculate nucleus. Visual loss is often central but can also be peripheral. There is central disc pallor; this can also be seen in normal subjects such as those with a large physiological cup and those who are short sighted or myopic. Optic atrophy can be distinguished by attenuation of the retinal vessels, poor colour vision, a central scotoma, atrophy in the nerve fibre layer of the retina and impaired afferent pupillary responses to light. Once established, the disc appearance will not return to normal despite relieving the cause, although vision may improve. It is rare to see persistent blindness in patients who have had optic neuritis due to MS, and vision often returns to a functional level, even though the disc is pale.

Causes of optic atrophy include:

- retinal disease: persistent central retinal artery occlusion, retinitis pigmentosa, toxins, e.g. quinine
- optic nerve neuropathy (Fig. 8.4)
- chiasmal and optic tract pathology, e.g. pituitary tumours and craniopharyngioma.

HINTS AND TIPS

Visual impairment due to ocular disease is likely to be painful. The pain is usually localized to the eye and there are accompanying signs in the eye. Headache and visual impairment are associated with:

- giant cell arteritis
- optic neuritis (pain on eye movement)
- glaucoma
- migraine (if transient)
- pituitary tumour.

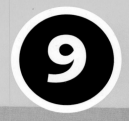
- Understand the anatomy of the sympathetic and parasympathetic innervation of the eye
- Describe the major causes of unilateral and bilateral miosis and mydriasis
- Understand the innervation and function of the extraocular muscles
- Describe the main causes of lesions affecting the third, fourth and sixth cranial nerves
- Understand the difference between jerky and pendular nystagmus, and the causes of central and peripheral nystagmus

The examination of the pupils provides important clinical information in patients with visual disturbance, abnormal eye movements and neurological disease.

PUPILLARY REFLEXES

The size of the pupils is determined by the balance between two groups of smooth muscle within the iris:

- Sphincter pupillae: a circular constrictor muscle innervated by the parasympathetic nervous system.
- Dilator pupillae: a radial dilator muscle innervated by the sympathetic nervous system.
- In order to understand the causes of pupillary abnormalities it is important to appreciate the relevant anatomical pathways.

Pupillary light reflex pathway – parasympathetic pathways

When light is shone into one eye, light information from the retinal ganglion cells travels through the optic nerves, to the chiasm and optic tract, to reach the pretectal nuclei of the dorsal midbrain. Each pretectal nucleus receives information from both eyes and sends axons to both Edinger–Westphal nuclei. From here parasympathetic fibres travel along the ipsilateral third cranial nerve to the ipsilateral ciliary ganglion within the orbit. Postganglionic parasympathetic fibres innervate the ciliary muscle (lens accommodation) and sphincter pupillae muscle (pupil constriction) (Fig. 9.1). Thus, when light is shone into one eye therefore, both pupils constrict symmetrically, and there is both a direct and indirect (consensual) response to light.

HINTS AND TIPS

Afferent pupillary fibres leave the optic tract before the lateral geniculate nucleus to reach the pretectal nuclei. This explains why lesions of the geniculate nucleus, optic radiations or visual cortex do not affect pupillary size or reactivity.

Pupillary light reflex pathway – sympathetic pathways

The sympathetic pathway responsible for pupillary dilation is composed of three neurons (Fig. 9.2):

- First-order neuron: sympathetic fibres arise in the hypothalamus and descend uncrossed to the midbrain, pons, medulla and lower cervical and upper thoracic spinal cord (C8–T2), where they synapse with the lateral or intermediate horn cells.
- Second-order neuron: these neurons travel from the sympathetic trunk, through the brachial plexus and over the lung apex to synapse in the superior cervical ganglion at the bifurcation of the common carotid artery.
- Third-order neuron: postganglionic fibres course along the adventitia of the internal carotid artery and through the cavernous sinus lying close to the sixth cranial nerve, and join the ophthalmic division of the fifth cranial nerve entering the orbit, where they innervate the dilator pupillae. Some fibres follow the external carotid artery and innervate the

Fig. 9.1 Pathway for the light reflex and pupillary constriction.

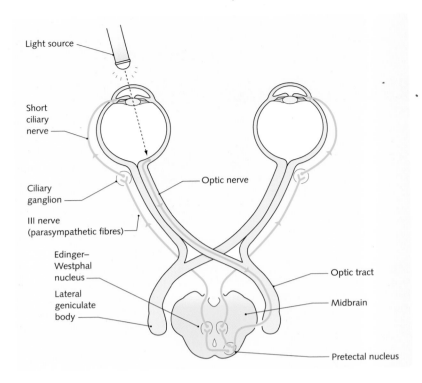

Light source

Short ciliary nerve

Ciliary ganglion

III nerve (parasympathetic fibres)

Edinger–Westphal nucleus

Lateral geniculate body

Optic nerve

Optic tract

Midbrain

Pretectal nucleus

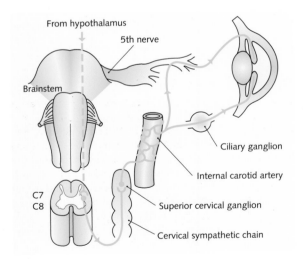

From hypothalamus

5th nerve

Brainstem

Ciliary ganglion

Internal carotid artery

C7
C8

Superior cervical ganglion

Cervical sympathetic chain

Fig. 9.2 The sympathetic pathway for pupillary dilatation.

blood vessels and sweat glands of the face, apart from fibres responsible for sweating of the medial aspect of the forehead, which follow the internal carotid artery.

The accommodation reflex

When looking at a near object, the eyes converge and no longer have parallel axes; the pupils constrict and the ciliary body contracts to increase the thickness of the lens and therefore its refractive power. This complex reflex probably involves coordination between several regions including the parieto-occipital cortex, the Edinger–Westphal nuclei (pupillary constriction) and medial recti components of the nuclei of the third cranial nerve in the midbrain (convergence). The distinction between light-reflex and near-reflex pathways forms the basis for pupils that do not react to light but react to near stimuli (light-near dissociation).

DIFFERENTIAL DIAGNOSIS OF PUPIL DISORDERS

Anisocoria

Anisocoria is inequality in the size of the pupils and can be a normal finding in 20% of the population, in whom the pupillary responses to light and accommodation are normal. In pathological anisocoria there is interruption of the pathways of the light and/or accommodation reflexes and these reflexes will be abnormal.

To identify which pupil is abnormal in a patient with anisocoria, the following should be assessed:

- Evaluate the pupillary response in the light and dark: the small pupil is abnormal if the anisocoria is greater in the dark than in the light. The large pupil is abnormal if the anisocoria is greater in the light than the dark.
- Look for associated features:
  - Ptosis on the side of a small pupil suggests a Horner syndrome
  - Diplopia, ptosis and impaired extraocular movements on the side of a large pupil suggest a third nerve palsy
  - An isolated large pupil without ptosis or diplopia suggests an Adie pupil or pharmacological mydriasis

Physiological anisocoria

There are a number of features that support a diagnosis:

- old photographs that show it is longstanding
- it is usually mild (<0.5 mm)
- the anisocoria is equal in light and dark.

Small constricted (miotic) pupil

This is caused by:

- ageing
- medications (topical or systemic)
- Horner syndrome
- Argyll Robertson pupils.

Old age

Both pupils are constricted, with absent or poor dilatation in the dark.

Medications

Both pupils are constricted and dilatation in the dark is absent or poor. Drugs include opiates and pilocarpine drops, which are used to treat chronic glaucoma.

Horner syndrome

Interruption of the sympathetic pathway gives rise to Horner syndrome. This is characterized by:

- unilateral miosis
- ptosis (usually partial)
- anhidrosis of the ipsilateral side of the face (lesion proximal to the carotid bifurcation) or medial side of the forehead only (lesion distal to the bifurcation)
- 'enophthalmos' (a sunken eye): this is apparent rather than actual; the eye appears sunken because of the narrowed palpebral fissure.

Horner syndrome occurs from a lesion at any of the levels of the sympathetic pathway (see Fig. 9.2). The most common causes of Horner syndrome in adults are shown in Figure 9.3.

An acute painful Horner syndrome is a dissection of the ipsilateral internal carotid artery until proven otherwise.

Argyll Robertson pupils

An Argyll Robertson pupil is small and irregular. There is no response to light but there is a response to accommodation (light-near dissociation). The lesion is thought to be within the midbrain. Argyll Robertson pupils are rare but occur with diabetes and tertiary neurosyphilis.

Fig. 9.3 Common causes of Horner syndrome based on level of sympathetic pathway lesion

Central (1st order)	Preganglionic (2nd order)	Postganglionic (3rd order)
Hypothalamus - stroke - tumour Brainstem - stroke - demyelination - tumour Spinal cord (cervicothoracic) - trauma - syringomyelia - tumour - demyelination - myelitis - arteriovenous malformation	Cervical spine disease Brachial plexus injury Pulmonary apical lesions (e.g. tumour, cervical rib) Iatrogenic (e.g. central line) Subclavian artery aneurysm Thyroid tumours	Superior cervical ganglion - trauma - iatrogenic (e.g. surgical neck dissection) Internal carotid artery - dissection - aneurysm - arteritis Skull base lesions (e.g. tumour) Cavernous sinus lesion - carotid aneurysm - inflammation - thrombosis

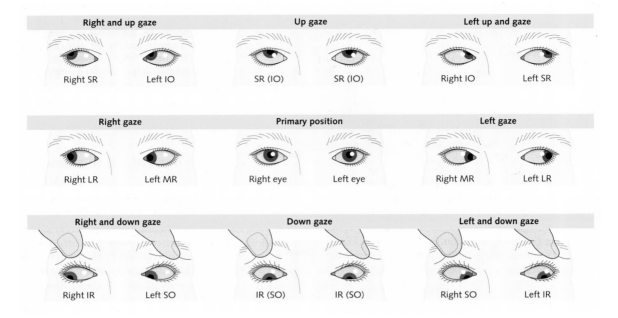

Fig. 9.5 Muscles responsible for eye movements. IO (inferior oblique), IR (inferior rectus), LR (lateral rectus), MR (medial rectus), SO (superior oblique), SR (superior rectus). The primary position refers to the position of the eyes when looking straight ahead.

Monocular diplopia is double vision that occurs in one eye when the other eye is covered. It is always due to a lesion of the eye itself. The most common organic causes are cataracts and corneal scarring. Some patients can present with monocular diplopia and no organic cause can be found.

Binocular diplopia

Binocular diplopia results from ocular misalignment secondary to dysfunction:

- or restriction of the extraocular muscles
- at the neuromuscular junction of the extraocular muscles
- of the ocular cranial nerves
- of the internuclear pathways of eye movement control.

Because of the ocular misalignment, images are projected onto different areas of the retina in both eyes, and two images of the same object are then perceived by the higher centres of the brain. Unlike monocular diplopia, the double vision resolves when one eye is covered.

Dysfunction of the extraocular muscles

Disorders of the extraocular muscles are often bilateral, involve the levator palpebrae and the orbicularis oculi, but never involve the pupil. The most common disorders are:

- Dysthyroid myopathy frequently involves the medial and inferior recti, although soft tissue infiltration is the most common cause of proptosis and mechanical disruption of the extraocular muscles. Patients typically have impaired upgaze and abduction.
- Inflammation of the extraocular muscles can occur in association with any orbital inflammatory syndrome (e.g. Wegener's granulomatosis, sarcoidosis).
- Oculopharyngeal muscular dystrophy causes diplopia from weakness of the extraocular muscles as well as ptosis. These patients also develop weakness of their bulbar musculature affecting speech and swallowing and weakness eventually progresses to involve the limb muscles.
- Mitochondrial disease can often affect the extraocular muscles and cause severe ptosis and ophthalmoplegia (e.g. chronic progressive ophthalmoplegia). There may be no family history and the weakness may be isolated to the eyes.

Dysfunction at the neuromuscular junction

Diplopia and ptosis are common presenting features of myasthenia gravis and both demonstrate fatigability on repetitive movements or may be worse at the end of the day. Ocular involvement may be the only manifestation of myasthenia gravis initially, although many of these patients eventually develop weakness elsewhere.

Dysfunction of the ocular cranial nerves

Lesions of the third (oculomotor) nucleus and nerve (see Figs 9.6 and 9.7)

The nucleus of the third cranial nerve is situated in the dorsal midbrain. It consists of a motor nucleus for the ocular muscles, and the Edinger–Westphal nucleus for pupillary constriction. The nerve emerges from the midbrain and enters the subarachnoid space, where it travels between the superior cerebellar artery and posterior cerebral artery next to the tip of the basilar artery. It then travels medially along the posterior communicating artery and lateral to the internal cartoid artery, to enter the cavernous sinus where it is enclosed within the lateral wall, superior to the fourth cranial nerve. It enters the orbit through the superior orbital fissure to supply part of levator palpebrae superioris; the inferior oblique; and the superior, inferior and medial recti muscles. A parasympathetic branch is also given off to supply the pupil and ciliary body.

With compressive lesions of the third nerve (e.g. aneurysms, tumours, herniation of the temporal lobe), the superficially sited pupillary constrictor fibres are affected early, causing a dilated pupil. By contrast, in diabetes, there is infarction of the centre of the nerve and the more superficial lying parasympathetic fibres may be unaffected, thus sparing the pupillary responses. In a patient with a third nerve palsy, visible intorsion (rotation inwards about an anterior-posterior axis) of the eye on attempted downwards and inwards gaze indicates that the fourth nerve is spared. If the fourth nerve is involved as well as the third nerve, then the paretic eye deviates in an 'out' position only, secondary to unopposed abducens action, and not in the 'down and out' position.

Lesions of the fourth (trochlear) nucleus and nerve (see Figs 9.8 and 9.9)

The nucleus of the fourth cranial nerve is in the lower dorsal midbrain. The fourth nerve arises from the nucleus and decussates as the nerve emerges from the dorsal midbrain to the contralateral side. It has a long intracranial course as it passes ventrally and enters the cavernous sinus with the third, sixth and ophthalmic and maxillary branches of the trigeminal (fifth) nerve. It enters the orbit through the superior orbital fissure to supply the superior oblique muscle contralateral to its nucleus (Fig. 9.8). Because of its long course, the fourth nerve is particularly susceptible to injury in the setting of head trauma.

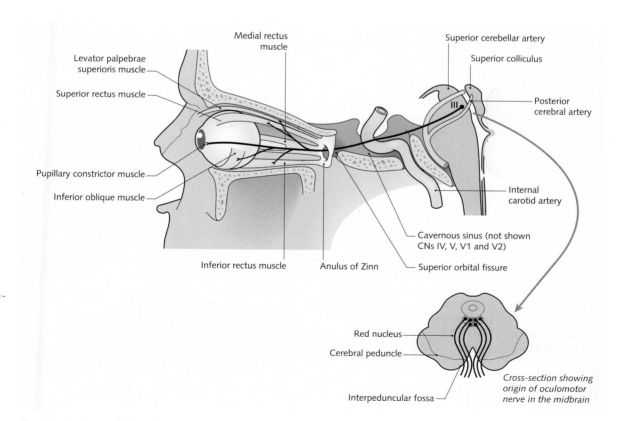

Fig. 9.6 Anatomy of the oculomotor nerve.

Fig. 9.7 3rd (oculomotor) cranial nerve lesions

3rd nerve and nucleus lesions give rise to
- Diplopia in all directions of gaze
- Lateral and downward deviation of the eye
- Ptosis (partial or full)
- A dilated pupil unresponsive to light and accommodation
- (There is often only partial involvement, and therefore the clinical signs may not include all of the features indicated above: e.g. partial ptosis, pupil-sparing, not all muscles supplied by the 3rd nerve affected)

Causes

3rd nerve lesions
- ICA/PcomA/Basilar/PCA/SCA aneurysm
- Cavernous sinus thrombosis
- Lesions of the superior orbital fissure (malignant infiltration)
- Microvascular – diabetes or vasculitis

Midbrain lesions affecting the 3rd nucleus
- Infarction
- Demyelination
- Glioma
- Metastasis

In midbrain lesions, also look for:
- A contralateral hemiplegia
- Ipsilateral limb ataxia
- Coarse rubral tremor (involvement of cerebellar and red nuclear fibres)

Patient looking forwards

Patient looking in the direction of the arrow

ICA, internal carotid artery; PcomA, posterior communicating artery; PCA, posterior cerebral artery; SCA, superior cerebellar artery

---

Lesions of the sixth (abducens) nucleus and nerve (see Figs 9.10 and 9.11)

The nucleus of the sixth cranial nerve lies in the floor of the fourth ventricle in the lower pons, encircled by the emerging fibres of the seventh nerve. The sixth nerve exits the brainstem, passes over the tip of the petrous temporal bone, and enters the cavernous sinus where it is freely situated lateral to the internal carotid artery, and closely related to the sympathetic fibres. It enters the orbit through the superior orbital fissure to supply the lateral rectus muscle (Fig. 9.9). Interneurons also leave the sixth nerve nucleus, crossing over to ascend within the contralateral medial longitudinal fasciculus to the medial rectus subnucleus of the third cranial nerve. The abducens nerve has an extremely long intracranial route from the nucleus to the lateral rectus muscle and is often damaged by compression against the tip of the petrous bone when there is raised intracranial pressure. This is called a false localizing sign because it does not mean the main pathology is affecting the sixth nerve or the pons but has caused the sixth nerve lesion usually through mass effect from anywhere in the skull.

Lesions of the brainstem and the internuclear pathways

Pathology involving the brainstem may involve one or more of the third, fourth and sixth ocular motor nuclei, as detailed individually (see Figs 9.7, 9.9 and 9.11). The blood supply to these nuclei is from the vertebrobasilar arterial tree, so occlusive vascular disease may cause transient or permanent diplopia due to involvement of all the ocular motor nuclei.

HINTS AND TIPS

If diplopia is due to a combined third, fourth and sixth nerve palsy, the differential diagnosis includes lesions of the:
- brainstem
- cavernous sinus
- superior orbital fissure.

If examination does not reveal the diplopia to be consistent with defined weakness of one or more of the extraocular muscles, look for proptosis and a mechanical aetiology, muscle disease (e.g. thyroid eye disease, mitochondrial cytopathy) or myasthenia gravis.

An internuclear ophthalmoplegia (INO) is caused by a lesion of the medial longitudinal fasciculus (Fig. 9.4). This results in paralysis of the medial rectus muscle on the ipsilateral side. There is failure of adduction of the eye on attempted lateral gaze away from the side of the lesion; this is can be associated with asymmetrical jerky nystagmus in the opposite abducting eye. Convergence may overcome the adduction deficit. Lesser degrees of INO may manifest simply as slowness of adduction compared with abduction on horizontal gaze, such that the adducting eye 'lags behind' the abducting eye. Though diplopia can result from an INO, it is not a common symptom. Brainstem lesions are more likely to give rise to the symptom of oscillopsia or the sensation that the outside world is moving up and down.

The most common cause of an INO is demyelination, and less commonly vascular lesions and tumours.

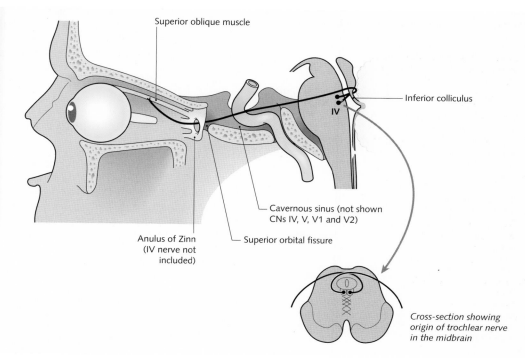

Superior oblique muscle

Inferior colliculus

IV

Cavernous sinus (not shown
CNs IV, V, V1 and V2)

Anulus of Zinn
(IV nerve not
included)

Superior orbital fissure

*Cross-section showing
origin of trochlear nerve
in the midbrain*

Fig. 9.8 Anatomy of the trochlear nerve.

Supranuclear lesions

Despite defects in gaze, the eyes remain conjugate in supranuclear palsies, and therefore diplopia does not occur. Patients with supranuclear gaze palsies for saccadic and pursuit movements often have an intact oculocephalic reflex (see Chapter 5). This reflex should be intact in supranuclear lesions as the afferent (information from vestibular apparatus and neck muscles) and the efferent (cranial nerves and muscles controlling eye movements) limbs of the reflex are intact.

Horizontal gaze palsy

The inability to move the eyes in a conjugate manner horizontally (a 'horizontal conjugate gaze palsy') is caused by a lesion in the contralateral frontal cortex or ipsilateral pons (in the horizontal gaze centre or the parapontine reticular formation). These structures are both anatomically close to the upper motor neurons and hemiparesis is therefore often seen in association with horizontal gaze palsy. The direction of deviation of the eye relative to the neurological deficit will aid localization of the lesion:

- Eyes deviating away from the hemiparetic side towards the side of the lesion: frontal lobe lesion contralateral to the hemiparesis.

- Eyes deviating towards the hemiparetic side away from the side of the lesion: pontine lesion contralateral to the hemiparesis.

During a focal seizure, the converse pattern is seen (i.e. in a frontal lobe seizure, the eyes deviate away from the side of the lesion and towards the convulsing limbs).

One-and-a-half syndrome

Lesions involving both the abducens nucleus and medial longitudinal fasciculus can cause a one-and-a-half syndrome. The 'one' refers to an ipsilateral conjugate gaze palsy due to damage to the abducens nucleus, and the 'half' refers to an ipsilateral internuclear ophthalmoplegia due to damage to the medial longitudinal fasciculus. Only abduction of the contralateral eye (which also has nystagmus) remains. The most common causes are demyelination or vascular.

Vertical gaze palsy

Vertical gaze control is not well localized in the cerebral cortex. Therefore, diffuse degeneration of the cortex (such as with dementia) can diminish the ability of the eyes to look vertically, especially upwards. The centres for conjugate vertical gaze in the brainstem lie in the midbrain and lesions at that site can cause impaired

Fig. 9.9 4th (trochlear) cranial nerve lesions

4th nerve and nucleus lesions give rise to paralysis of the superior oblique muscle:
- Vertical and oblique diplopia on looking down and inwards
- The eye sits rotated slightly outwards and upwards (extorsion)
- The patient tries to compensate by tilting the head away from the affected eye

Causes

4th nerve lesions
- Isolated 4th nerve lesions are rare and usually due to diabetes (ischaemic infarction of the nerve) or trauma
- Lesions of the cavernous sinus and superior orbital fissure will involve the 3rd and 6th nerves, and branches of the 5th nerve

Midbrain lesions affecting the 4th nucleus
- Infarction
- Demyelination
- Glioma
- Metastasis

Patient looking forwards

Patient looking in the direction of the arrow
- The right eye fails to depress and adduct.

Note: The weakness of the superior oblique muscle is contralateral to the side of a lesion at nuclear level. Many patients show a head tilt to the side opposite to that of the defective eye

upgaze. These include rare degenerative conditions such as progressive supranuclear palsy and strokes affecting the dorsum of the midbrain (Parinaud syndrome). The brainstem centres for downgaze are less well localized, but lesions at the midbrain and the level of the foramen magnum can both produce limitation of voluntary downgaze.

Nystagmus

Nystagmus is an involuntary oscillatory movement of the eyes. There are two types:

1. Jerky nystagmus is characterized by a slow pathological phase and a fast corrective phase in the opposite direction. The direction of the nystagmus is described in terms of the direction of the fast component. This type of nystagmus can be pathological or non-pathological and will be discussed in further detail below.
2. Pendular nystagmus is characterized by equal oscillations in both directions as occurs in a swinging pendulum.

Pendular nystagmus due to visual impairment

An acquired pendular nystagmus occurs in patients with marked visual impairment or visual loss in early life (e.g. albinism, congenital cataracts). Here, nystagmus is always in the horizontal plane whether the eye movements are vertical or horizontal and jerk nystagmus may be seen at the extremes of gaze.

Congenital nystagmus

Congenital nystagmus is a pendular nystagmus present in all positions of gaze, often including the resting position. The condition is present from birth and has an autosomal dominant inheritance. The patient is unaware of the movement due to synchronized oscillations of the head in the opposite direction, which steadies the image.

Jerky nystagmus

The causes of jerky nystagmus can be subdivided into central and peripheral groups. It can be important to differentiate the side on which the fast-phase nystagmus occurs because this points towards the lesion if it is central and away from the lesion if it is peripheral.

The central pathways involve:

- vestibular nuclei in the brainstem and their connections
- cerebellar disease and its brainstem connections. Nystagmus from cerebellar disease is uncommon and usually involves the brainstem connections.

The peripheral pathways include the:

- vestibulocochlear, or eighth cranial nerve
- inner ear vestibular apparatus.

It is first important to establish non-pathological from pathological nystagmus.

Physiological nystagmus

'Nystagmoid jerks'
Physiological nystagmus can be seen if eye movements are tested too fast or at the extremes of lateral gaze beyond the range of binocular vision.

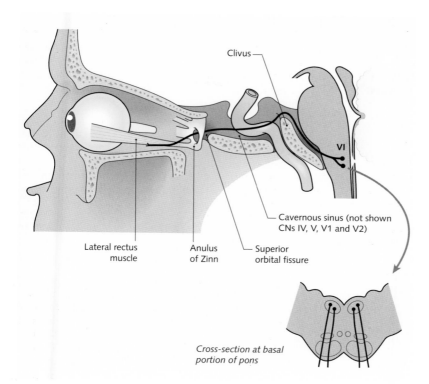

Fig. 9.10 Anatomy of the abducens nerve.

Clivus

VI

Cavernous sinus (not shown
CNs IV, V, V1 and V2)

Lateral rectus
muscle

Anulus
of Zinn

Superior
orbital fissure

Cross-section at basal
portion of pons

Optokinetic nystagmus

When we follow a moving object (e.g. trees from a moving train or vertical stripes on a rotating optokinetic drum) jerky nystagmus occurs. The slow component represents normal pursuit movements to the limit of conjugate gaze and the fast component in the opposite direction represents rapid saccadic movements with subsequent fixation on a new object entering the field of view. Optokinetic nystagmus (OKN) is interrupted in lesions of the ipsilateral parietal cortex and its connections to the brainstem centres involved in conjugate gaze. If a striped drum is rotated towards the side of the lesion, OKN is lost or reduced and if rotated in the opposite direction, OKN is normal. OKN is normal in disorders of the peripheral vestibular system and in non-organic blindness (i.e. hysterical blindness).

Pathological nystagmus

Central nystagmus

Lesions of the brainstem, including the vestibular nuclei, as well as the cerebellum and its connections to the brainstem usually cause central nystagmus. Vertigo and ataxia may be present, but nausea and vomiting are less common than in peripheral nystagmus. The nystagmus is frequently vertical as well as horizontal, and its direction may change with the direction of gaze (multidirectional). Symptoms may improve with eye closure. There may also be associated pursuit or saccadic defects in eye movements, or associated cranial nerve or long tract signs.

Asymmetrical nystagmus mainly occurs in internuclear ophthalmoplegia associated with lesions of the pons.

Vertical nystagmus is less common in brainstem disease and there are two types:

1. Upbeat nystagmus is seen in lesions of the midbrain, e.g. in multiple sclerosis, vascular disorders or tumours.
2. Downbeat nystagmus is characteristic of lesions in the cerebellum or at the foramen magnum/craniocervical junction, e.g. Arnold–Chiari malformation, foramen magnum meningioma.

Both types of vertical nystagmus are seen in Wernicke's disease following vitamin B_1 insufficiency.

'Ocular bobbing' may be seen in comatose patients with extensive pontine lesions and absent horizontal eye movements. This is fast, jerky, downward movements followed by a slow drift upwards.

Peripheral nystagmus

Peripheral nystagmus is characterized by marked vertigo, nausea and vomiting. The nystagmus is typically horizontal or rotatory, and the fast phase is away from

Fig. 9.11 6th (abducens) cranial nerve lesions

6th nerve and nucleus lesions give rise to paralysis of the lateral rectus muscle:

- Horizontal diplopia maximal on lateral gaze to the side of the lesion. A convergent strabismus may be evident in the primary position, but becomes more apparent on abduction of the affected eye

Causes

6th nerve lesions
- Microvascular – diabetes or vasculitis
- Trauma
- Vertebral or basilar aneurysm
- Gradenigo's syndrome – due to infection of the petrous temporal bone
- Cavernous sinus thrombosis
- Fracture or malignant infiltration (nasopharyngeal carcinoma) of the skull base
- Lesions of the superior orbital fissure

Pontine lesions affecting the 6th nucleus
- Infarction
- Demyelination
- Glioma
- Metastasis

In pontine lesions, also look for:

- A contralateral hemiplegia
- Ipsilateral weakness of the upper and lower face (7th nerve fibres hooking around the 6th nucleus)

Patient looking forwards

Patient looking in the direction of the arrow

the side of the lesion in all positions of gaze (unidirectional). It is most marked when gaze is directed away from the abnormal ear. There may be unsteadiness of gait (ataxia) towards the side of lesion, as well as deafness and tinnitus on the affected side. It is independent of vision and it persists or is worse if the eyes are shut.

Causes include:

- labyrinthine disease (common): benign positional vertigo, Ménière's disease, repeated ear infections, head trauma
- vestibular nerve lesion (rare): acoustic schwannoma (vertigo is uncommon), aminoglycoside toxicity, herpes zoster infection.

Facial sensory loss and weakness (10)

● **Objectives**

- Understand the basic anatomy of the fifth and seventh cranial nerves
- Describe the neurology of lesions along the course of the trigeminal nerve
- Understand the difference between upper and lower motor neuron facial weakness
- Describe the causes and associated differentiating features of types of facial weakness

Facial sensory disturbance may result from disorders affecting the trigeminal (fifth cranial) nerve or its central connections within the brainstem, high cervical cord, thalamus, internal capsule and sensory cortex. The upper cervical nerves (C2, C3) supply sensation over a small part of the face, along the lower jaw, as well as the back of the head to the vertex and under the chin.

Facial weakness may result from lesions involving the seventh cranial nerve and its central connections in the brainstem, internal capsule and motor cortex, as well as from disease of the neuromuscular junction (myasthenia) or of muscle (myopathies).

THE TRIGEMINAL NERVE

The trigeminal or fifth cranial nerve is the largest cranial nerve and is a mixed motor and sensory nerve. It arises from the lateral aspect of the pons and passes forwards across the subarachnoid space to form a large ganglion over the tip of the petrous bone where it divides into three parts:

1. Ophthalmic branch (V_1): this traverses the lateral wall of the cavernous sinus and enters the orbit through the superior orbital fissure. Its cutaneous distribution is shown in Figure 10.1; it also supplies the cornea (supplying most of the afferent limb of the corneal reflex), mucosae of the nasal cavity and frontal sinuses, dura mater of the falx, and the superior surface of the tentorium.
2. Maxillary branch (V_2): this traverses the lower lateral wall of the cavernous sinus and exits the skull in the foramen rotundum. It enters the floor of the orbit via the inferior orbital fissure. In addition to supplying the skin (see Fig. 10.1), it supplies the floor of the middle cranial fossa, the upper teeth and gums, and the adjacent palate. It contributes secretomotor parasympathetic fibres to the lacrimal gland.
3. Mandibular branch (V_3): this carries the motor component of the nerve that supplies the muscles of

mastication (chewing) including masseter and temporalis. It exits the skull via the foramen ovale. Its sensory supply is to the lower face (see Fig. 10.1), mucosa of the cheek, lower lip, jaw, incisor and canine teeth, floor of the mouth, lower gums and anterior two-thirds of the tongue.

The proximal axons of the somatic sensory Gasserian ganglion cells divide in the pons into short ascending and long descending branches. The short fibres carry light touch and deep pressure to the main sensory nucleus, and proprioception to the mesencephalic nucleus in the mid pons. The long descending fibres form the spinal trigeminal tract and carry information about pain and temperature. The nucleus of the spinal trigeminal tract extends from the junction of the pons and medulla to C2 of the spinal cord and fibres cross to the opposite side and ascend to the thalamus in the trigeminothalamic tract (Fig. 10.2).

The motor nucleus of the fifth nerve is in the mid pons. The fibres from the motor root pass below the Gasserian ganglion to join the sensory fibres in the mandibular nerve (V_3) and innervate the muscles of mastication.

DIFFERENTIAL DIAGNOSIS OF FACIAL SENSORY LOSS

The wide anatomical distribution of the fifth nerve means that complete motor and sensory lesions of the fifth nerve are uncommon. The sensory component is mostly affected and the motor component is often spared.

On examination look for:

- Sensory deficit in the distribution of the three branches of the fifth nerve: loss of the corneal reflex is an early sign of damage to the ophthalmic branch as seen in lesions at the cerebellopontine angle, e.g. acoustic schwannoma. Lesions of the lower pons, medulla or upper cervical cord produce dissociated sensory loss of pain and temperature, with normal light touch, vibration and proprioception in a

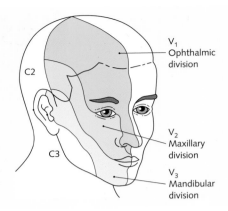

Fig. 10.1 The cutaneous distribution of the trigeminal nerve. Note that the upper cervical dermatomes (C2, C3) extend onto the face, above the angle of the jaw, and onto the back of the head to the vertex.

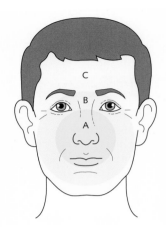

Fig. 10.3 Low pontine (A), medullary (B) and cervical lesions (C) produce an 'onion skin' distribution of pin-prick (pain) and temperature loss due to lesions in the descending trigeminal tract and nucleus (see also Fig. 10.2).

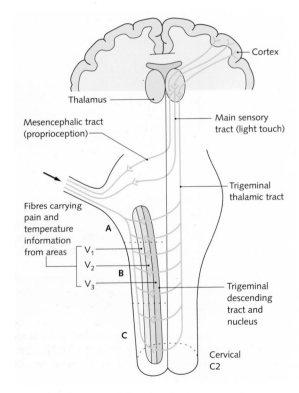

Fig. 10.2 Anatomy of the trigeminal sensory pathways.

'Balaclava' distribution (Fig. 10.3). As the lesion extends up the brainstem, the sensory deficit spreads towards the nose

- Motor involvement: this may be manifested by weakness of the muscles of mastication and deviation of the jaw towards the side of the lesion because of weakness of the pterygoid muscles

- The jaw jerk (a trigeminal pontine reflex): this is brisk in upper motor neuron lesions above the motor nucleus of the fifth nerve.

Facial sensory loss can be caused by a lesion anywhere from the cerebral cortex to the cranial nerve and its terminal branches. The site of the lesion can be determined by the associated neurological signs.

A supranuclear lesion is contralateral to the facial sensory loss because the sensory fibres cross the midline after they synapse in the brainstem. Lesions at all other sites are therefore ipsilateral to the facial sensory loss.

Supranuclear lesions

These include lesions to the primary sensory cortex, internal capsule and upper brainstem. There may be associated:

- ipsilateral 'pyramidal' weakness
- ipsilateral lower facial weakness (upper motor neuron)
- other cortical signs such as dysphasia, inattention, apraxia, hemianopia.

Causes:

- Cerebral infarction/haemorrhage
- Demyelination, e.g. multiple sclerosis
- Neoplasms (glioma, metastatic deposits).

Brainstem lesions

These include lesions of the pons for all sensory modalities and the medulla/upper cervical cord for pain and temperature sensation only. There may be:

- contralateral 'pyramidal' weakness

- ipsilateral cranial nerve lesions in close proximity to the fifth nerve nuclei
- horizontal conjugate gaze palsies if the pons is involved
- lesions of the lower pons, medulla or upper cervical cord can produce dissociated sensory loss due to involvement of the descending trigeminal spinal tract and/or nucleus. There is ipsilateral loss of pain and temperature in an 'onion skin' distribution with preservation of light touch, vibration and proprioception.

  Causes:

- Infarction
- Demyelination
- Neoplasia (glioma, metastatic disease)
- Syringobulbia and syringomyelia.

Cerebellopontine angle lesions

Lesions at the cerebellopontine angle (CPA) are often associated with a disturbance in ipsilateral facial sensation and a reduced corneal reflex early in the disease before the onset of facial weakness. There may be:

- contralateral 'pyramidal' weakness
- damage of the ipsilateral seventh and eighth cranial nerves with late involvement of the sixth, ninth and tenth nerves
- ipsilateral cerebellar signs in the limbs.

  Causes:

- Vestibular schwannoma (acoustic neuroma)
- Meningioma
- Metastatic deposits
- Trigeminal neuroma
- Arteriovenous malformation
- Basilar artery aneurysm.

Cavernous sinus lesions

Patients with pathology in the cavernous sinus may have signs of third, fourth and sixth cranial nerve palsies, as well as the ophthalmic branch, and occasionally the maxillary branch, of the fifth nerve (see Fig. 10.4). Proptosis, eyelid and conjunctival oedema and papilloedema may be present if there is venous obstruction or a carotico-cavernous fistula (also pulsating exophthalmos and orbital bruit).

Causes can be divided into several groups:

Vascular:
- Aneurysm of the intracavernous portion of the internal carotid artery
- Carotico-cavernous fistula
- Cavernous sinus thrombosis.

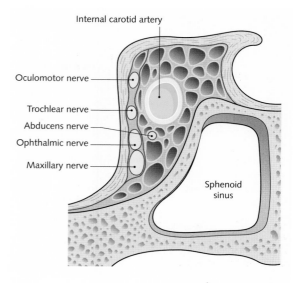

Fig. 10.4 A coronal section through the cavernous sinus.

Inflammation:
- Sarcoidosis
- Meningitis (acute and chronic).

Neoplasms:
- Meningioma of sphenoid wing
- Metastatic infiltration
- Extension of a pituitary tumour.

Lesions of the trigeminal root, ganglion and peripheral branches of the nerve

These lesions include:

- herpes zoster: this manifests as a vesicular rash in the cutaneous distribution of the nerve (usually the ophthalmic division)
- skull fractures affecting the superficial branches of the trigeminal nerve (cutaneous deficit) or at the skull base (additional cranial nerve palsies)
- neoplastic infiltration or compression: from tumours of the sinuses, cholesteatoma, fifth nerve neuroma, nasopharyngeal carcinoma at the skull base or lesion of the superior orbital fissure (third, fourth and sixth nerve palsies)
- malignant and infective infiltration of the meninges affecting the skull base
- Guillain–Barré syndrome and other peripheral neuropathies
- granulomatous disease: tuberculosis, sarcoidosis
- connective tissue disease: Sjögren's syndrome, scleroderma and systemic lupus erythematosus
- trigeminal neuralgia
- isolated trigeminal sensory neuropathy.

FACIAL NERVE

Facial nerve anatomy

- The seventh cranial nerve is composed of motor fibres, which innervate the muscles of facial expression, and the nervus intermedius, which carries taste fibres from the anterior two-thirds of the tongue and parasympathetic fibres to the salivary glands and stapedius.
- The motor nucleus of the facial nerve lies in the lateral pons and its intrapontine fibres hook around the nucleus of the sixth nerve (abducens) before emerging from the pons at the cerebellopontine angle.
- The facial nerve enters the internal auditory meatus with the nervus intermedius and the eighth nerve.
- The eighth nerve subsequently dives deep within the petrous bone to the middle ear and the nervus intermedius and facial nerve enter the geniculate ganglion. This contains the cell bodies of taste fibres subserving the anterior two-thirds of the tongue.
- The greater petrosal nerve comes off the geniculate ganglion and carries parasympathetic fibres to the lacrimal gland.
- The seventh nerve then courses through the facial canal in the petrous temporal bone and gives off two important branches within the canal. The first is a small branch to the stapedius muscle, which is involved in controlling the sensitivity of the ossicles

to sound. If it is damaged then sounds become louder (hyperacusis). The second branch is the chorda tympani, which subserves taste to the anterior two-thirds of the tongue as well as parasympathetic fibres to the submandibular and sublingual glands.

- The main facial nerve continues in the facial canal and leaves the skull through the stylomastoid foramen. It enters the parotid gland and divides into branches that supply the muscles of facial expression (Fig. 10.5).

Upper and lower motor neuron facial weakness

- The facial motor nucleus is supplied by upper motor neurons from the primary motor cortex, which travel in the corticobulbar pathway in the internal capsule to synapse on the lower motor neurons in the facial nerve nucleus in the pons.
- The lower facial muscles receive input from the contralateral hemisphere only, whereas the upper facial muscles have input from both cortices. Consequently, a supranuclear (upper motor neuron) lesion will cause contralateral weakness of only the lower facial muscles, because the upper facial muscles remain innervated by the intact ipsilateral pathway. In contrast, a lower motor neuron lesion will cause ipsilateral weakness involving both the upper and lower facial muscles.

Fig. 10.5 The anatomy of the facial nerve and its branches. The chorda tympani supplies taste sensation to the anterior two-thirds of the tongue. GPN, greater petrosal nerve to lacrimal gland.

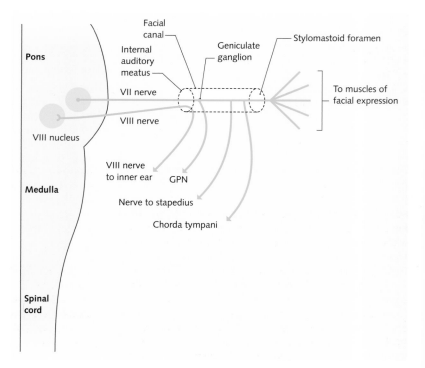

Fig. 10.6   Differential diagnosis of facial weakness

Syndrome	Clinical features and causes
Unilateral upper motor neuron facial weakness	**Unilateral weakness of the lower face** Unilateral weakness of the lower face is due to a contralateral supranuclear (upper motor neuron) lesion. It is usually caused by a contralateral stroke or tumour. Associated symptoms may include ipsilateral hemiparesis, hemisensory loss, hemineglect or hemianopia.
Unilateral lower motor neuron facial weakness	**Unilateral weakness of the upper and lower face** Unilateral weakness of the upper and lower face is due to disorder of the nucleus of the 7th nerve, the geniculate ganglion, or the peripheral nerve; additional clinical features aid lesion localization; lesions may occur at the following sites: • Pons–ipsilateral 6th nerve lesion, contralateral 'pyramidal' weakness (recall that the intrapontine fibres hook around the nucleus of the 6th nerve), ipsilateral limb ataxia, facial numbness, gaze palsy to the side of the facial weakness, e.g. infarction, demyelination, tumour deposits • Cerebellopontine angle: ipsilateral facial sensory loss, loss of corneal reflex, ataxia and sensorineural hearing loss e.g. cerebellopontine angle tumours • Facial canal–hyperacusis (denervation of nerve to stapedius) and loss of taste in the anterior two-thirds of the tongue (involvement of the chorda tympani), e.g. middle ear infection, Bell's palsy, tumour deposits, fracture of the skull base, (carcinomatous) basal meningitis. Lacrimation is often spared • Geniculate ganglion, e.g. herpes zoster infection of the ganglion; look for pain and vesicles in the auditory canal • Peripheral branches of the nerve, e.g. parotid gland lesions (tumour, infection), trauma • Facial mononeuropathy, e.g. small vessel disease (vasculitis), sarcoidosis, Behçet's or Sjögren's syndrome, syphilis, Lyme disease
Bilateral lower motor neuron facial weakness	**Bilateral weakness of the upper and lower face** If a patient presents with bilateral upper and lower facial weakness (i.e. bilateral lower motor neuron facial weakness), the following differential diagnoses should be borne in mind: • Guillain–Barré syndrome • Myasthenia gravis • Myopathies-dystrophia myotonica, facio-scapulo-humeral dystrophy Rarer differentials include: • Lyme disease • Sarcoidosis • (Carcinomatous) basal meningitis

Differential diagnosis of facial weakness

Facial weakness arises from a lesion anywhere from the motor cortex to the seventh cranial nerve and its distal connections (including the neuromuscular junction and muscle).

To differentiate the site of the lesion, the first step is to determine whether the weakness involves the upper and lower or only the lower part of the face, and then whether it involves one side or both. Lesions of the neuromuscular junction and muscle itself cause weakness of the upper and lower face as in a lower motor neuron lesion, but it is bilateral and usually symmetrical. A summary of the differential diagnosis of facial weakness is shown in Figure 10.6.

COMMUNICATION

When a patient presents with unilateral lower motor neuron facial weakness it is important to ask about associated neurological symptoms such as loss of taste, perception of loud sounds and a dry eye. If these symptoms are absent, then be suspicious that the lesion may be distal to the facial canal, e.g. tumour within the parotid gland.

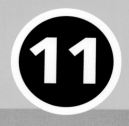
● Objectives

- Understand the basic anatomy of the auditory and vestibular systems
- Define the Rinne's and Weber's tests and how you may differentiate between conductive and sensorineural hearing loss
- Describe the common causes of deafness and tinnitus
- Understand how you may localize the lesion in a patient with vertigo

DEAFNESS AND TINNITUS

Deafness and tinnitus usually result from diseases of the cochlea and patients are generally seen by ear, nose and throat (ENT) surgeons. A vestibular schwannoma (previously referred to as an acoustic neuroma) is a rare but important 'neurological' cause of deafness, and the eighth (vestibulocochlear) cranial nerve may be involved in other conditions affecting the brainstem or multiple cranial nerves.

The eighth cranial nerve comprises the cochlear nerve, which subserves hearing, and the vestibular nerve, which is concerned with maintenance of balance (Fig. 11.1). Deafness and tinnitus arise from damage to the auditory apparatus and its central connections via the eighth nerve.

THE AUDITORY SYSTEM

Sound waves are channelled through the external auditory meatus to the tympanic membrane and the auditory ossicles to the oval window setting up waves in the perilymph of the cochlea. The waves in the perilymph are transduced into nerve impulses by the end organ of hearing, the spiral organ of Corti (Figs 11.1 and 11.2):

- These nerve impulses travel in the cochlear nerve, which, together with the vestibular and facial nerves, passes through the internal auditory canal within the temporal bone to enter the posterior fossa. It then synapses in the cochlear nuclei in the lower pons.
- Fibres from the cochlear nuclei project to the superior olives bilaterally from where fibres ascend in the lateral lemniscus to the inferior colliculus (midbrain) on both sides.
- These fibres project to the medial geniculate nucleus of the thalamus.

- Fibres then pass from the thalamus through the internal capsule to the auditory cortex in the superior temporal gyrus.
- The bilateral nature of the connections ensures that unilateral central lesions do not cause lateralized hearing loss.

DIFFERENTIAL DIAGNOSIS OF DEAFNESS

There are two types of deafness:

1. Conductive: there is failure of transmission of sound from the outer or middle ear to the cochlea.
2. Sensorineural: this is due to disease of the cochlea, cochlear nerve, cochlear nuclei and their supranuclear connections.

Clinically, conductive and sensorineural deafness can be distinguished by the Rinne and Weber tests.

Rinne's test

The base of a vibrating 512 Hz tuning fork is held first against the mastoid process, and then, when the tone has disappeared, in front of the external auditory meatus. Normally the transmission of sound through the outer and middle ear to the cochlea is better than transmission through bone to the cochlea, which bypasses the middle ear apparatus. Thus, in normal ears, air conduction is better than bone conduction.

In conductive deafness, this ability is impaired due to disease of the outer or middle ear and bone conduction is better. In sensorineural deafness, there is impairment of sound perception whether transmitted through air or bone. However, with the latter, the sound may be transmitted through bone to the normal contralateral ear, giving a false positive result.

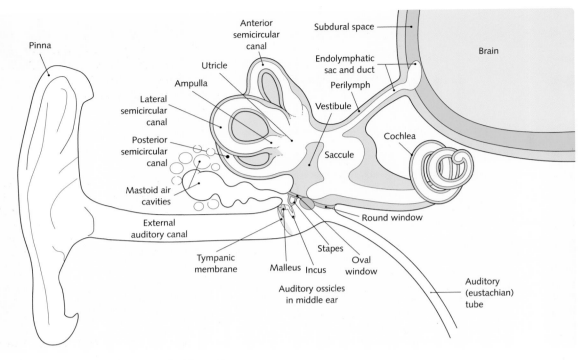

Fig. 11.1 Components of the outer, middle and inner ear.

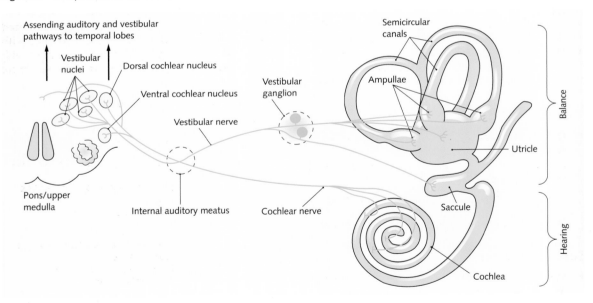

Fig. 11.2 The auditory and vestibular system.

Weber's test

When a vibrating tuning fork is placed in the middle of the forehead, sound is normally heard equally in both ears. In conductive deafness, the sound localizes to the affected ear (due to lack of competitive sounds that would normally be heard on that side). By contrast, in sensorineural deafness, the sound lateralizes to the normal ear.

Conductive deafness

In conductive deafness, there is impaired perception, especially of low-pitched sounds.

Conductive deafness can be caused by:

- disorders of the outer ear: the build up of wax in the external auditory canal is the commonest cause
- disorders of the middle ear: otitis media, cholesteatoma, otosclerosis, rupture of the tympanic membrane.

Sensorineural deafness

In sensorineural deafness, there is often preferential impairment of perception of high-pitched sounds. Sensorineural deafness can be caused by a variety of disorders:

Disorders of the cochlear apparatus

- Congenital disorders: from rubella or syphilis in the pregnant mother
- Infection: basal meningitis, spread of infection from the middle to the inner ear, mumps or measles
- Medication: aminoglycosides, diuretics, salicylates, quinine. (Deafness is transient with the last two but can be permanent with aminoglycosides)
- Presbycusis: neuronal degeneration in the elderly causing high-frequency hearing loss
- Noise-induced disorders: high-frequency hearing loss from, e.g. gun blasts, industrial machinery
- Ménière's disease: vertigo, fluctuating tinnitus and deafness
- Head injury: fractures through the base of the skull and petrous temporal bone can lead to damage to the cochlea and eighth nerve.

Disorders of the cochlear nerve

- Lesions of the cerebellopontine angle, e.g. vestibular schwannoma, other tumours, granulomatous disease, arteriovenous malformation, stroke (anterior inferior cerebellar artery)
- Lesions of the base of the skull e.g. infective, inflammatory such as sarcoidosis, carcinomatous meningeal seeding such as nasopharyngeal carcinoma

Disorders of the brainstem

- Multiple sclerosis: plaques of demyelination involving the cochlear nuclei
- Infarction
- Neoplastic infiltration.

Disorders of the supranuclear connections

Unilateral lesions of the supranuclear pathways will not cause deafness as the cochlear nuclei on each side have bilateral connections projecting to the temporal cortices.

HINTS AND TIPS

Sensorineural deafness can be associated with other features if there is involvement of adjacent neurological structures in the brainstem, cerebellopontine angle, or inner ear (e.g. trigeminal nerve, facial nerve, vestibular nerve)

Investigations for deafness

Several audiometric procedures can distinguish deafness caused by cochlear lesions from those caused by lesions of the eighth nerve. Auditory evoked potentials test the integrity of the pathway from the cochlea to the auditory cortex in the temporal lobe; this does not need the cooperation of the patient (i.e. it can be done in a comatose patient).

DIFFERENTIAL DIAGNOSIS OF TINNITUS

Tinnitus is the sensation of ringing, buzzing, hissing, chirping or whistling in the ear. It is a manifestation of disease of the middle ear, inner ear or cochlear component of the eighth nerve, and is usually accompanied by some degree of deafness. The causes are summarized in Figure 11.3. Conductive deafness is associated with low-pitched tinnitus, and sensorineural deafness with high-pitched tinnitus (except Ménière's disease, where

Fig. 11.3 Causes of deafness and tinnitus

Site of damage	Cause
Outer ear	Wax, foreign body
Middle ear	Trauma, e.g. fracture of temporal bone Infection, e.g. suppurative otitis media Otosclerosis
Cochlea	Age (presbycusis) Infection, e.g. purulent meningitis Noise induced Drugs, e.g. aminoglycosides Ménière's disease
8th nerve	Lesions of the cerebellopontine angle, e.g. acoustic neuroma, Basal meningitis, e.g. TB, sarcoid, malignant infiltration
Brainstem (rare)	Multiple sclerosis Neoplasia Infarction
Cerebral hemisphere (rare)	Bilateral lesions of the temporal lobes, e.g. infarction, neoplasia

the tinnitus is low pitched). Vibratory mechanical noises in the head can be mistaken for tinnitus. The most common is a bruit from turbulent blood flow in the great vessels of the neck. This may occur as a result of high cardiac output (e.g. febrile or anaemic state) or mechanical obstruction within the lumen of an artery (e.g. arteriovenous malformation or carotid artery stenosis), when the noise heard is in time with the pulse.

THE VESTIBULAR SYSTEM

The sensory feedback from the vestibular, visual and proprioceptive systems is required to maintain balance. The labyrinthine—vestibular apparatus lies in each inner ear. It consists of the utricle, saccule and semicircular canals. There are three semicircular canals (lateral, anterior, and posterior), each positioned perpendicularly with respect to one another (see Fig. 11.2). They respond to rotational acceleration of the head. The utricle and saccule respond to linear acceleration, including gravity.

Afferent information from the labyrinth is relayed by the vestibular component of eighth cranial nerve, the vestibular nerve. The vestibular and cochlear nerves follow the same route from the inner ear through the internal auditory meatus to the cerebellopontine angle before entering the brainstem at the lower pons. The vestibular fibres synapse in the four vestibular nuclei located at the junction of the pons and medulla. From here there are connections to the:

- anterior horn cells of the spinal cord, via the vestibulospinal tract
- flocculonodular lobe of the cerebellum
- third, fourth and sixth ocular motor nuclei, via the medial longitudinal fasciculus
- pontine reticular formation
- temporal cortex.

COMMUNICATION

The vestibular nucleus has vertical ramifications over much of the brainstem from the midbrain down to the cervical cord. Therefore, vestibular features are often associated with brainstem pathology but not of significant localizing value.

DIFFERENTIAL DIAGNOSIS OF DIZZINESS AND VERTIGO

Dizziness is a very common symptom but is non-specific, and can be used by patients to refer to vertigo, but also feelings of faintness, disorientation, drowsiness, visual disturbance or even unsteadiness in the legs (imbalance).

It is important to separate all of these from the phenomenon of vertigo, which is best defined as an illusion of movement. This perceived movement may be described as to-and-fro, up-and-down or spinning, but often it has a swaying, rocking or heaving quality. It is often associated with nausea and vomiting. The patient might veer to one side when walking and the gait is more unsteady in the dark or with the eyes closed. Nystagmus usually accompanies vertigo. Vertigo may arise from a lesion of the labyrinth, vestibular nerve, cerebellopontine angle, brainstem, cerebellum or, rarely, the supranuclear connections (Fig. 11.4).

Clinical features of labyrinthine failure

- Vertigo: occurs in attacks of 1–2 hours duration; there may be accompanying nausea and vomiting.
- Nystagmus: there is horizontal and/or rotary nystagmus with the fast phase opposite to the side of the lesion.
- Gait: the patient may veer towards the side of the lesion when walking.
- Hearing: there may be conductive or sensorineural deafness and tinnitus if the auditory pathway is involved.
- Neurological signs: none apart from nystagmus.

Examples of labyrinthine failure

Ménière's disease

Ménière's disease is characterized by recurrent attacks of vertigo, deafness, tinnitus and a feeling of pressure or fullness in the ears. It occurs in middle age and the vertigo is usually self-limiting. It is thought to arise from excessive accumulation of endolymphatic fluid and degeneration of the organ of Corti. Permanent deafness may occur after repeated attacks.

Benign paroxysmal positional vertigo

Benign paroxysmal positional vertigo (BPPV) arises from dislocation of particulate material from the otoliths, usually into the posterior semicircular canals. Sudden paroxysms of vertigo occur with movements of the head, particularly lying down, rolling over in bed, bending forward, straightening up and extending the neck. The vertigo lasts less than a minute and is fatigable with recurrent movements. The accompanying nystagmus is torsional and similarly fatigable. Symptoms may be present for several days or months at a time. Some cases follow head trauma or a viral infection of the labyrinth. The Hallpike manoeuvre (see below) can make the diagnosis and a similar manoeuvre can sometimes be therapeutic (Epley's manoeuvre) (Fig. 11.5).

Fig. 11.4 Differential diagnosis of vertigo and dizziness

		PERIPHERAL		CENTRAL	
	Labyrinthine failure	Vestibular nerve lesion	Cerebellopontine angle lesion	Brainstem lesions	Cerebellar lesions
Vertigo	Common short attacks which may be triggered or worsened by head movements	May be short or prolonged	Rare	May be prolonged	Brainstem connections involved
Nystagmus	Horizontal and/or rotary and suppressed with visual fixation	Horizontal and/or rotary and suppressed with visual fixation	Horizontal	Vertical/ horizontal and may persist despite visual fixation	Horizontal and may persist despite visual fixation
Fast phase	Opposite to lesion	Opposite to lesion	Towards lesion	Towards lesion	Towards lesion
Gait	Veers towards lesion	Veers towards lesion	Ataxia towards lesion; hemiparetic	Hemiparetic	Ataxia towards lesion
Hearing	Conductive or Sensorineural loss	Sensorineural loss	Sensorineural High-frequency loss early	Unaffected	Unaffected
Other neurological signs	May have positive Hallpike test	± 7th, 5th nerve lesions Ipsilateral cerebellar signs Contralateral 'pyramidal' signs	5th, 7th, 9th, 10th nerve lesions Contralateral 'pyramidal' weakness Ipsilateral ataxia	Ipsilateral cranial nerve palsies	Unilateral cerebellar signs from an ipsilateral cerebellar Hemisphere lesion

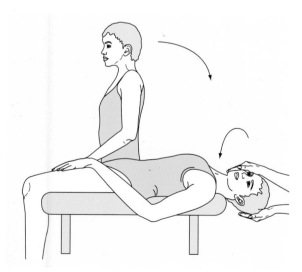

Fig. 11.5 Technique for exhibiting positional nystagmus (Hallpike's manoeuvre).

Other causes

Other causes of labyrinthine dysfunction include purulent labyrinthitis following meningitis, motion sickness, and toxic effects from alcohol, quinine and aminoglycosides.

Vestibular nerve lesions

- Vertigo: this may be severe in vestibular neuronitis (see below)
- Nystagmus: there is horizontal and/or rotary nystagmus with the fast phase opposite to the side of the lesion
- Gait: the patient may veer towards the side of the lesion
- Hearing: sensorineural deafness and tinnitus may occur if there is also involvement of the cochlear nerve
- Neurological signs: depending on the aetiology there may be involvement of adjacent cranial nerves, e.g. fifth and seventh.

The vestibular nerve may be damaged in the petrous temporal bone or the cerebellopontine angle. The latter is dealt with below. Trauma or infection of the petrous temporal bone may involve the seventh and fifth cranial nerves, as may occur with a herpes zoster infection of the nerve or ganglion. Purely vestibular dysfunction occurs in vestibular neuronitis.

Vestibular neuronitis

Vestibular neuronitis manifests as a single severe paroxysm of vertigo without deafness and tinnitus, usually in young or middle-aged adults. Symptoms usually subside within several days, but may persist for weeks. An inflammatory aetiology is presumptive rather than proven but the condition frequently follows an upper respiratory tract infection, thus a viral cause has been postulated.

Cerebellopontine angle lesions

The cerebellopontine angle (CPA) is the junction between the pons and cerebellum where the seventh and eighth nerve exits the brainstem. Both brainstem and cranial nerve involvement occurs:

- Vertigo: rarely occurs in the early stages
- Nystagmus: horizontal, coarse and towards the side of the lesion
- Gait: ataxic towards the side of the lesion
- Hearing: high-frequency deafness is often one of the first symptoms
- Neurological signs: loss of corneal reflex (early sign), larger lesions may cause fifth, seventh, ninth and tenth nerve palsies, ipsilateral cerebellar signs and contralateral 'pyramidal' weakness.

Causes to consider are vestibular schwannoma, other tumours, granulomatous disease and vascular lesions.

Brainstem lesions

- Vertigo: this may be severe and prolonged
- Nystagmus: often vertical or multidirectional nystagmus
- Hearing: usually unaffected since the cochlear and vestibular fibres separate before entering the brainstem
- Neurological signs: ipsilateral cranial nerve palsies, contralateral 'pyramidal' weakness, and often ipsilateral 'cerebellar' ataxia.

Causes include infarction, demyelination, primary brainstem tumour or metastatic infiltration. Episodes of vertigo may arise from transient vertebrobasilar ischaemia, but it is rarely the only manifestation of brainstem transient ischaemic attacks.

Cerebellar lesions

- Vertigo: particularly if the lesion is acute and involving brainstem vestibular connections to the flocculonodular lobe
- Nystagmus: horizontal, coarse and mainly towards the side of the lesion
- Gait: ataxia of gait with unsteadiness towards the side of the lesion
- Hearing: unaffected
- Neurological signs: unilateral cerebellar signs from an ipsilateral lesion.

Causes of cerebellar dysfunction are considered in Chapter 10.

Vertigo may occur as part of the aura of temporal lobe seizures. Uncommonly, it arises from the neck or from ocular motor disorders (ophthalmoplegia).

Other types of dizziness

Patients use the word 'dizziness' can be used to describe a wide range of symptoms such as: light-headedness, a feeling of being on a ship and faintness. Other causes must be considered in the history and examination:

- Anxiety with hyperventilation – 'light-headed'
- Anaemia
- Postural hypotension: in the elderly, due to drugs, usually antihypertensives, or as part of an autonomic neuropathy
- Cardiac: low-output cardiac failure and arrhythmias
- Vasovagal pre-syncope/syncope
- Iatrogenic: with or without hypotension.

INVESTIGATIONS FOR VERTIGO

Hallpike manoeuvre

The Hallpike manoeuvre is performed with the patient sitting on a bed. The patient's head is positioned 30° to the affected side and taken to 30° below bed level. After a latent period of a few seconds, vertigo is experienced. There is accompanying torsional nystagmus with upper pole beating towards the floor; the direction of vertigo and nystagmus are reversed on sitting up again. With peripheral (labyrinthine) lesions, symptoms and signs last for about 30 seconds and fatigues with repetition such that they cannot then be reproduced (see Fig. 11.5).

Caloric test

The caloric test is a test of vestibular function. With the patient lying supine, the head is raised 30° from horizontal so that the horizontal canals are vertical. Each external meatus is irrigated for 30 seconds with water, first at 30°C, and then, about 5 minutes later, at 44°C. The normal response is summarized by the acronym 'COWS': Cold water results in nystagmus, with the fast phase Opposite to the side irrigated; Warm water results in nystagmus, with the fast phase to the Same side irrigated.

Two pieces of information can be obtained from the caloric test:

1. Canal paresis: there is no response to irrigation of the external meatus with either cold or warm water; this occurs in peripheral lesions, i.e. the labyrinth, or vestibular ganglion or nerve.

2. Directional preponderance: cold water in the left ear and warm in the right will both result in nystagmus to the right. If this response is greater than left-sided nystagmus produced by cold water in the right ear and warm in the left, a right directional preponderance exists. This usually implies a lesion of the brainstem vestibular nuclei on the left.

Consider the following when assessing a patient with vertigo:
- Vertigo is either peripheral or central in origin
- Vertigo from a supranuclear lesion is uncommon, therefore the main differential is between a peripheral (labyrinth, vestibular ganglion/nerve) lesion and a brainstem or cerebellar lesion
- Vertigo is rarely the sole manifestation of brainstem disease: look for symptoms and signs of additional ipsilateral cranial nerve palsies and contralateral 'pyramidal' limb weakness. Vertigo is typically less prominent than ataxia and nystagmus in central compared to peripheral lesions
- In vertigo from a cerebellar lesion there might be signs of cerebellar dysfunction; these are absent in vertigo from a lesion of the peripheral vestibular system.

Dysarthria, dysphonia and dysphagia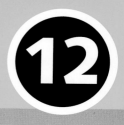

Objectives

- Understand the motor pathways responsible for articulation, phonation and swallowing
- Describe the types and common causes of dysarthria, dysphagia and dysphonia

DEFINITIONS

- Dysarthria is a disorder of articulation of speech; there is no difficulty in comprehension or expression of language.
- Dysphonia is a disorder of vocalization, i.e. strength or quality of spoken words.
- Dysphagia is difficulty with swallowing.

Dysarthria, dysphonia and dysphagia may result from lesions at all levels from the motor cortex down to the numerous muscles involved in articulation, phonation and swallowing. The intervening pathways include the basal ganglia, cerebellum, brainstem, cranial nerves and the neuromuscular junctions (Fig. 12.1).

Non-neurological local pathology can sometimes account for these symptoms (e.g. dysarthria due to absence of dentures, dysphagia due to oesophageal stricture, dysphonia due to lesions of the vocal cords).

Knowledge of the motor pathways responsible for articulation, phonation and swallowing enable localization of the site of the lesion.

DYSARTHRIA

Articulation involves the use of the respiratory musculature, larynx, pharynx, palate, tongue and lips. When a word is heard, signals from the primary auditory cortex are received by Wernicke's area (comprehension of speech), from where the signal is transmitted to Broca's area (expression of speech), and thence to the motor area of the precentral gyrus (primary motor cortex), which controls the speech muscles. The motor pathways for articulation arise from the left (dominant hemisphere in most people) precentral gyrus and cross to the opposite motor cortex as well, then descend in both corticobulbar tracts to the nuclei of the seventh (motor fibres to the facial muscles, including those of the lips), tenth (nucleus ambiguus: motor fibres to the pharynx, larynx and soft palate), and twelfth (motor fibres to the tongue) cranial nerves and in the corticospinal tracts

to the diaphragm and intercostal muscles. The nuclei of the seventh, tenth and twelfth cranial nerves receive corticobulbar fibres from both the ipsilateral and contralateral hemispheres. As with all movements, articulation is modulated by the cerebellum and by the basal ganglia (see Fig. 12.1).

Dysarthria can be caused by a lesion at any level in these pathways. Clinical features of lesions at each level are described below.

Upper motor neuron lesions

The muscles of articulation are bilaterally innervated and a unilateral lesion may be asymptomatic. A bilateral lesion is usually required to produce significant dysarthria. This may occur at the same event or at separate times. A lesion may interrupt the corticobulbar tract at the level of the motor cortex, internal capsule, midbrain or pons before the fibres synapse in the cranial nerve nuclei with the lower motor neurons. An upper motor neuron disorder of articulation may be part of a 'pseudobulbar palsy', which can be found in generalized degenerative conditions such as motor neuron-disease. Pseudobulbar palsy is caused by disruption of both the right and left corticobulbar fibres supplying the motor nuclei of the brainstem. It results in a spastic dysarthria, slow movements of the face with a staring gaze and emotional lability due to the loss of the connections from the frontal cortex to the brainstem that suppress emotional output. Facial, palatal and jaw reflexes are brisk, and primitive reflexes are often present. A spastic dysarthria consists of slow, indistinct and strained speech. On examination, the tongue may appear contracted, with limited protrusion. It is often associated with upper motor neuron signs, especially spasticity in the limbs, brisk reflexes, clonus and extensor plantar responses.

Causes of bilateral upper motor neuron lesions include:

- multiple sclerosis
- motor neuron disease
- bilateral subcortical ischaemic lesions/stroke

Fig. 12.1 Structures and pathways involved in articulation of speech.

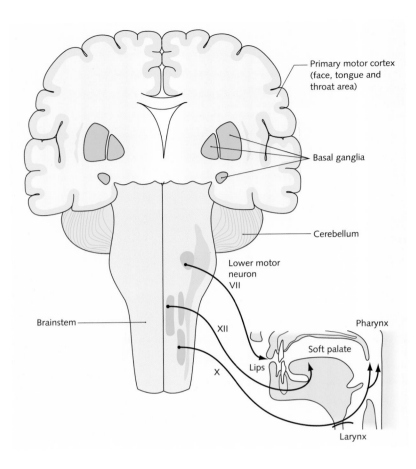

- as part of rare neurodegenerative disorders, e.g. progressive supranuclear palsy
- central pontine myelinolysis.

Lower motor neuron lesions

Lower motor neuron lesions result from damage to the motor nuclei of the seventh, tenth and twelfth cranial nerves, or their peripheral extensions (the corresponding cranial nerves) and give rise to a 'bulbar palsy'. Speech is slurred and indistinct. Labial and lingual sounds are affected. With bilateral paralysis of the soft palate, the speech gains a nasal quality and there may be nasal regurgitation with choking and aspiration. The tongue becomes wasted and may fasciculate. The facial muscles may also be weak. Other signs that may be present in a bulbar palsy include an absent gag reflex, hoarse voice, weak cough and occasionally stridor.

Causes of bilateral lower motor neuron lesions include:

- Guillain–Barré syndrome
- motor neuron disease

- medullary tumours
- syringobulbia
- subacute/chronic infective, inflammatory or malignant meningitis
- poliomyelitis.

Basal ganglia lesions

Parkinson's disease

The speech in Parkinson's disease is often low volume, monotonous and without inflection; it often trails off at the end of sentences. There may be alternating acceleration and stuttering pauses in the speech analogous to the 'festinating' gait.

Chorea

The speech in chorea (e.g. Huntington's disease) is hyperkinetic. It is loud and harsh, intonation is variable, and there is poor coordination of the diaphragm and respiratory muscles. This results in short, breathless sentences.

Athetosis

In patients with athetosis, such as in athetoid cerebral palsy, the speech is loud and slow, and consonants are indistinctly pronounced; the speech is sometimes described as 'dystonic'.

With the above syndromes, the diagnosis is often made by the accompanying characteristic movement abnormalities.

Cerebellar lesions

Cerebellar lesions cause ataxic dysarthria. The speech is slow and slurred with abnormally long pauses between syllables. This arises from impaired coordination of articulation, which is evident on attempted rapid side-to-side movements of the tongue. Other cerebellar signs are usually present. If there is also involvement of the corticobulbar tracts, the speech may be 'scanning', with words broken up into syllables, which are spoken with varying force.

Causes of cerebellar lesions include:

- multiple sclerosis
- vascular lesions, e.g. infarcts and haemorrhages
- tumours
- inherited ataxias, e.g. spinocerebellar dysarthrias
- alcoholic cerebellar degeneration.

Myopathies and disorders of the neuromuscular junction

Myopathies and disorders of the neuromuscular junction give rise to a dysarthria similar to that of a bulbar palsy.

In a neuromuscular junction problem there may be evidence of fatigability, characterized by deterioration of the dysarthria at the end of the day and subsequent improvement the following morning (e.g. myasthenia gravis). If the patient has a myopathic dysarthria there may be a family history of a muscle disorder. There is often prominent wasting and weakness of the facial muscles, involvement of the proximal limbs and myotonia may be present (e.g. dystrophia myotonica).

Oropharyngeal lesions

Local lesions of the oropharynx can cause difficulty with articulation. Examples include:

- multiple mouth ulcers, e.g. following chemotherapy
- oral candidiasis
- quinsy
- dental abscess
- loose dentures.

DYSPHAGIA

The descending motor pathways for swallowing closely follow those for articulation. Dysarthria is therefore often accompanied by dysphagia. Corticobulbar fibres travel bilaterally to the nuclei of both ninth and tenth cranial nerves. Motor fibres from the tenth nucleus (nucleus ambiguus) supply the soft palate and pharynx, which are required for swallowing. The adjacent ninth nucleus (also the nucleus ambiguus) sends motor fibres to the middle constrictor of the pharynx and stylopharyngeus but the ninth nerve is mostly involved in the sensory component of the swallowing reflex and supplies the sensation to the back of the tongue and oropharynx as part of the gag reflex.

Lesions that bilaterally interrupt these pathways will initially cause difficulty with swallowing liquids and subsequently solids. By contrast, lesions causing obstruction of the oesophagus initially tend to cause difficulty with swallowing solids, and then, as the obstruction progresses, difficulty swallowing liquids.

Dysfunction of the swallowing mechanism can be confirmed by videofluoroscopy, when a radio-opaque dye is swallowed and real-time radiographs are taken at each step of swallowing.

Causes of dysphagia overlap with those for dysarthria and the two symptoms often coexist.

Sites of lesions causing dysphagia

Dysphagia can be caused by lesions of:

- both cerebral hemispheres (vascular, trauma, motor neuron disease, multiple system atrophy)
- brainstem (multiple sclerosis, vascular, tumours, syringobulbia)
- cranial nerves (ninth and tenth e.g. Guillain–Barré syndrome)
- neuromuscular junction (myasthenia)
- muscle (polymyositis)
- pharynx and oesophagus (local pathology).

DYSPHONIA

Dysphonia is alteration of the volume or quality of vocal sound. Phonation is a function of the larynx and the vocal cords. Sound is produced by air passing over the vocal cords. The pitch is altered by changes in tension of the membranous part of the vocal cords. This is performed by the intrinsic laryngeal muscles, which are supplied by the laryngeal branches of the tenth cranial nerve which arise from the nucleus ambiguus in the medulla. The nucleus ambiguus has bilateral supranuclear innervation from the corticobulbar fibres

Fig. 12.2 Causes of dysarthria, dysphagia and dysphonia

Site	Example
Bilateral upper motor neuron pathways	Disorders affecting primary motor cortex, e.g. motor neuron disease Internal capsule vascular disease
Basal ganglia Cerebellum (often midline) Brainstem nuclei (VII, X, XII)	Parkinson's disease, Huntington's disease Multiple sclerosis Motor neuron disease
Seventh, tenth, and twelfth cranial nerves Neuromuscular junction Muscle	Bell's palsy, malignant, chronic infective or inflammatory meningitis Myasthenia gravis Dystrophia myotonica, rare inherited muscle disorders
Oropharynx	Tongue or laryngeal tumours

arising in the primary motor cortex. Lesions in this pathway will cause dysphonia (the voice having a husky quality) or aphonia (the inability to produce any sound). There may be impairment of coughing, which requires normal vocal cord function. Paralysis or a local lesion of the vocal cord can be visualized by indirect laryngoscopy. The paralysed cord fails to abduct and adduct during attempted phonation.

Causes of dysphonia include:

- medullary lesions involving the nucleus ambiguus: infarction, tumour, demyelination
- recurrent laryngeal nerve palsy: following thyroid surgery, bronchial carcinoma, aortic aneurysm
- vocal cord lesions: polyps, tumour
- functional (psychogenic aphonia).

The proximity of the motor pathways controlling articulation, swallowing and phonation often leads to impairment of one or more of these functions at the same time (e.g. a patient with a bulbar palsy may present with dysarthria and nasal intonation, drooling due to difficulty swallowing, and a hoarse voice with poor cough).

The causes of dysarthria, dysphagia and or dysphonia are summarized in Figure 12.2.

HINTS AND TIPS

It is always wise to inspect the oropharynx first to exclude a local cause for dysarthria/dysphagia.

Cerebellar dysfunction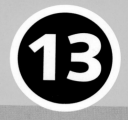

Objectives

- Understand the basic anatomy and function of the cerebellum
- Describe the clinical features associated with cerebellar hemisphere and vermis dysfunction
- Describe the main causes of cerebellar dysfunction

The cerebellum and its connections are responsible for the coordination of skilled voluntary movement, posture and gait.

The cerebellum can be divided into three functional units (Figs 13.1 and 13.2):

1. The flocculonodular lobe (vestibulocerebellum) and inferior vermis, which are mainly involved in controlling information from the vestibular system.
2. The small anterior lobe and the anterior superior vermis (spinocerebellum), which are mainly involved in receiving proprioceptive information from the limbs.
3. The large posterior lobe and the middle part of the vermis (neocerebellum), which are mainly involved in receiving inputs from the contralateral cerebral cortex via pontine nuclei. They are involved in fine motor control, e.g. finger movements.

Efferent pathways pass from the cerebellum to the deep cerebellar and brainstem nuclei and enable coordination of skilled movements.

CLINICAL FEATURES OF CEREBELLAR DYSFUNCTION

HINTS AND TIPS

Cerebellar dysfunction is characterized by:
- ataxia of limbs and gait
- dysarthria
- nystagmus
- dysdiadochokinesis (impaired rapid alternating movements)
- pendular reflexes and the rebound phenomenon may also be present (secondary to hypotonia).

Incoordination of movement

Cerebellar dysfunction causes impairment of the process of controlling movements once they have been initiated. This gives rise to ataxia (incoordination) as manifested by the following signs:

- Intention tremor: there is no tremor at rest. When the patient moves a limb towards a target a tremor develops, e.g. abnormal finger–nose test.
- Dysdiadochokinesia: the inability to carry out rapid alternating movements with regularity.
- Dysmetria: the inability to control smooth and accurate targeted movements. The movements are jerky, with overshooting of the target as manifested in the finger–nose and heel–shin tests.

Ataxic gait

The patient walks with a staggering gait and may later develop a wide-based gait to improve stability. In mild cases, the unsteadiness may be apparent only when walking heel-to-toe (tandem walking). In a unilateral cerebellar hemisphere lesion, there is unsteadiness towards the side of the lesion. In truncal ataxia, there is difficulty sitting or standing without support.

Ataxic dysarthric speech

Speech can be slow, slurred and scanning in quality. In scanning speech, there is loss of variation of intonation and the words may be broken up into syllables.

Abnormal eye movements

- Jerky pursuits: pursuit movements are slow, with catch-up saccadic movements on attempting to maintain fixation on the moving target or 'saccadic intrusions'.
- Dysmetria of saccades: when trying to fixate on a target, the eyes overshoot and oscillate several times before fixation is achieved.
- Nystagmus: this is maximal on gaze towards the side of the lesion. Nystagmus results from damage of the vestibular connections of the cerebellum.

Fig. 13.1 Posterior aspect of the cerebellum.

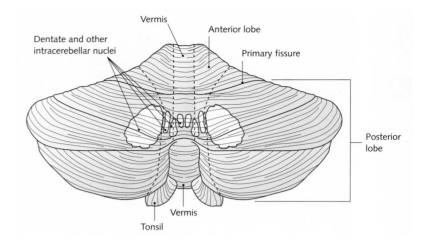

Fig. 13.2 The major phylogenetic subdivisions of the cerebellum.

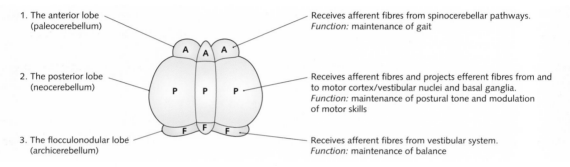

1. The anterior lobe (paleocerebellum) — Receives afferent fibres from spinocerebellar pathways. *Function:* maintenance of gait

2. The posterior lobe (neocerebellum) — Receives afferent fibres and projects efferent fibres from and to motor cortex/vestibular nuclei and basal ganglia. *Function:* maintenance of postural tone and modulation of motor skills

3. The flocculonodular lobe (archicerebellum) — Receives afferent fibres from vestibular system. *Function:* maintenance of balance

Titubation

Nodding tremor of the head may occur. This is mainly in the anterior–posterior plane.

Altered posture

A unilateral cerebellar lesion may cause the head and – when the lesion is recent and severe – the body, to tilt towards the side of the lesion. Head tilt may also be due to a fourth nerve palsy, which can accompany a lesion of the superior medullary vellum (Fig. 13.3).

Hypotonia

Hypotonia is a relatively minor feature of cerebellar disease, resulting from depression of alpha and gamma motor neuron activity. Hypotonia can sometimes be demonstrated clinically by decreased resistance to passive movement (e.g. extension of a limb), by 'pendular' reflexes, or by the rebound phenomenon. This occurs when the patient's outstretched arms are pressed down for a few seconds and then abruptly released by the examiner. The arms rebound upwards much further than would be expected in the presence of cerebellar

hypotonia. The reflexes are poorly checked so that when testing the patellar reflex, for example, the leg may swing to and fro (like a pendulum).

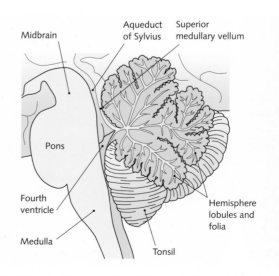

Fig. 13.3 Sagittal section though the cerebellum and brainstem.

Fig. 13.4   Causes of cerebellar dysfunction

Cause	Additional clinical characteristics
Tumours	Type of tumour – metastatic disease, meningioma, acoustic neuroma, medulloblastoma, haemangioblastoma, paraneoplastic syndrome with bronchial, ovarian, uterine carcinomas and lymphomas
Multiple sclerosis	Pyramidal, brainstem and dorsal column signs; optic atrophy
Vascular	
Haemorrhage	History of hypertension, bleeding disorder, on anticoagulants
Infarction	History of hypertension, ischaemic heart disease, atrial fibrillation, diabetes, hyperlipidaemia
Infections	
Abscess	Infection or abscess elsewhere, fever, unwell, IV drug abuser
Prion disease	Dementia, myoclonus, characteristic EEG changes
Viral encephalitis	Notably chickenpox within 3 weeks of initial infection
Toxins	
Anticonvulsants	History of epilepsy; signs of acute toxicity or past history of recurrent toxicity
Alcohol	Acute intoxication; history of chronic abuse, signs of alcoholic liver disease
Metabolic	
Myxoedema	Myxoedematous facies, dry skin and hair, increased weight, cold intolerance, slow-relaxing reflexes, bradycardia
Vitamin deficiency (B_1, B_{12}, E)	See Chapter 34
Trauma	Head injury
Neurodegenerative conditions	
Multiple system atrophy (MSA)	Atypical parkinsonism, and primary autonomic failure in addition to ataxia (see Chapter 21)
Developmental deformities	
Arnold–Chiari malformation	Pyramidal signs, lower cranial nerve palsies, occipital headache, ± signs associated with a syrinx
Congenital aqueduct stenosis	6th nerve palsies, deafness, papilloedema, intellectual decline
Dandy–Walker syndrome	Large cystic fourth ventricle resulting in hydrocephalus
Inherited cerebellar ataxias	Early onset (< 25 years) – tend to be autosomal recessive: - Friedreich's ataxias, ataxia telangiectasia (see Chapter 35), ataxia with oculomotor apraxia, metabolic ataxias including vitamin E deficiency and mitochondrial disorders, progressive myoclonic ataxias Late onset (>25 years) – tend to be autosomal dominant: - Spinocerebellar ataxias (see Chapter 35), episodic ataxias, dentatorubropallidoluysian atrophy (DRPLA)

The causes of cerebellar dysfunction are listed in Figure 13.4.

LOCALIZATION OF A CEREBELLAR LESION

Cerebellar hemisphere

A lesion of the cerebellar hemisphere causes ataxia in the limbs ipsilateral to the lesion. The gait is ataxic, with a tendency to fall towards the affected side. There may be nystagmus maximal towards the side of the lesion and the speech may be slurred.

Cerebellar vermis

Lesions of the midline vermis cause truncal ataxia (imbalance of gait and stance) typically without the classic triad of limb ataxia, dysarthria and nystagmus.

Lesions of the flocculonodular lobe cause truncal ataxia, vertigo (damage to the vestibular reflex pathways), vomiting (involvement of the floor of the fourth ventricle) and nystagmus.

Space-occupying lesions at midline sites can cause early obstruction of the cerebral aqueduct in the midbrain or the fourth ventricle. This results in hydrocephalus with dilated third and lateral ventricles as well as headache, vomiting and, eventually, papilloedema.

Movement disorders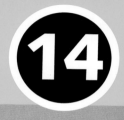

- Classify movement disorders into two main groups and subdivisions
- Differentiate the non-jerky hyperkinesias (tremor and dystonia)
- Differentiate the jerky hyperkinesias (chorea, tics and myoclonus)

THE ANATOMICAL BASIS AND CLASSIFICATION OF MOVEMENT DISORDERS

The basal ganglia are symmetrical groups of grey matter or 'nuclei' deep within the cerebral hemispheres and brainstem. The main components are the caudate nucleus, globus pallidus, putamen, substantia nigra and subthalamus. These nuclei are mostly concerned with controlling movement, especially the initiation and termination of movement.

Movement disorders can be classified into two main categories with additional subdivisions. The akinetic or hypokinetic disorders are characterized by an insufficient or a loss of movement. These include akinetic rigid disorders with parkinsonism as the main feature, and Parkinson's disease is the most common hypokinetic movement disorder.

Hyperkinetic disorders have additional or excessive movements and these can be subdivided into non-jerky (tremor or dystonia) and jerky hyperkinetic movements (chorea, tics or myoclonus). This chapter will mostly focus on the hyperkinetic movement disorders. The hypokinetic disorders are discussed in detail in Chapter 21.

THE HYPERKINETIC MOVEMENT DISORDERS: TREMOR AND DYSTONIA

The non-jerky hyperkinetic movement disorders include tremor and dystonia.

Tremor

Tremor is an involuntary and rhythmic (refers to a regular oscillatory) movement of one or more body parts. All tremors should disappear during sleep. Tremor may be normal (physiological) or abnormal (pathological), and are described as 'fine' if they are low amplitude and 'coarse' if they are high amplitude. The positions in which a tremor can occur are at rest, on posture (e.g. holding the arms outstretched) or during movement (kinetic tremor). Tremors should therefore be assessed by observing the patient at rest, during maintenance of a posture (e.g. holding the arms outstretched), and during volitional, kinetic movements of the limbs. The term intention tremor refers to a tremor that increases throughout the movement, whereas terminal tremor refers to a tremor that occurs at the end of the movement. Both are forms of a kinetic tremor (Fig. 14.1). Some people also use the term action tremor, which refers to all tremors that do not occur at rest, but for simplicity this term is best avoided.

A physiological tremor affects all muscle groups, although it is most commonly noted in the hands. The tremor is present during waking. It is usually bilateral, worse on maintaining a posture, fine in character and fast in rate (8–14 Hz). Patients often do not notice their own tremor.

A pathological tremor often occurs at rest or with movement, is slower (4–7 Hz), coarse in character, proximal as well as distal and often asymmetrical. This tremor often interferes with everyday activities.

Resting tremor

The most common cause of a resting tremor is Parkinson's disease. The parkinsonian tremor is a coarse 'pill-rolling' tremor and disappears during voluntary movement. It is usually observed in the hands and arms and is asymmetrical, being worse on one side more than the other (see Ch. 21). The tremor may affect other parts of the body, including the jaw and feet. The patient may have other signs of Parkinson's disease (e.g. a shuffling gait, stooped posture, reduced or loss of arm swing; immobile facies as well as rigidity and bradykinesia with fatiguing of the limbs) (see Ch. 21). The tremor may respond to anticholinergic or dopaminergic medication.

Fig. 14.1 Summary of hyperkinetic movement disorders

Tremor		
Rhythmic, oscillatory, involuntary movements	Resting	Tremor of parkinsonism/Parkinson's disease (note parkinsonian tremor can also have postural component)
	Postural	Physiological Essential tremor Dystonia (also has rest component) Neuropathy (also has rest component)
	Kinetic	Cerebellar (intention tremor) Rubral tremor (also has rest and postural components)
	Focal syndromes	Orthostatic tremor (high-frequency tremor of both legs present on standing) Palatal tremor (tremor of the soft palate which can be essential or symptomatic) Head tremor (common causes include cerebellar disease, Parkinson's disease and dystonia)
Chorea		
Abrupt, irregular, jerky movements		Medication, e.g. levodopa, neuroleptics, OCP Neurodegenerative disorders, e.g. Huntington's disease, Wilson's disease Infectious, e.g. Sydenham's chorea, HIV Autoimmune, e.g. antiphospholipid syndrome Metabolic, e.g. hyperthyroidism Haematological, e.g. polycythaemia rubra vera Structural, e.g. vascular, demyelination, tumour
Ballism		
Large amplitude proximal form of chorea – can be hemiballism or monoballism		Infarction of subthalamus Tumour
Dystonia		
Twisting movements and abnormal postures	Primary generalized	Dystonia musculorum deformans
	Primary focal	Spasmodic torticollis, blepharospasm oromandibular dystonia, writer's cramp
	Dystonia plus	Dopa responsive dystonia
	Secondary	Brain injury Drugs Neurodegenerative diseases
Tic		
Stereotyped movements or vocalisations	Primary	Simple tics of childhood Gilles de la Tourette syndrome
	Secondary	Neurodegenerative disease, developmental disorders, infection, structural, pharmacological
Myoclonus		
Brief shock-like movements	With epilepsy	Myoclonus with epilepsy Progressive myoclonic epilepsy and ataxia
	Symptomatic	With encephalopathy: – liver failure, renal failure, drug intoxication, post-hypoxia Without encephalopathy: – plus dementia (Alzheimer's disease, Creutzfeldt–Jakob disease, dementia with Lewy bodies) – plus parkinsonism (corticobasal degeneration, multiple system atrophy) – focal/segmental (spinal cord/ root/plexus injury)

Postural tremor

A postural tremor occurs when a body part assumes a position against gravity and is usually physiological but can occur in essential, dystonic and neuropathic tremor.

1. Physiological tremor

Physiological tremor may be exaggerated by:

- anxiety
- metabolic disturbances: hyperthyroidism, phaeochromocytoma
- alcohol withdrawal
- drugs: lithium, sodium valproate, sympathomimetics, tea and coffee.

Beta-blockers may diminish a physiological tremor.

2. Essential tremor

Essential tremor may be difficult to distinguish from an exaggerated physiological tremor. It is coarser and slower (8 Hz), affecting the upper limbs, and can spread to the head, trunk and legs. It can be inherited in an autosomal dominant manner in about 50% of patients, in which case it presents in childhood or early adulthood. Otherwise its incidence increases with age. On movement (finger–nose testing) the tremor may worsen terminally (terminal tremor), but does not progressively worsen throughout the movement. The tremor can progress to be disabling and there is often temporary improvement with alcohol intake. This can be used as a diagnostic and therapeutic manoeuvre. Essential tremor may partially respond to beta-blockers, anticholinergics (e.g. trihexyphenidyl) and primidone, and sometimes to barbiturates or benzodiazepines.

3. Neuropathic tremor

Peripheral neuropathies can cause a postural tremor which is distinct from pseudo-athetoid movements that can be seen with proprioceptive loss. Signs of the underlying neuropathy are typically present when the tremor presents, and treatment of the neuropathy may improve the tremor.

4. Dystonic tremor

A tremor that involves a body part affected with dystonia is called a dystonic tremor. Dystonic tremor can mimic the tremor seen in Parkinson's disease and many cases of true dystonic tremor are misdiagnosed as essential tremor. Dystonic tremor is often position and task specific, and is typically asymmetrical and of large amplitude when compared to essential tremor.

Kinetic tremor

A kinetic tremor is a tremor that occurs during movement.

1. Cerebellar tremor (intention tremor)

Cerebellar dysfunction (see Ch.13) gives rise to a coarse, often slow (4–6 Hz), action or 'intention' tremor. It is absent at rest and becomes apparent on movement. On performing the finger–nose test, the finger oscillates with increasing amplitude on approaching the target. Rhythmic oscillation of the head and trunk (titubation) may occur and there may be other signs of cerebellar dysfunction such as nystagmus, dysarthria, dysdiadochokinesis and an ataxic gait.

2. Red nuclear 'rubral' tremor

This tremor is present at rest, deteriorates with posture, but is worst during movement. It is caused by damage to the cerebellar–brainstem connections, typically from multiple sclerosis, but also from vascular lesions and tumours. It is an unusually coarse and often violent tremor. Slight movement of the arm may precipitate a wide-amplitude tremor of the limb. Stereotactic surgical lesions of the contralateral ventrolateral thalamus may abolish pathological tremors.

Mixed tremors

Combinations of rest, postural and kinetic tremor may be present in severe essential tremor, dystonic tremor and rubral tremor.

DYSTONIA

Dystonia is a hyperkinetic movement disorder characterized by involuntary and repetitive contractions of opposing muscles, causing twisting movements and abnormal postures. Dystonias can affect one or more parts of the body. In addition, tremor often occurs with dystonia and tends to affect the same body part. Dystonias can be classified in a variety of ways. They may affect only one part of the body (focal dystonia), two or more contiguous body parts such as the head and neck (segmental dystonia), non-contiguous body regions such as laryngeal with limb dystonia (multifocal), one-half of the body (hemidystonia), or the whole of the body (generalized dystonia). The focal dystonias tends to be idiopathic or secondary to lesions often within the basal ganglia, whereas generalized dystonia tends to have a genetic basis. Adult-onset dystonia affects those >25 years old, and young-onset dystonia those <25 years old. Dystonia can also be classified according to aetiology (see Fig. 14.1).

1. Primary dystonia

Patients have no features of neurodegeneration or secondary causes of dystonia. Dystonia is the only clinical feature except for perhaps a dystonic tremor. There is no underlying or secondary disorder, although there may be a genetic aetiology. The most common primary forms are the late-onset, focal dystonias, which are also the most common form of all dystonias, accounting for 90% of all cases. Late-onset dystonia usually starts in mid-adulthood and often has a focal onset without a tendency to spread to other body parts (cervical dystonia such as torticollis, writer's cramp, blepharospasm or isolated laryngeal dystonia). The most effective treatment for focal dystonia is botulinum toxin injections into the affected muscles at approximately 3-monthly intervals:

- **Focal dystonia:** typically late in onset and sporadic:
  Cervical dystonia ('spasmodic torticollis'): usually occurs in the third to fifth decades of life. There are involuntary movements of the neck: laterally towards one side (laterocollis) or rotating around to one side (torticollis), in extension (retrocollis) or flexion (anterocollis). The overactive muscles such as sternomastoid, trapezius and splenius are most affected, can be painful and may eventually hypertrophy. Women are affected more than men. Patients often demonstrate a 'geste antagonist', which is a manoeuvre that stops the involuntary movement (e.g. gentle pressure with the hand on the side of the jaw). Cervical dystonia may be complicated by a jerky postural and kinetic tremor referred to as a 'dystonic tremor'. Response to anticholinergics is often poor. Botulinum toxin injections to overactive muscles can provide good relief.
  Blepharospasm: involuntary contractions of the eyelid muscles where the eyes screw up and remain closed with a 'shampoo in the eyes' effect.
  Oromandibular dystonia: involuntary dystonic movements of the mouth, tongue and jaw can affect women in the sixth decade of life. Speech and swallowing may also be affected. It may also occur in patients on long-term neuroleptic therapy and the elderly.
  Writer's cramp: attempts at writing triggers a task-specific, focal hand dystonia which may be painful but resolves on cessation of writing. The symptoms can spread to the forearm and shoulders. There is a specific inability to perform a previously highly developed skilled movement, in this case writing, due to dystonic posturing of the

affected hand when a pen is gripped. It usually occurs in middle or late life, and does not typically progress to involve other parts of the body. Other skilled functions of the hands are usually normal. Some patients respond to anticholinergics or to selective botulinum injections to affected muscles. Other focal, occupational, task-specific dystonias occur in musicians and sportsmen.

- **Early-onset generalized dystonia:** typically early in onset and genetic. Historically, this was previously described as idiopathic torsion dystonia and dystonia musculorum deformans. It is rare, but is the most common hereditary dystonia and is caused by mutations in the gene DYT1. There is an autosomal dominant pattern of inheritance with incomplete penetrance as only 40% of patients with a mutation develop the disease. At its onset there appears to be focal dystonia that often starts in the legs and usually spreads over months to years, resulting in generalized dystonia, often with sparing of the head and neck. Treatment consists of the anticholinergics clonazepam and baclofen. Surgery is confined to patients who are severely affected and consists of deep brain stimulation to the globus pallidus.

2. Dystonia-plus syndromes – dopa-responsive dystonia

Patients have no features of neurodegeneration or secondary causes of dystonia. However, other signs may occur with the dystonia. Dopa-responsive dystonia is the main example in this group. This is a rare disorder in which there is progressive dystonia that initially affects the lower limbs in early childhood. There is marked diurnal variation, with symptoms worsening as the day progresses but improving with rest and sleep. Patients also have parkinsonism and spasticity. There is a striking response to small doses of L-dopa, which treats many of the symptoms of the disease. This disease is also familial and inherited in an autosomal dominant manner with incomplete penetrance.

3. Secondary dystonia

There is a clear secondary cause of the dystonia and other signs may be apparent. The most common cause of secondary dystonia is due to the side effects of medication. The dopamine-receptor blocking drugs, particularly the neuroleptics, cause acute transient dystonic reactions or a persistent dystonic disorder referred to as tardive dystonia. Tardive dystonia can persist despite discontinuing medication and often occurs after several years of treatment with neuroleptics. It typically manifests as axial dystonia with hyperextension of the spine and neck referred to as retrocollis. Treatment can have limited success and prevention is the most important method of avoiding all of the tardive movement disorders. Other causes of secondary dystonia include:

- **Brain injury:** cerebral palsy, following hypoxic damage or kernicterus
- **Neurodegenerative diseases:** e.g. Parkinson's disease, corticobasal degeneration, progressive supranuclear palsy, multiple system atrophy, Huntington's disease, Wilson's disease.

4. Paroxysmal dystonia

These are a group of familial conditions which consist of brief attacks of dystonic posturing provoked by sudden noise, movement, emotional stimuli or exercise. There may be no clinical signs between attacks.

The most effective treatment for focal dystonias is botulinum toxin injections into the affected muscles at approximately 3-monthly intervals.

THE HYPERKINETIC MOVEMENT DISORDERS: CHOREA, TICS AND MYOCLONUS

Chorea

Chorea, from the Greek word for 'a dance', consists of involuntary movements that are non-rhythmic, abrupt and jerky and that randomly move from one body part to another. It can affect the face, trunk and limbs or be generalized. The causes of chorea are wide ranging:

- Medications: levodopa, neuroleptics (e.g. phenothiazines, butyrophenones), oral contraceptives, anticonvulsants and calcium antagonists
- Inherited/degenerative disorders: Huntington's disease, Wilson's disease
- Autoimmune/post-infectious: systemic lupus erythematosus, antiphospholipid syndrome, vasculitis, Hashimoto's thyroiditis and Sydenham's chorea (post-streptococcal infection)
- Infections: HIV, CJD
- Metabolic disorders: disorders of thyroid, parathyroid, glucose, sodium, calcium and magnesium
- Haematological disorders: polycythaemia rubra vera
- Structural disorders: vascular, demyelination, tumour.

Huntington's disease (Huntington's chorea)

Huntington's disease is clinically characterized by progressive personality/behavioural changes, generalized chorea and eventually dementia. Towards the end of the disease, chorea diminishes and parkinsonism and dystonia dominates the clinical picture. It typically manifests in the fourth decade and progresses to death within 12–15 years. Management includes dopamine-blocking or -depleting drugs to reduce the chorea by causing parkinsonism. Patients often have tic disorder that may also require treatment. Huntington's disease is a hereditary condition caused by an expanded trinucleotide repeat (CAG) on chromosome 4. It shows genetic anticipation, such that with each generation the repeat increases in length, manifesting with a younger age of onset. About 6% of cases start before 21 years of age, and are dominated by an akinetic rigid syndrome (Westphal variant). There is neuronal loss initially in the caudate nucleus and putamen, as well as other areas such as the cerebral cortex. There is no effective treatment, although dopamine-blocking or -depleting drugs may reduce the chorea by causing parkinsonism.

> ### COMMUNICATION
>
> It is essential to counsel patients prior to performing genetic tests. The patients should understand what are the implications of a positive and negative test on other relatives, including those who may have inherited the mutation but have not shown the signs (asymptomatic carriers). Many relatives decide not to undergo presymptomatic testing.

Ballism

Ballism, which is derived from the Greek word 'to throw', and is an additional term that describes chorea when it is severe, proximal and of large amplitude. In these cases it can appear as a violent flinging movement of the proximal limb. Hemiballism, the commonest presentation, affecting an arm and ipsilateral leg, is due to a stroke in the contralateral subthalamic nucleus. If the amplitude of limb movements is small, it is referred to as hemichorea, and if a single limb is affected, it is called monoballism.

> ### HINTS AND TIPS
>
> Clinically, it can be difficult to differentiate chorea, tremor, dystonia and myoclonus because they often occur together. In these cases you should try to decide which movement disorder is predominant.

Tics

A tic is an involuntary, stereotyped movement or vocalization, which can be suppressed for periods of time by patients, but at the cost of mounting inner tension. Tics can be motor or vocal, and simple (e.g. one discrete movement or unarticulated sounds) or complex (e.g. combination of movements or words or phrases). Tics can be primary (e.g. simple tics of childhood or Giles de la Tourette syndrome) or secondary to a variety of neurodegenerative, structural, developmental (e.g. Down's syndrome), infective (e.g. streptococcal infection) or pharmacological causes.

Gilles de la Tourette syndrome is a rare disease in which multiple motor and, in particular, vocal tics develop before the age of 18 years. There may be psychiatric and behavioural disorders including attention-deficit hyperactivity disorder, depression or obsessive compulsive disorder. The caudate nucleus has been implicated in the pathology of the condition and treatment is symptomatic. The syndrome is characterized by involuntary snorting, grunting, shouting of verbal obscenities, and aggressive and sexual impulses. It may respond to dopamine-blocking neuroleptic drugs (e.g. sulpiride).

Myoclonus

Myoclonus are sudden, brief and shock-like involuntary movements. It can be a normal experience in healthy individuals. For example, the jerks that can occur on falling asleep and hiccups are both forms of myoclonus. Pathophysiological myoclonus can occur in the same muscle (focal myoclonus) or affect many different parts at different times (multifocal myoclonus) or affect all of the body (generalized myoclonus). Myoclonus may also be sensitive to a variety of stimuli (e.g. a sudden noise, light, touch, or voluntary movement). Generalized myoclonus arises from the cerebral cortex, whereas focal myoclonus can arise from cerebral cortex, brainstem, spinal cord or even peripheral nerves and roots.

Myoclonus can be classified according to the underlying cause.

1. Myoclonic epilepsy

Myoclonus may be a feature of many different forms of epilepsy (e.g. juvenile myoclonic epilepsy, Lennox–Gastaut syndrome).

2. Progressive myoclonic epilepsy

Myoclonus may be combined with epilepsy and progressive dementia in several rare inherited metabolic diseases, e.g. Lafora body disease, lipid-storage diseases (Gaucher's disease).

3. Symptomatic myoclonus

Myoclonus can occur in the context of conditions causing an encephalopathy. It can therefore be seen in patients with liver failure, renal failure, drug intoxication (alcohol lithium) and post-hypoxia. Asterixis is the sporadic 'flapping tremor' of the hands observed with arms outstretched and hands dorsiflexed. These brief, non-rhythmic movements are not actually a tremor. It is actually a form of 'negative' myoclonus (sudden involuntary relaxation of a muscle group) and is seen in metabolic encephalopathies. Post-anoxic action myoclonus occurs following severe cerebral anoxia (e.g. after cardiorespiratory arrest) and is known as 'Lance Adams syndrome'. Symptomatic myoclonus can also be seen in diseases without encephalopathy. This includes those that cause dementia (e.g. Alzheimer's disease, Creutzfeldt–Jakob disease) or atypical parkinsonism (e.g. corticobasal degeneration, multiple system atrophy). Focal myoclonus can be seen in spinal cord/root/plexus injuries. Myoclonus may respond to benzodiazepines such as clonazepam.

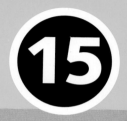
- Understand the neuroanatomy of the motor system from cerebral cortex to muscle
- Describe the symptoms and signs associated with upper and lower motor neuron syndromes
- Define the upper and lower motor neuron pathways and how lesions along the course of each pathway are differentiated

Weakness in the limbs can result from pathology at any level of the motor pathway:

- Pathology anywhere along the upper motor neuron (UMN) pathway (from motor cortex to the spinal cord)
- A lesion of the lower motor neuron (LMN) pathway (from the anterior horn cell to the peripheral nerve)
- Disorders of the neuromuscular junction
- Muscular disorders.

The distribution and pattern of weakness, together, with associated physical signs, usually allows determination of the level of the motor pathway affected, and therefore possible differential diagnoses.

> **COMMUNICATION**
>
> Many patients use the word 'weakness' to describe other deficits that are not actually characterized by a lack of power, such as stiffness, slowness, ataxia, fatigue and clumsiness due to sensory loss.

NEUROANATOMY

The upper motor neuron pathway

UMN cell bodies are arranged in a homuncular distribution in the primary motor cortex, at the posterior limit of the frontal lobe (Fig. 15.1):

- The axons of the UMNs descend through the subcortical white matter (corona radiata and then internal capsule).
- The axons descend in the midbrain as the cerebral peduncles and then in the anterior pons and medulla where they cross as the pyramidal decussation.
- During their brainstem course, some of the UMN axons synapse in motor nuclei (cranial nerve nuclei III, IV, V, VI, VII, X, XI, XII). These axons are called the corticobulbar fibres because the motor nuclei in the brainstem are known as the 'bulbar nuclei'.
- The remaining axons form the corticospinal tracts and descend in the lateral white matter of the spinal cord.

The lower motor neuron pathway

- At each spinal level, some of the corticospinal fibres enter the anterior horn of the grey matter and synapse with cell bodies of the LMN, the anterior horn cells or motor neurons.
- When these cell bodies are damaged, the syndrome is referred to as an **anterior horn cell disorder**.
- Each LMN sends out an axon in the ventral (motor) root which joins a dorsal (sensory) root at each spinal level in the intervertebral foramen to form a spinal segmental or mixed nerve. When this nerve is damaged, it is called a **radiculopathy**.
- The spinal nerve in the cervical and lumbosacral regions joins other adjacent spinal nerves in a junctional network referred to as a plexus. If these structures are damaged, the clinical syndrome is a **plexopathy**.
- From the plexi emerge peripheral nerves and, when these are damaged, the patient develops a **neuropathy**.
- The axons in the peripheral nerves split into many fibres just before synapsing with muscle fibres.

The neuromuscular junction and muscle pathway

- One axon innervates from 10 to 10 000 muscle fibres, depending on whether fine motor control or a coarser antigravity use of the muscle is required. The group of muscle fibres innervated by one axon is called a motor unit. When the synapses are damaged, the condition is called a **neuromuscular junction disorder**.
- Finally, the muscle itself can be damaged and this is termed a **myopathy**.

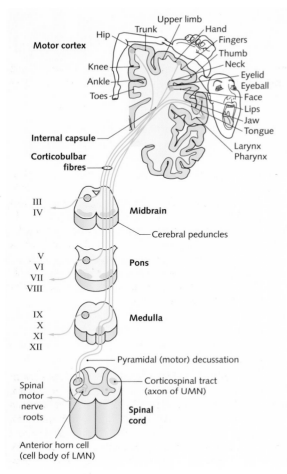

Fig. 15.1 Descending motor pathways from the cortex to the brainstem, cranial nerves and spinal cord.

Any disorder affecting the UMN, LMN, neuromuscular junction or the muscle can give rise to the symptom of weakness and/or the sign of loss of power (Fig. 15.2).

TERMINOLOGY

Paralysis is the complete loss of voluntary movement. The words 'plegia', 'palsy' and 'paresis' are sometimes used interchangeably to describe weakness, although 'paresis' is the correct term to describe incomplete paralysis. 'Plegia' means complete paralysis and the word 'palsy' is used when the paralysis affects cranial motor nerves (e.g. Bell's palsy, pseudobulbar palsy) or when one is referring to a static weakness (e.g. cerebral palsy). There are several specific terms used to describe the anatomical distribution of weakness:

- **Pyramidal weakness:** loss of power is most marked in the extensor muscles in the arms and the flexors in the legs. This is characteristic of UMN lesions involving the pyramidal tract within the brain or spinal cord (see further details below).
- **Proximal weakness,** affecting the shoulders, hips, trunk, neck and sometimes face. This is characteristic of muscle disease (myopathy) and also a common pattern in myasthenia gravis (neuromuscular junction).
- **Distal weakness,** affecting the hands and feet. This is typical of peripheral motor neuropathy, often affecting the lower limbs first and more severely.
- **Global weakness:** this term is used to describe generalized weakness in a limb (both proximal and distal), which may result from severe pathologies affecting any level within the motor system.

UPPER MOTOR NEURON WEAKNESS

UMN weakness results from damage of the corticospinal tract at any point from the motor cortex to the spinal cord (see Fig. 15.1). If the lesion occurs above the pyramidal decussation at the level of the lower medulla, the weakness is contralateral to the site of the lesion. If it occurs below this level, the weakness is ipsilateral to the lesion.

	Fig. 15.2 Anatomical sites of weakness	
	Site of pathology	**Clinical syndrome**
UMN pathway	Motor cortex, corona radiata, internal capsule, brainstem	Hemisphere or brainstem (pyramidal weakness)
	Spinal cord (corticospinal tract)	Myelopathy (pyramidal weakness)
LMN pathway	Anterior horn or motor neuron cell body	Motor neuronopathy or 'anterior horn cell disease'
	Spinal nerve root	Radiculopathy
	Brachial or lumbosacral plexus	Plexopathy
	Peripheral nerve	Neuropathy
Neuromuscular junction	Synapse	Neuromuscular junction disorder
Muscle	Muscle	Myopathy

The following clinical features characterize a UMN lesion.

Increased tone (spasticity)

Initially, UMN weakness may be flaccid, with absent or diminished deep tendon reflexes. There is little understanding of the reasons behind this initial flaccidity and it is often referred to as 'shock'. Increased tone of a UMN type is called spasticity. It may develop several hours, days, or even weeks after the initial lesion has occurred. Spasticity is manifested by:

- 'spastic catch': mild spasticity may be detected as a resistance to passive movement or 'catch' in the pronators on passive supination of the forearm and in the flexors of the hand/forearm on extension of the wrist/elbow
- the 'clasp-knife' phenomenon: in more severe lesions, following strong resistance to passive flexion of the knee or extension of the elbow, there is a sudden relaxation of the extensor muscles of the leg and flexor muscles in the arm
- clonus: rhythmic involuntary muscular contractions follow an abruptly applied and sustained stretch stimulus, e.g. at the ankle following sudden passive dorsiflexion of the foot.

'Pyramidal-pattern' weakness

The antigravity muscles are preferentially spared and stronger (i.e. the flexors of the upper limbs and the extensors of the lower limbs). The patient can develop a characteristic posture of flexed and pronated arms with clenched fingers, and extended and adducted legs with plantar flexion of the feet.

Absence of muscle wasting and fasciculations

Focal muscle wasting and fasciculations are features of an LMN lesion. With chronic disuse, some loss of muscle bulk can occur after a UMN lesion, but this is rarely severe or focal.

Brisk tendon reflexes and extensor plantar responses

The tendon reflexes are brisk. The cremasteric and abdominal or 'cutaneous' reflexes are depressed or absent. The plantar responses are extensor ('upgoing toes' or 'positive Babinski sign').

UPPER MOTOR NEURON SYNDROMES

The common UMN syndromes are hemiparesis and paraparesis. Tetraparesis and monoparesis are less common.

Hemiparesis – unilateral arm and leg weakness

Hemiparesis results from unilateral lesions of the contralateral cerebral hemisphere or brainstem (when the face is usually also affected) or from an ipsilateral lesion below the pyramidal decussation in the lower medulla or high cervical cord (when the face is spared) (Fig. 15.3).

The clinical features associated with the hemiparesis usually enable a more accurate localization of the site of the pathology. The most common cause of hemiparesis is a stroke involving the contralateral cerebral cortex or internal capsule (see Fig. 15.3).

Tetraparesis – weakness in all four limbs

Pyramidal (UMN) weakness of all four limbs may result from lesions in the brainstem or high cervical cord. When the UMNs are damaged, the condition is called a 'spastic' tetraparesis (or sometimes quadraparesis). Tetraparesis caused by spinal cord pathology is most commonly due to cervical spondylosis, multiple sclerosis and traumatic cord lesions, and less often from neoplasms, arteriovenous malformations (AVMs) or rheumatoid arthritis affecting the atlantoaxial (C1/C2) joint. Cervical spondylotic myelopathy is usually associated with a cervical radiculopathy affecting one or more spinal nerves, usually C6 and/or C7. The patient will therefore have UMN signs in the legs and predominantly LMN signs in the arms, a syndrome referred to as a myeloradiculopathy. Extensive bilateral pathology in the cerebral hemispheres can occasionally cause tetraparesis. Brainstem pathology is usually associated with additional cranial nerve symptoms such as diplopia, facial numbness, vertigo, dysarthria, dysphagia and signs such as ocular, facial or bulbar weakness. The most common brainstem pathologies to cause tetraparesis include stroke, neoplasms and multiple sclerosis.

Weakness of all four limbs may also result from several LMN disorders, e.g. some types of motor neuron disease and polio, motor neuropathies, disorders of the neuromuscular junction (e.g. myasthenia gravis) and muscle disease (e.g. polymyositis). The pattern of weakness and associated signs would be typical of that of lower motor neuron syndromes. Tetraparesis in motor neuron disease is usually due to a combination

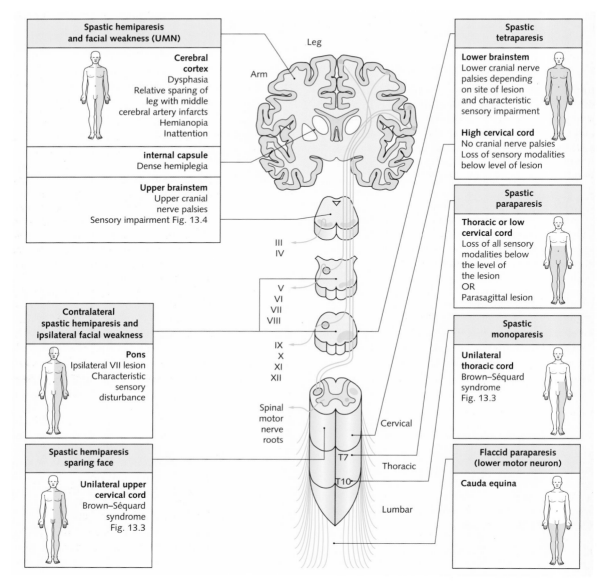

Fig. 15.3 Patterns of motor weakness. Note that these are all upper motor neuron lesions except for pathology in the cauda equina, which damages multiple lumbar and sacral nerve roots.

of UMN (corticospinal pathway) and LMN (anterior horn cell) involvement (see Ch. 24).

Paraparesis – weakness in both legs

Paraparesis is usually due to spinal cord disease and is consequently a UMN syndrome, characterized by spasticity, pyramidal weakness, brisk reflexes and extensor plantar responses in the legs. This syndrome is called 'spastic paraparesis'. The most common causes are multiple sclerosis or extrinsic compression in the cervical region

between C3 and C6, due to cervical spondylosis. This is a degenerative osteoarthritis associated with osteophytes and disc prolapse which causes cord compression. Spastic paraparesis is often encountered in clinical exams as well as in the clinic setting, and a systematic approach to the numerous causes is important (Fig. 15.4).

A much rarer cause of bilateral UMN symptoms and signs in the legs, resembling a spinal cord syndrome, is a cerebral lesion involving both cortical leg areas in the parasagittal region of the brain. A parasagittal meningioma classically causes this syndrome but sagittal sinus thrombosis with subsequent venous infarction and

Fig. 15.4 Causes of spastic paraparesis	
Spinal cord compression	Cervical spondylosis Cervical or thoracic disc herniation Metastatic tumour Primary tumour (e.g. meningioma, neurofibroma) Infective (e.g. epidural abscess, spinal TB) Epidural haematoma
Inflammatory disorders	Multiple sclerosis Idiopathic transverse myelitis Sarcoidosis Infections (e.g. Lyme, zoster, TB, HIV, syphilis, HTLV-1)
Degenerative disorders	Motor neuron disease Syringomyelia
Vascular	Spinal cord infarction Vasculitis, systemic lupus erythematosus (SLE) Spinal arteriovenous malformation
Trauma	Cord contusion, laceration or transection Displaced vertebral fracture or disc Traumatic epidural haematoma
Metabolic/ nutritional	Vitamin B$_{12}$ deficiency (subacute combined degeneration)
Rare hereditary conditions	Friedreich's ataxia Hereditary spastic paraparesis
Parasagittal brain lesions	Meningioma Cerebral venous sinus thrombosis Congenital spastic diplegia (cerebral palsy)

the form of cerebral palsy known as 'congenital spastic diplegia' are other causes.

Paraparesis can also be associated with low tone in the legs when it is called 'flaccid paraparesis'. This usually results from lesions in the cauda equina such as central lumbar disc prolapse or infiltrating neoplasms. A cauda equina syndrome is usually associated with severe and early sphincter dysfunction and sensory impairment over sacral and lower lumbar dermatomes or 'saddle anaesthesia' (see Fig. 15.3). Lower back pain accompanied by pain radiating into one ot both legs may also be present in a cauda equina syndrome. The radicular pain reflects involvement of the dorsal nerve roots. The cauda equina is made up of the spinal nerves that exit at the inferior pole of the spinal cord called the conus medullaris. The conus is a highly compacted region of the spinal cord containing many spinal levels. The clinical signs of a conus lesion are therefore often mixed between UMN and LMN, such as brisk knee jerks and extensor plantar responses, but with flaccid tone and absent ankle jerks. Other causes of a flaccid

paraparesis include a polyradiculopathy or a peripheral neuropathy.

Monoparesis – weakness of a single limb

A stroke in one of the distal branches of the middle cerebral artery (MCA) is the most common cause of an isolated upper limb monoparesis. More usually, the MCA is blocked more proximally and there is weakness in the contralateral upper limb with some UMN facial weakness and relative sparing of the leg. This is in contrast to anterior cerebral artery occlusion, which often spares the face and arm and causes contralateral leg weakness.

Other localized cerebral cortical lesions may cause weakness confined to one contralateral limb. This typically affects the leg and foot and occurs with cortical tumours but occasionally with multiple sclerosis, abscesses and granulomas.

A unilateral thoracic cord lesion may also occasionally present with monoparesis of the leg (see Fig. 15.3). There will usually be reflex and sensory findings of a Brown–Séquard syndrome (see Ch. 23) to clarify the diagnosis. This is usually caused by a demyelinating plaque in multiple sclerosis. Monoparesis is a more typical presentation of lower motor neuron weakness than upper motor neuron weakness.

COMMUNICATION

Upper motor neuron signs are often absent in the earliest stages of a stroke and the patient may have a flaccid hemiparesis. Extensor plantar responses and brisk reflexes often occur within 24–48 hours but spasticity may take weeks to develop. The most important key to the diagnosis is therefore the history of an abrupt onset with possible vascular risk factors.

LOWER MOTOR NEURON WEAKNESS

LMNs extend from the anterior horn cell in the spinal cord to the neuromuscular junction in the muscles. Lesions to the LMNs are characterized by a constellation of typical clinical signs, which vary in their presence and degree by the anatomical site of damage to the LMN in its course from the spinal cord to the muscles. There are typically four different types of LMN lesion (anterior horn cell, spinal nerve, plexus and peripheral nerve – see below). Although the neuromuscular junction and muscle are not strictly a part of the LMN, disorders of these structures are also considered in the differential diagnosis of LMN syndromes because they produce similar signs and symptoms.

LMN syndromes are characterized by the following features.

Decreased tone

Tone is typically reduced, particularly when muscle wasting has occurred.

Focal pattern of weakness and wasting

LMN weakness can occur in individual muscles and in groups of muscles if more than one level of LMN is involved. The denervated muscle becomes atrophied and wasting is evident within days to weeks after the onset. The pattern of weakness and wasting depends on the site of the lesion:

- **Anterior horn cell disease** (see Ch. 24): eventually causes generalized weakness and wasting; however, it can begin distally in either a hand or foot and it may mimic a peripheral nerve lesion, e.g. an ulnar neuropathy, common peroneal nerve palsy (foot drop).
- **Radiculopathies** (see Ch. 25): result in weakness and wasting in the respective myotomes, i.e. the group of muscles innervated by a single spinal nerve root.
- **Plexopathies** (see Ch. 25): cause weakness and wasting in the distribution of more than one spinal nerve root, e.g. C8 and T1 in lesions of the lower cord of the brachial plexus.
- **Peripheral neuropathies** (see Ch. 26):
  - Mononeuropathy: a single peripheral nerve is affected, e.g. ulnar mononeuropathy
  - Multiple mononeuropathies or 'mononeuritis multiplex': many single nerves are involved, e.g. ulnar, radial and common peroneal nerves
  - Polyneuropathy: the longest axons in all the nerves are affected. This typically causes symmetrical distal wasting and weakness affecting the feet, leg and hands, with loss of all tendon reflexes. If there is also sensory involvement, there will be impairment of sensation in a 'glove and sock' distribution affecting the hands and the legs below the knees.
- **Neuromuscular junction disorders**, such as myasthenia gravis: typically cause weakness in muscles of the head and neck as well as proximal upper limbs. The weakness is characteristically fatigable, i.e. worsens quickly with exercise, and there is little or no muscle wasting (see Ch. 27).

- **Myopathies:** usually cause symmetrical wasting and weakness in the proximal limb girdles (shoulders, hips and thighs), although distal muscles can be involved, depending on the cause of the myopathy (see Ch. 28).

Fasciculations

Fasciculations are brief, flickering contractions of individual motor units in a denervated muscle, of which patients are usually not aware. They may be present in weak and wasted muscles but can also occur in muscles that appear unaffected. Fasciculations are particularly prevalent in motor neuron disease and motor neuropathies. Benign fasciculations are common in normal individuals. These are typically infrequent, localized to one muscle at a time, fast, and may be noticed by the individual when associated with triggers such as stimulants, e.g. caffeine.

Pain and sensory disturbance

Sensory changes often occur in lesions of the spinal nerve roots, plexii and peripheral nerves. It should be noted that anterior horn cell disease, diseases of the neuromuscular junction and myopathies do not have objective sensory signs. Pain accompanies the sensory disturbance when the lesion is caused by infiltrating tumour, vasculitis or by some toxins, e.g. alcohol. There are no sensory signs in motor neuron disease, but patients can experience sensory symptoms such as muscle cramps.

Reduced tendon reflexes and flexor plantar responses

Tendon reflexes may be reduced or lost depending on the severity and distribution of the LMN lesion. Abdominal and cremasteric reflexes are unaffected. Plantar responses are flexor unless there is severe loss of sensation or power to the big toe when the reflex may be completely absent.

LOWER MOTOR NEURON SYNDROMES

1. **Anterior horn cells**, e.g. polio, motor neuron disease and syringomyelia
2. **Spinal nerves** or 'nerve roots', e.g. L5 radiculopathy
3. **Plexopathy**, e.g. brachial plexopathy (e.g. brachial neuritis)
4. **Peripheral neuropathy**, e.g. ulnar mononeuropathy or generalized polyneuropathy.

Anterior horn cell disease

There are usually prominent fasciculations, especially in motor neuron disease. Causes:

- Motor neuron disease, e.g. amyotrophic lateral sclerosis
- Infective, e.g. poliomyelitis
- Toxic, e.g. triorthocresyl phosphate
- Local structural pathology, e.g. syringomyelia or intrinsic cord tumours.

Radiculopathy and plexopathy

A knowledge of the myotomes is necessary to differentiate the site of a radiculopathy or plexopathy. A radiculopathy will cause muscle weakness and wasting in the myotome supplied by the affected single nerve root, with loss of the segmental tendon reflex, if there is one, and sensory loss in the corresponding dermatome (see Ch. 16). A polyradiculopathy is rare in isolation and indicates a lesion involving many roots, but can be found in infiltrative processes such as a malignant radiculopathy. It may be differentiated from many peripheral neuropathies as it produces a more proximal weakness. It is often found in Guillain–Barré syndrome, which is also known as acute demyelinating polyradiculoneuropathy (AIDP) because it involves demyelination within multiple roots as well as nerves.

A plexus lesion will cause weakness and wasting in muscles innervated by several of the spinal nerves that form the plexus, as well as loss of corresponding reflexes. There may be accompanying sensory loss over several dermatomes (see Fig. 15.7). Only part of the plexus is usually involved, although characteristic patterns can often be seen.

Brachial plexopathy

The brachial plexus is illustrated in Figure 15.5 and is discussed in detail in Chapter 25. The following are examples of brachial plexus syndromes:

- Neuralgic amyotrophy
- Tumour infiltration
- Radiotherapy-induced plexopathy
- Pancoast tumour
- Thoracic outlet syndrome, e.g. cervical rib
- Erb's palsy (lateral cord: C5, C6)
- Klumpke's palsy (medial cord: C8, T1).

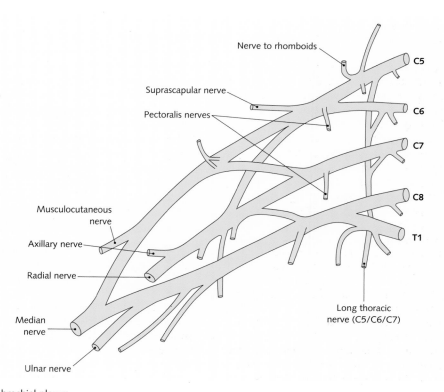

Fig. 15.5   The brachial plexus.

Lumbosacral plexopathy

In general, lesions of the lower plexus cause weakness and wasting of the hamstrings and foot muscles with loss of the ankle jerk and sensory loss on the posterior leg, whereas upper plexus lesions cause failure of hip flexion and adduction with anterior leg sensory loss (Fig. 15.6). Causes:

- Trauma following abdominal or pelvic surgery, e.g. hysterectomy
- Infiltration by neoplasia, e.g. cervical, ovarian and colorectal carcinoma, or granulomatous disease
- Compression from an abdominal aortic aneurysm.

Neuropathy

There are several types of peripheral neuropathy:

- **Mononeuropathy:** disease of a single peripheral nerve, e.g. lesion of the median nerve from compression in the carpal tunnel, lesion of the common peroneal nerve from trauma involving the fibular head.
- **Multiple mononeuropathy** or 'mononeuritis multiplex': this term is used when many single nerves are involved, such as in diabetes, sarcoid, leprosy and vasculitic disease, especially polyarteritis nodosa and neoplasia.
- **Polyneuropathy:** this is the more widespread involvement of the peripheral nerves and typically occurs in a symmetrical distal distribution, starting

in the lower limbs, e.g. diabetic neuropathy, vitamin B_{12} deficiency, drugs such as isoniazid. Other polyneuropathies may exhibit some proximal signs as well as having a distal distribution, e.g. Guillain–Barré syndrome. Patterns of weakness caused by these disorders are shown in Figure 15.7. See also Chapter 26.

DISORDERS OF THE NEUROMUSCULAR JUNCTION

These include myasthenia gravis, Eaton–Lambert syndrome and iatrogenic syndromes.

Myasthenia gravis is the most common disorder of the neuromuscular junction and the extraocular muscles are almost always affected at some point in the disease; they may be the only feature at presentation. There may also be weakness of the bulbar and respiratory muscles as well as proximal muscles, especially in the upper limbs.

The characteristic feature is fatigability of muscle strength, which can often be demonstrated clinically. Wasting is uncommon and rarely severe unless the patient has had prolonged immobilization or malnutrition. Reflexes are usually normal and plantar responses are flexor. There is no sensory involvement or fasciculations. See also Chapter 27.

MYOPATHY

The limb weakness is usually bilateral and proximal in the shoulder and pelvic girdles and patients complain of an inability to stand from sitting, climb stairs, brush their hair or reach for objects above their head. Involvement of the face, neck and trunk occurs in many myopathic disorders. Dysphagia and respiratory muscle weakness might also occur and can be life threatening (e.g. polymyositis). Muscle pain (myalgia) and cramps can occur, especially after exercise. Muscle wasting might be severe and tone is reduced. Reflexes are reduced in advanced myopathy but unaffected in the

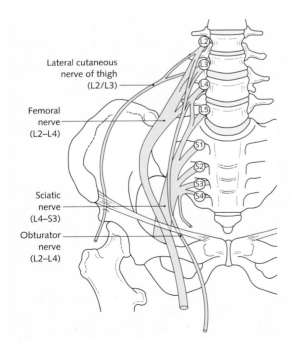

Lateral cutaneous nerve of thigh (L2/L3)

Femoral nerve (L2–L4)

Sciatic nerve (L4–S3)

Obturator nerve (L2–L4)

Fig. 15.6 The lumbosacral plexus.

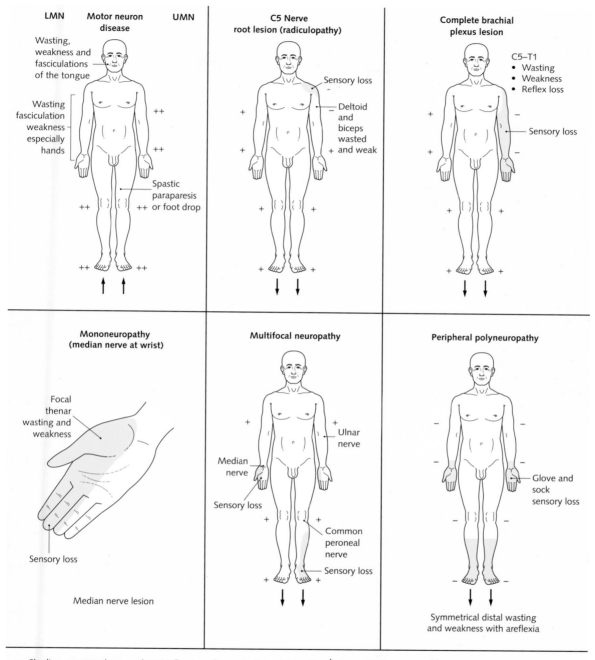

Shading = sensory loss, −, absent reflex; +, reflex present; ++, brisk reflex; ↓, flexor plantar response; ↑, extensor plantar response

Fig. 15.7 Patterns of weakness and sensory loss due to lower motor neuron lesions. The shaded areas indicate sensory loss.

early stages. Plantar responses are flexor if there is enough power in the big toe to elicit the reflex. There is no sensory disturbance.

Dystrophia myotonica is a genetic disorder involving many organs. It is associated with a myopathy and a distinctive failure of relaxation of muscles following contraction or 'myotonia'. The myopathy is not only proximal but also involves the head and neck as well as forearms and legs. Myopathies are discussed in more detail in Chapter 28.

Limb sensory symptoms (16)

● Objectives

- Define the two main neuroanatomical pathways responsible for sensation and the sensory modalities that are transmitted
- Describe how to differentiate between the distribution of sensory symptoms caused by diseases of the peripheral nerves, spinal cord, brainstem and cerebral cortex
- Understand and learn to sketch the clinically important dermatomes (C5, C6, C7, C8, T1 in the arm and L4, L5, S1 in the leg) and the territories of the most commonly affected peripheral nerves (median, ulnar, radial, common peroneal)

Sensory symptoms can arise from lesions at various levels within the central nervous system (cortex, subcortex, thalamus, brainstem, spinal cord) or from lesions of the peripheral sensory pathways (spinal nerve root, plexus, peripheral nerve). The anatomical distribution of sensory disturbance and the finding of other physical signs may help point towards a diagnosis. The knowledge of the anatomy of the main sensory pathways is an essential prerequisite for this diagnostic process.

Nerve endings in skin, joints, ligaments, tendons and muscle contain different receptors adapted to respond to a variety of sensory stimuli. The sensory information gathered by these receptors is carried back to the spinal cord by sensory nerves. There are two main pathways for the appreciation of different modalities of sensation:

1. Dorsal (posterior) column pathway (see Fig. 16.1)
2. Spinothalamic pathway (see Fig. 16.1).

DORSAL (POSTERIOR) COLUMN PATHWAY

The dorsal column pathway carries information concerned with light touch, two-point discrimination, vibration and proprioception. Fibres carrying this information travel from the cutaneous nerves to the dorsal root ganglia, where their cell bodies lie and relay the information via the dorsal nerve roots to enter the spinal cord. These fibres ascend the spinal cord ipsilaterally in the dorsal columns and synapse in the gracile and cuneate nuclei of the lower medulla in the brainstem. They then decussate in the medulla and travel upwards as the medial lemniscus to synapse in the thalamus and then the parietal cortex. A somatotopic order is maintained throughout the pathway from the spinal cord to parietal cortex.

When pathology affects the dorsal column pathway, the patient may complain of numbness, 'pins and needles' or incoordination of the hands or gait due to loss of proprioceptive information.

SPINOTHALAMIC PATHWAY

The spinothalamic pathway carries information about pain and temperature; itch and tickle are also carried by this pathway. The fibres travel within the peripheral nerves to the dorsal root ganglia and dorsal nerve roots (see Fig. 16.1). The fibres ascend or descend for one or two segments before synapsing in the dorsal horn. At this level, they decussate and ascend in the contralateral spinothalamic tract. In the brainstem, the tract becomes the lateral lemniscus and these fibres synapse in the thalamus and ultimately the parietal cortex. A somatotopic order is maintained throughout the central pathway with the sacral fibres being outermost and the cervical fibres innermost.

Clinical manifestations of lesions of this pathway may include pins and needles, pain and impaired pain perception leading to painless burns and excessive wearing of the joints (which may become deformed and then called a 'Charcot joint').

Light touch is mediated by both the spinothalamic tract and dorsal columns.

TROPHIC SKIN CHANGES AND ULCERS

When patients lose the sensory supply to limbs, they are less able to prevent trauma and are less aware of the effect of prolonged pressure to their skin. This may

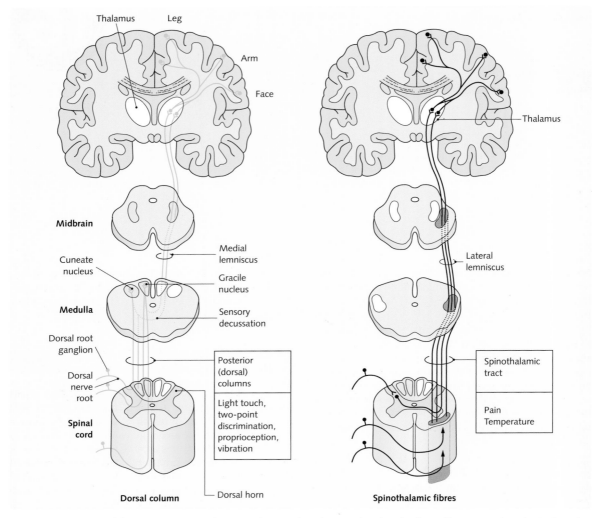

Fig. 16.1 Anatomy of the main sensory pathways in the spinal cord. Note that dorsal column fibres ascend on the ipsilateral side of the spinal cord and decussate in the medulla, whereas spinothalamic fibres cross the central grey matter of the spinal cord (after synapsing in the dorsal horn) and ascend on the opposite side of the cord.

result in ulcers, especially at pressure points, e.g. heels and sacrum. There is also loss of the autonomic supply to piloerector muscles, sweat glands and blood vessels. This can lead to a dry, pale, hairless skin that can become atrophic, swollen and shiny.

SENSORY SYNDROMES

Sensory symptoms may arise from a lesion involving the peripheral nerves, spinal nerves and dorsal roots ganglia, or the central pathways. Lesions of the central pathways can be considered at the level of the spinal cord, brainstem, thalamus and parietal cortex. The

distribution and pattern of sensory loss, together with associated physical signs, usually allows determination of the level of the sensory pathway affected and, therefore, possible differential diagnoses.

Lesions of peripheral nerves

Mononeuropathy

A lesion affecting sensory fibres in a peripheral nerve is accompanied by sensory impairment of all modalities in the corresponding anatomical distribution (Fig. 16.2). If a mixed motor and sensory nerve is involved, there will also be weakness of the muscles

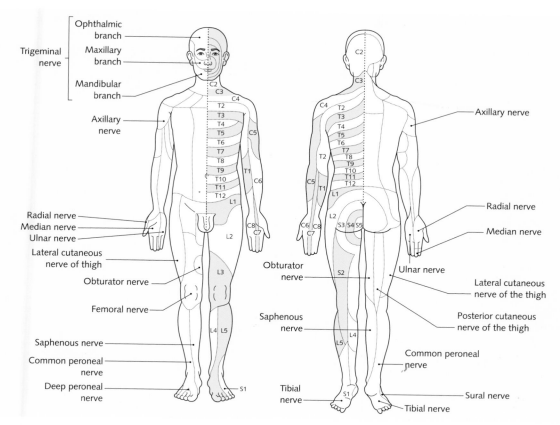

Fig. 16.2   Distribution of sensory dermatomes and the territories of individual peripheral nerves.

supplied by the nerve (see Ch. 26). The most common cause is an entrapment neuropathy, e.g. median nerve at the wrist causing carpal tunnel syndrome.

Multiple mononeuropathy

Mononeuritis multiplex involves a number of individual nerves and occurs in diabetes, sarcoidosis, vasculitis, leprosy, amyloidosis and carcinomatous disease.

Polyneuropathy

Polyneuropathy most commonly results in a symmetrical impairment of all sensory modalities involving the feet and legs first, followed by hands and arms, due to length-related axonal loss; this is characteristically termed a 'glove and sock' sensory loss. The reflexes are diminished or lost and, more rarely, there may be accompanying muscle weakness. Causes of a polyneuropathy include diabetes, chronic alcohol abuse, vitamin B_{12} deficiency, paraproteinaemia and drugs (isoniazid, heavy metals, chemotherapeutic agents). Rarer causes may be inherited (e.g. Charcot–Marie–Tooth disease),

or more asymmetrical (e.g. vasculitis), or demyelinating (e.g. Guillain–Barré syndrome).

Lesions of the spinal nerve roots, dorsal roots and ganglia

Each dorsal nerve root carries sensory fibres of all modalities from an area on the skin called a dermatome (Fig. 16.2). The overlap of input from adjacent roots means that lesions of a single nerve root do not result in complete loss of sensation within the defined dermatome. The corresponding tendon reflexes may be diminished or lost. LMN muscle weakness occurs if the anterior roots are also involved and is especially common in plexus lesions.

Reactivation of the herpes zoster virus (shingles) and prolapsed intervertebral discs can cause damage to the spinal nerves and dorsal roots.

Lesions of the spinal cord

Sensory disturbances arising from lesions of the spinal cord are illustrated in Figure 16.3.

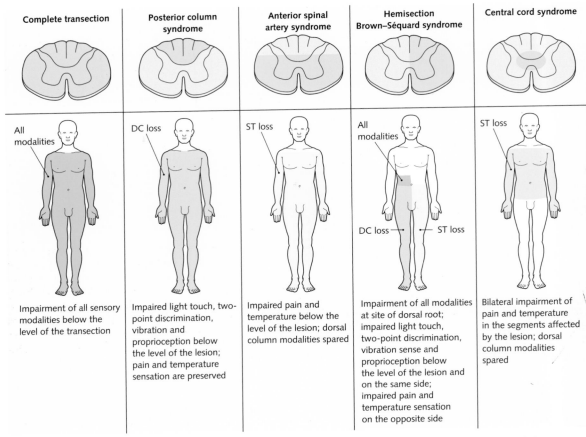

Fig. 16.3 Distribution of sensory disturbance caused by lesions of the spinal cord. DC, dorsal column; ST, spinothalamic.

Transection of the cord

Transection of the cord causes bilateral impairment of all sensory modalities below the level of transection (as defined by the dermatomal pattern in Fig. 16.2). There is initially a flaccid and, eventually, a spastic paraplegia (thoracic and lumbar cord) or tetraplegia (cervical cord). Traumatic transection is the most common cause, e.g. road traffic accident.

Lesion of the posterior spinal cord

A lesion of the posterior spinal cord affects the dorsal columns, with sparing of the spinothalamic and corticospinal fibres. There is impaired light touch, two-point discrimination, vibration and proprioception below the level of the lesion. Motor function and perception of pain and temperature are spared unless the lesion progresses to involve the anterior part of the cord. Isolated loss of dorsal column function is rare but can occur in multiple sclerosis, spondylosis or prolapsed intervertebral discs, and vitamin B_{12} deficiency.

Lesion of the anterior cord

A lesion of the anterior cord affects the spinothalamic and corticospinal tracts, with sparing of the dorsal columns. There is bilateral impairment of pain and temperature perception and a spastic paraplegia or tetraplegia below the level of the lesion. Anterior spinal artery occlusion is the commonest cause of this syndrome.

Hemisection of the cord (Brown–Séquard syndrome)

Hemisection of the cord causes impairment of light touch, two-point discrimination, vibration and proprioception below the level of the lesion on the same side (dorsal column); and impaired perception of pain and temperature on the opposite side (spinothalamic). Involvement of one or more nerve roots at the site of the lesion will result in impairment of all sensory modalities on that side within the distribution of the dermatomes affected. Upper motor neuron

(UMN) weakness is present on the side of the lesion, due to the disruption of the corticospinal tracts prior to their decussation. Demyelination due to multiple sclerosis and asymmetrical central disc prolapse are the most common causes.

Central cord lesion

A central cord lesion affects the spinothalamic fibres and spares the dorsal columns. There is bilateral loss of pain and temperature perception in the segments affected by the lesion. Only the crossing fibres are involved so that a 'cape-like' distribution of sensory loss occurs, e.g. a syrinx within the cervical cord. More commonly, a 'belt-like' loss of sensation can occur and is often due to a multiple sclerosis plaque in the thoracic cord. The loss of spinothalamic sensation with preservation of dorsal column function is called a 'dissociated' sensory loss. Wasting and weakness and loss of reflexes may occur from involvement of anterior horn cells and fibres subserving the reflex arc within the cord at the level of the lesion. If the lesion expands sufficiently it may eventually involve the corticospinal tracts and cause UMN signs below the lesion.

HINTS AND TIPS

A dissociated pattern of sensory loss comprises loss of pain and temperature sensation (spinothalamic) with preservation of light touch, two-point discrimination, vibration and proprioception (dorsal columns). It can occur in:
- Central cord lesions
- Hemisection of the cord
- Lateral medullary lesions
- B12 deficiency
- Anterior cord syndrome.

Lesions of the brainstem

- Lower medulla: a unilateral lesion of the lower medulla (Fig. 16.4) causes impairment of pain and temperature perception of the face on the side of the lesion, and on the opposite side of the body (Harlequin syndrome). Light touch, two-point discrimination, vibration and proprioception could be impaired on the side of the lesion, but this is usually spared in a lateral medullary infarction. This

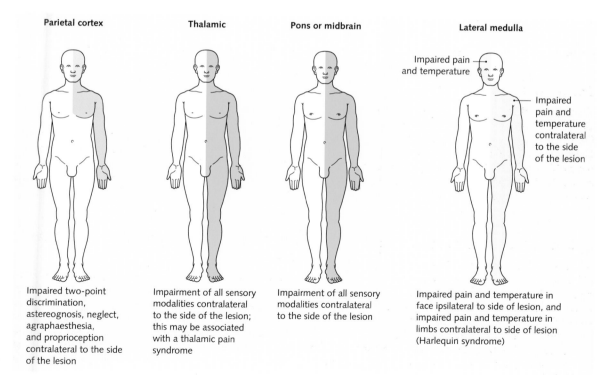

Parietal cortex — Impaired two-point discrimination, astereognosis, neglect, agraphaesthesia, and proprioception contralateral to the side of the lesion

Thalamic — Impairment of all sensory modalities contralateral to the side of the lesion; this may be associated with a thalamic pain syndrome

Pons or midbrain — Impairment of all sensory modalities contralateral to the side of the lesion

Lateral medulla — Impaired pain and temperature. Impaired pain and temperature contralateral to the side of the lesion. Impaired pain and temperature in face ipsilateral to side of lesion, and impaired pain and temperature in limbs contralateral to side of lesion (Harlequin syndrome)

Fig. 16.4 Distribution of sensory disturbance caused by cerebral and brainstem lesions.

lesion involves the ipsilateral spinal trigeminal nucleus and tract and the spinothalamic tract subserving contralateral sensation.

- Pons and midbrain: a unilateral lesion of the pons or midbrain causes impairment of all sensory modalities on the opposite side of the body, including the face, because all the sensory tracts have already crossed, including the spinal nucleus and tract of the trigeminal nerve.

The brainstem syndromes discussed above can be accompanied by cranial nerve palsies and cerebellar signs ipsilateral to the lesion, and by contralateral hemiparesis. In practice, brainstem lesions are often bilateral and, therefore, affect sensation in the face and all four limbs. In younger patients multiple sclerosis is the most common cause of a brainstem pattern of sensory loss, while in older patients stroke and tumours are common causes.

Lesions of the thalamus

A thalamic lesion (see Fig. 16.4) causes impairment of all sensory modalities on the opposite side of the body, including the face. There may be spontaneous pain and dysaesthesia on the affected side – the 'thalamic pain syndrome'. The most common causes of a thalamic pattern of sensory loss are stroke, tumours, multiple sclerosis and trauma.

Lesions of the parietal lobe

A parietal lobe lesion (see Fig. 16.4) causes:

- loss of discriminative sensory function of the opposite side of the face and limbs. There is impaired two-point discrimination, lack of recognition of objects by touch (astereognosis) or figures drawn on the hand (agraphaesthesia), and loss of perception of limb position. However, the primary modalities of pain, temperature, touch and vibration are relatively preserved.
- sensory inattention: this is usually caused by lesions of the non-dominant parietal cortex. The patient fails to perceive stimuli on the opposite side of the body when the stimulus is applied bilaterally. However, when applied on the affected side only, the same stimulus is perceived normally. This inattentive defect or 'neglect' may also apply when testing the visual fields, the phenomenon of visual inattention.

COMMUNICATION

Testing sensation can be difficult. However, sensation is typically tested at the end of a neurological examination, by which point an examiner should have an idea of whether any sensory loss is likely to be present and, if so, the type and distribution of sensory loss.

Disorders of gait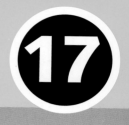

Objectives

- How to examine and define the common abnormalities of gait
- Describe the main causes of gait disorders

A patient's gait is a coordinated action requiring integration of motor and sensory functions. It therefore often provides clues to a patient's underlying diagnosis, and is a critical part of any neurological examination. The most common gaits are:

- cerebellar ataxia
- spastic paraparesis
- hemiparetic
- parkinsonian
- sensory ataxia
- steppage
- myopathic
- apraxic
- antalgic (painful)
- functional (non-organic).

PRACTICAL APPROACH TO THE ASSESSMENT OF GAIT

Always ensure the patient is safe to walk unaided prior to assessment. Watch the patient walk away from and back towards you along a stretch of corridor if possible. Analyse the gait in a systematic fashion, starting with an overall impression and then carefully assessing the gait from the feet upwards. Observe the upper and lower half of the patient's body, respectively, from the front and back as they walk, and watch how the patient turns:

- Does the patient walk with an aid – stick, crutches, rollator?
- Does the patient walk in a straight line? Patients who have impairment of cerebellar or vestibular function, or of postural sensation (sensory ataxia), are unsteady and may be unable to tandem walk, i.e. 'heel-to-toe' walking. Patients who have apraxic gaits appear as if they have forgotten how to walk and may often appear rooted to the spot.
- Look at the size of the paces the patient uses – if small, this is typically seen in extrapyramidal syndromes or an apraxic gait.

- Look at the lateral distance between the feet. They may be widely separated in a broad-based gait, which is present in cerebellar or sensory ataxia or apraxic gaits. In a scissoring gait of a severe spastic paraparesis, the lateral distance is reduced and the legs may cross over with toe dragging.
- Look at the knees – in a high-stepping gait they are lifted off the floor more than normal due to foot drop.
- Look at the pelvis and shoulders. In a waddling gait of proximal myopathies, there is marked rotation of both.
- Does the patient have normal arm swing? Arm swing may be reduced in patients who have an extrapyramidal syndrome. This is often more marked on one side than the other, especially in idiopathic Parkinson's disease.
- How well does the patient turn around? Patients who have a extrapyrimidal syndrome or ataxia perform this with difficulty. Patients with idiopathic Parkinson's disease turn in a series of movements or 'en bloc'.
- Ask the patient to walk on the toes (S1) and then heels (L5). Patients with a common peroneal nerve palsy and L5 or S1 radiculopathy will find this difficult.
- Perform Romberg's test. Ask the patient to stand with feet together and eyes closed. The test is positive if the patient is more unsteady with eyes closed than with eyes open. This occurs in patients with a sensory ataxia who have impaired proprioception or, more rarely, vestibular dysfunction.

HINTS AND TIPS

Romberg's is a test of impaired proprioception, and is not a test of cerebellar dysfunction. In addition, it cannot be tested reliably in patients with a cerebellar or vestibular disorder, or moderate-to-severe weakness from any cause, as the patient will be unsteady irrespective of whether there is a sensory ataxia.

Gait of cerebellar ataxia

Patients with cerebellar ataxia stand and walk unsteadily, as if they are drunk. They soon begin to compensate for this by adopting a broad base with feet further apart. The gait is unsteady, with irregularity of stride. The trunk sways and the patient may veer towards one side. In mild cases, the only manifestation of gait disturbance may be difficulty walking heel-toe in a straight line (i.e. tandem walking).

On neurological examination there may also be nystagmus, dysarthria and cerebellar signs in the limbs. Ataxia may be absent in the limbs and apparent only in the gait when the lesion is in the midline (cerebellar vermis.), so-called 'truncal ataxia'.

Causes include:

- multiple sclerosis
- vascular disease, e.g. ischaemic, haemorrhagic, AVMs
- alcoholic cerebellar degeneration
- anticonvulsant therapy, e.g. phenytoin, carbamazepine
- posterior fossa tumours
- cerebellar paraneoplastic syndrome
- hereditary cerebellar ataxias.

Hemiparetic gait

Patients with a hemiparetic gait have a characteristic posture on one side, of flexion and internal rotation of the upper limb and extension of the lower limb. The leg moves stiffly and is swung around in a semicircle to avoid scraping the foot across the floor. However, such scraping does occur to some extent and the toe and outer sole of the shoe become worn.

Causes include:

- cortical or internal capsular strokes
- cerebral hemispheric tumour
- traumatic lesions.

Spastic gait

A spastic gait is seen in patients who have a spastic paraparesis. The legs move slowly and stiffly and the thighs are strongly adducted such that in severe cases the legs may even cross as the patient walks ('scissor gait'). The feet may be plantar flexed and inverted, and the toes may scuff the ground.

Causes include:

- spinal cord compression
- trauma/spinal surgery

- birth injuries or congenital deformities: cerebral palsy
- multiple sclerosis
- motor neuron disease
- parasagittal meningioma
- subacute combined degeneration of the cord.

Parkinsonian gait

The patient often has a stooped and flexed posture with loss of arm swing, which is almost always more marked on one side in idiopathic Parkinson's disease. The steps are short and the patient shuffles. There may be difficulty starting and stopping. Turning may occur as multiple small steps or 'en bloc' (i.e. not smoothly but in stiff, stuttering movements). Having started to walk, the patient leans forward and the pace quickens, as though the patient is attempting to catch up on himself (festinant gait).

Gait of sensory ataxia

Sensory ataxia arises from impaired proprioception caused by a lesion of the peripheral nerves, posterior roots, dorsal columns in the spinal cord or, rarely, the ascending afferent fibres to the parietal lobes. The gait is unsteady and wide-based, and often 'stamping'. Romberg's test is positive and there is impaired perception of joint position on examination of the lower limbs.

Causes include:

- posterior spinal cord lesions:
  - multiple sclerosis
  - cervical spondylosis
  - tumours
  - vitamin B_{12} deficiency
  - tabes dorsalis (tertiary syphilis).
- sensory peripheral neuropathies:
  - hereditary: Charcot–Marie–Tooth disease
  - metabolic: diabetes
  - inflammatory: Guillain–Barré syndrome
  - malignancy: myeloma, paraneoplastic syndrome
  - toxic: alcohol, drugs (e.g. isoniazid).

Steppage gait

Steppage gait arises from weakness of the pretibial and peroneal muscles of lower motor neuron type. The patient has foot drop and is unable to dorsiflex and evert the foot. The leg is lifted high on walking so that the toes clear the ground, and there is, therefore, exaggerated hip flexion. On striking the floor again, there is a slapping noise. Shoe soles are worn on the anterior and lateral aspects.

Causes include:

- Charcot–Marie–Tooth disease (bilateral foot drop)
- Common peroneal nerve palsy, e.g. from a fibular fracture (unilateral foot drop)
- Anterior horn cell disease, e.g. polio, motor neuron disease (often asymmetrical foot drop).

Myopathic gait

The myopathic gait is often called a 'waddling gait' and is caused by weakness of the proximal muscles of the lower limb girdle. The weight is alternately placed on each leg, with the opposite hip and side of the trunk tilting up towards the weight-bearing side. However, the weak gluteal muscles cannot stabilize the weight-bearing hip, which sways outward, with the opposite pelvis and trunk dropping. The patient will shift their weight over the weight-bearing leg so that the shoulders will drop on the side opposite to the hip drop.

Causes include:

- muscular dystrophies: Duchenne's, Becker's, limb-girdle, facio-scapulo-humeral
- metabolic myopathies: periodic paralysis, hypo- and hyperkalaemia, hypo- and hypercalcaemia
- endocrine myopathies: Cushing's disease, Addison's disease, hypo- and hyperthyroidism
- inflammatory myopathies: polymyositis and dermatomyositis.

Apraxic gait

Disease of the frontal lobes gives rise to an apraxic gait. The patient walks with feet placed apart and with small, hesitant steps, which may be described as 'walking on ice' or *marche au petit pas*. There is difficulty with initiation of walking and, in advanced cases, it may seem as though the patient's feet are stuck to the floor. There are no abnormalities of power, sensation or coordination. There may be other signs of frontal cortical dysfunction (e.g. a grasp or rooting reflex); the tendon reflexes may be brisk and the plantar responses extensor.

Causes include:

- subcortical ischaemic leucoencephalopathy 'small vessel disease'
- hydrocephalus including normal pressure hydrocephalus

- frontal lobe tumours, e.g. meningioma
- frontal subdural haematomas (bilateral)
- frontal contusions post-head injury.

Antalgic gait

The antalgic gait arises from pain (e.g. a painful hip or knee due to arthritis). The patient tends to bear weight mainly on the unaffected side, only briefly putting weight onto the affected side.

Functional gait

A 'functional', 'hysterical' or 'non-organic' gait arises from psychological or behavioural disturbance. It does not conform to any of the descriptions given above. It can take a number of forms and is variable in character. There are no objective abnormal neurological signs on formal examination. There are often other positive features of an underlying psychiatric disturbance. However, the only manifestation of a midline cerebellar lesion may be severe ataxia of gait, with normal limb signs on formal examination and this can sometimes be mistaken for a non-organic illness.

HINTS AND TIPS

The character of a patient's gait will provide clues to the clinical signs that might be expected on further neurological examination. The abnormal types of gait are summarized below:

- Ataxic: broad-based and unsteady
- Hemiplegic: unilateral flexed posture of the upper limb and extended posture of the lower limb
- Spastic paraparesis: stiff, slow movements of the legs; 'scissoring' posture of the legs if severe
- Parkinsonian: flexed posture, shuffling small stepped gait with loss of arm swing
- Sensory ataxia: high stepped 'stamping' gait
- Steppage: foot drop
- Myopathic: 'waddling' gait
- Apraxic: hesitant 'walking on ice' gait
- Non-organic: bizarre and variable.

PART III
DISEASES
AND DISORDERS

18. Dementia 125

19. Epilepsy 131

20. Headache and craniofacial pains 139

21. Parkinson's disease and other extrapyramidal disorders 145

22. Cranial nerve lesions 153

23. Diseases affecting the spinal cord (myelopathy) 159

24. Motor neuron disease 169

25. Radiculopathy and plexopathy 173

26. Disorders of the peripheral nerves 177

27. Disorders of the neuromuscular junction 189

28. Disorders of skeletal muscle 193

29. Vascular diseases of the nervous system 201

30. Neuro-oncology 215

31. Infections of the nervous system 223

32. Multiple sclerosis 237

33. Systemic disease and the nervous system 243

34. The effects of vitamin deficiencies and toxins on the nervous
    system 247

35. Hereditary conditions affecting the nervous system 251

- Define the term 'dementia'
- Describe different causes of dementia
- Describe the features in the history and examination that enable the differentiation of dementias
- Understand the investigations required in patients with dementia
- Describe the main primary neurodegenerative dementias – how would you differentiate these?

DEFINITION

Dementia is a syndrome and not a single disease entity. It refers to progressive impairment of higher cortical functions, including memory, orientation, comprehension, calculation, learning capacity, language and judgement. The dominant symptoms depend on the brain region most affected by disease. Often it is accompanied, or preceded by, deterioration in emotional control, social behaviour or motivation. In the initial stages, there are often focal cortical deficits, and as it progresses it is eventually associated with diffuse involvement of both cerebral hemispheres. The patient is often alert in the early and middle stages of the disease. This is in contrast to delirium (acute confusional state), in which alteration of level of consciousness is a defining feature. There are many causes of dementia, but the most common are degenerative.

DIFFERENTIAL DIAGNOSES

- Primary neurodegenerative diseases, e.g. Alzheimer's disease, dementia with Lewy bodies, Parkinson's disease dementia, frontotemporal lobar degeneration (including Pick's disease), Huntington's disease
- Vascular, e.g. small vessel disease, multiple cortical infarcts
- Metabolic/storage disorders, e.g. hypothyroidism, vitamin B_{12} and folate deficiency, mitochondrial cytopathies, Wilson's disease and leucodystrophies
- Infections, e.g. HIV, prion disease, syphilis, progressive multifocal leucoencephalopathy (PML), subacute sclerosing panencephalitis (SSPE)
- Inflammatory disorders, e.g. CNS vasculitis, neurosarcoidosis, Behçet's, multiple sclerosis
- Neoplastic/paraneoplastic, e.g. tumour (primary or secondary), limbic encephalitis

- Normal pressure hydrocephalus
- Epilepsy, e.g. non-convulsive status epilepticus
- Head injury, e.g. chronic subdural haematoma
- Repeated exposure to toxins, e.g. alcohol, heavy metal poisoning, organic solvents
- Depression: pseudodementia – patients who are depressed may appear demented.

EPIDEMIOLOGY

The most common causes of dementia are Alzheimer's disease and vascular dementia, and these are predominantly diseases of the elderly.

The prevalence of dementia in persons aged between 50 and 70 years is about 1% and in those approaching 90 years it reaches 50%. The annual incidence rate is 190/100 000 and, with an increasing ageing population, it is expected to rise even further.

GENERAL CLINICAL FEATURES

In the assessment of a patient with dementia, several key factors should be addressed in order to aid diagnosis. Firstly, dementia must be distinguished from acute confusional states (delirium) and psychiatric disorders (Fig. 18.1). The earliest symptoms and length of the history, along with the tempo of the disease should be elicited. Is the tempo fluctuant, gradually or rapidly progressive, or a stepwise deterioration. Finally, the impact on the social and occupational functioning should be explored. In the examination, one should try to distinguish the pattern of cognitive impairment and look for any other abnormalities apart from dementia.

Fig. 18.1 Differentiating dementia from delirium and depression as causes of cognitive impairment

	Dementia	Delirium	Depression
Conscious state	Alert	Impaired	Alert
Onset	Insidious/gradual	Abrupt	Variable
Course tempo	Gradually progressive	Fluctuant – may be circadian disruption	Fluctuant
Orientation	Initially preserved	Early prominent disorientation	Variable
Hallucinations	Late feature	Prominent	Rare (auditory typically)
Behaviour	Depends on cause	Restless	Withdrawn

HISTORY

It is essential to obtain a history from a relative or friend, as well as from the patient, to gauge the following:

- Rate of intellectual decline
- Activities of daily living and social interaction
- Nutritional status
- Medication history
- Alcohol and smoking history
- General health and relevant disorders, e.g. stroke, head injury
- Family history of dementia, or other neurological/psychiatric disorders.

The rate of progression of dementia depends on the underlying cause:

- Alzheimer's disease: slowly progressive over years
- Vascular dementia: repeated large vessel occlusion causes stepwise deterioration, whereas small vessel disease causes a progressive decline without steps. Both often coexist
- Prion disease or a CNS vasculitis: progressive over months
- Encephalitis: over days to weeks
- It should be noted that all dementias tend to be accelerated by a change in environment, intercurrent infection or surgical procedures.

The earliest symptoms described tend to correlate with the area of the brain first affected. As disease spreads through the brain, other symptoms develop. Therefore, in Alzheimer's disease, recent memory impairment is the most common initial complaint and reflects early degeneration of the hippocampal areas. In frontotemporal dementia, changes in personality can often be reported, reflecting early involvement of frontal structures.

EXAMINATION

A careful neurological examination may reveal clues as to the aetiology, and should specifically look for evidence of:

- focal signs
- involuntary movements
- pseudobulbar signs
- primitive reflexes, e.g. pout, grasp and rooting reflexes
- gait disorder.

Formal assessment by a clinical psychologist is advisable, but a bedside 'mini-mental' test may allow initial assessment of the pattern of cognitive impairment. These tests are designed to test memory, abstract thought, judgement and specific higher cortical functions, and should include questions similar to those listed in Chapter 2.

COMMUNICATION

It is vital to take a history from a relative or friend who knows the patient well. Patients with dementia, especially with frontal lobe disease, are often completely unaware of any problem. The relative should ideally be interviewed separately from the patient, as personality change, especially when related to disinhibiton, can be difficult for the relative to talk about in front of the patient.

INVESTIGATIONS

It is important to carry out a number of investigations to exclude potentially treatable causes of dementia.

Blood tests

Routine blood tests may be necessary to exclude:

- hypothyroidism
- vitamin B_{12} and folate deficiency
- syphilis.

Specific blood tests should be performed to screen for rarer causes of dementia:

- metabolic disorders, e.g. Wilson's disease, leucodystrophies
- HIV: 'AIDS dementia'
- vasculitis and inflammatory diseases
- limbic encephalitis.

Imaging of the brain

Imaging of the brain is obligatory in a patient with dementia and can be performed using computed tomography (CT), and preferably magnetic resonance imaging (MRI). The primary goal is to exclude:

- space-occupying lesions: especially chronic subdural haematoma in the elderly following a fall
- normal-pressure hydrocephalus: dilated ventricles without cortical atrophy. This presents with cognitive decline, urinary incontinence and gait apraxia. The diagnosis is supported by a lumbar puncture removing of up to 50 mL of CSF, which should result in improvement in the clinical features. It can be treated by ventriculoperitoneal shunting.

Typically, variable degrees of cerebral atrophy with enlarged ventricles are seen with most forms of dementia. However, MRI can also be used to allow assessment of signal change and patterns of atrophy consistent with specific forms of dementia. For example increased T2 signal in the thalami is characteristic of variant Creutzfeldt–Jakob disease (CJD). Bilateral hippocampal and temporal lobe atrophy is seen in Alzheimer's disease and asymmetrical anterior hippocampal, amygdala and temporal lobe atrophy is seen in frontotemporal lobar degeneration (FTLD). In cerebrovascular disease imaging can demonstrate multiple infarcts or significant small vessel disease.

Lumbar puncture

NICE guidelines recommend the use of cerebrospinal fluid (CSF) examination in those patients under 65 years, in order to exclude potentially treatable causes of dementia. For example, a lymphocytic CSF may point to an infective, or an inflammatory disorder. The presence of oligoclonal bands may suggest an immune process (e.g. limbic encephalitis). The CSF levels of tau (increased) and a beta 42 (decreased) can sometimes help with the diagnosis of Alzheimer's disease, but tend to be measured only in specialist centres. Similarly, elevated S100 and protein 14-3-3 are supportive of a diagnosis of CJD.

Neuropsychometry

Neuropsychologists test the different domains of cognitive function in considerable detail. Formal neuropsychometry is especially useful when performed at intervals. This enables comparison of intellectual function within a patient over time. It can be a reliable indicator of either progression in disease (suggesting an organic dementia) compared to improvement or plateau in decline of intellectual function which can be seen in patients with treated depression or functional memory loss.

Electroencephalography

Electroencephalography (EEG) traces rarely demonstrate specific changes in dementia. The most common finding is widespread delta waves. These changes can be seen earlier in Alzheimer's disease than in FTLD. There is often a loss of the responsive alpha rhythm in Alzheimer's disease which is often preserved in FTLD. Periodic complexes on the EEG tracing may indicate prion disease such as CJD. This group of disorders is associated with a rapidly progressive course, which is usually an important diagnostic feature.

Genetic testing

The following genetic mutations can be associated with dementia:

- Huntington mutation: Huntington's chorea
- Alzheimer's disease: amyloid precursor protein (APP), presenilin 1 and 2, and apoliprotein E4 mutations
- familial Creutzfeldt–Jakob disease: prion protein gene mutation
- FTLD: tau, progranulin and C9orf72 mutations.

Brain biopsy

Brain biopsy is rarely performed but may be indicated when a disease is rapidly progressive or a treatable cause of dementia is suspected and other investigations fail to reach a diagnosis (e.g. cerebral vasculitis).

MANAGEMENT

Treatable causes of dementia should be addressed. Some of these are potentially reversible or their clinical course can be stabilized (e.g. vasculitis, hydrocephalus and depressive pseudodementia).

In other cases such as Alzheimer's disease, depression and any underlying systemic disorders should be treated to maximize cognitive function. The use of centrally acting cholinergic drugs for primary neurodegenerative dementias is discussed below.

Neuroleptic medication may be required for behavioural disturbance but can exacerbate extrapyramidal features, such as slowing of movements, but the risk of this is diminished by using atypical neuroleptics.

Management of most cases of dementia requires careful advice and counselling of the patient and family, and shared care involving the family, carers, hospital specialists, GP and community psychiatric services. Long-term residential care is often required.

PRIMARY NEURODEGENERATIVE DEMENTIAS

Alzheimer's disease

Alzheimer's disease is the most common cause of dementia in the developed world. There are approximately 500 000 cases in the UK at any one time. It is rarely seen in persons under the age of 45 years, except in familial cases, and the incidence increases dramatically with age, especially in patients over 70 years.

Familial Alzheimer's disease is rare. Mutations in the amyloid precursor protein (APP) gene on chromosome 21, presenilin 1 and 2 genes is associated with young-onset AD. There is also an association of late-onset disease with the apolipoprotein E4 genotype. Individuals with Down syndrome develop the full neuropathological and clinical changes of Alzheimer's disease by their fourth to fifth decade of life, probably as a consequence of the excessive APP produced by a 50% increase in gene dosage due to the extra chromosome 21.

Pathology

Alzheimer's disease is identified by the presence of extracellular amyloid plaques and intracellular neurofibrillary tangles in the brain. The plaques consist of dystrophic neurites clustered round a core of β-amyloid protein, which is derived from the larger precursor protein, APP. Amyloid can also be deposited in cerebral blood vessels, leading to amyloid angiopathy.

Neurofibrillary tangles are derived from the micro-tubule-associated protein tau, which is in an abnormally hyperphosphorylated state and causes protein aggregation. The majority of the pathology affects the hippocampus, temporal and parietal lobes. Typically, the primary motor and sensory cortex are spared.

Clinical features

Alzheimer's disease presents with features of progressive episodic (knowledge of events) memory loss and evolves over many years. Patients may become repetitive in their questioning, forget to pass on messages and misplace items around the house. Dysphasia, apraxia, visuo-spatial deficits and topographical disorientation are also common early features reflecting involvement of the parietal lobes. Patients may fail to recognize previously familiar environments and faces. They may have difficulty with naming, and using common household objects or dressing. There my be problems in executive function such as planning, decision making and sequencing. Seizures and myoclonus are relatively common in late disease. Agitation and delusions (often paranoid in ideation) can also occur late in disease. Pyramidal and extrapyramidal features rarely occur.

There are several rarer, atypical presentations of Alzheimer's disease. These include: posterior cortical atrophy, where visuospatial problems predominate; language-dominant presentations; and frontal variants, where behavioural problems are seen early.

Diagnosis

A definite diagnosis of Alzheimer's disease can be made only from pathological findings. In practice, a typical history with progressive episodic memory loss and negative routine tests will allow a diagnosis of probable Alzheimer's disease.

CT scans show non-specific generalized cerebral atrophy with a compensatory enlargement of ventricles due to loss of brain tissue rather than hydrocephalus. The temporal lobes may be more severely atrophic. Serial volumetric analysis of the temporal lobes and hippocampi using MRI may show atrophy of these areas and may enable a more specific diagnosis.

Drug treatment

The acetylcholinesterase inhibitor tacrine is licensed in the USA and France, and donepezil, galantamine and rivastigmine have been licensed in the UK. In general, these arrest symptoms by approximately 6 months, but do not alter the course of the neurodegenerative process. NICE recommend their use in patients with mild-to-moderate disease, and they need to be monitored carefully for cholinergic side-effects (e.g. bowel disturbance).

Memantine has also been demonstrated to improve symptoms in advanced disease and may have an additional benefit in combination with anticholinesterase inhibitors. NICE recommends its use in patients with moderate disease who are intolerant of acetylcholinesterase inhibitors, or in patients with severe disease.

Prognosis

In spite of recent advances in our understanding and treatment, the prognosis of Alzheimer's disease is very poor, with relentless progression to death, which is often due to bronchopneumonia. The mean survival is 8 years from the onset of the disease.

Dementia with Lewy bodies

Dementia with Lewy bodies (DLB) has only been recognized as a separate clinical entity within the past 15 years. It is associated with prominent early visual hallucinations, memory disturbance and fluctuations in the clinical course even from day to day. The visual hallucinations often do not upset patients (compared with drug-induced visual hallucinations in idiopathic Parkinson's disease), and need to be directly asked about as patients may not volunteer information about them. The extrapyramidal features in DLB are similar to those in idiopathic Parkinson's disease, except the characteristic resting tremor may be absent, there is a poor response to L-dopa therapy and the clinical signs are often symmetrical. In contrast to dementia seen in the later stages of idiopathic Parkinson's disease, the dementia often predates the onset of parkinsonism in DLB. Together, DLB and Parkinson's disease dementia make up the third most common cause of dementia in later life. The neuropathology is a mixture of that seen in Parkinson's disease with Lewy bodies (eosinophilic intraneuronal inclusions containing alphasynuclein, aggregated with abnormally phosphorylated neurofilaments and ubiquitin) in the substantia nigra, but also in the cerebral cortex, as well as Alzheimer's disease type pathology such as amyloid plaques and neurofibrillary tangles. The patients often develop prominent psychiatric side-effects with dopamine agonists, such as confusion and hallucinations. Patients are also very sensitive to neuroleptics, developing profound rigidity and akinesia. Clinical trials have shown that acetylcholinesterase inhibitors can produce significant improvement in the symptoms of DLB, including non-cognitive symptoms for which NICE recommends their use.

Frontotemporal lobar dementia

Frontotemporal lobar dementia (FTLD) is a relatively rare cause of dementia, accounting for 20% of young-onset dementia, and 5–10% dementia overall. It is accompanied by marked cerebral atrophy in the frontal and anterior temporal lobes with relative sparing of the parietal lobes in contrast to Alzheimer's disease. The neuropathology of FTLD is heterogeneous. Some cases demonstrate argyrophilic inclusions (i.e. pieces of protein that stain with silver), which are called Pick bodies. They are found within the neuronal cytoplasm and contain the protein tau. Some cases have inclusions which contain tau but are not Pick bodies and other cases contain inclusions which are ubiquitin positive and tau negative.

The disease is more common in women: and up to 50% are genetic (see above). It tends to occur between the ages of 50 and 65 years, which is younger than sporadic Alzheimer's disease.

FTLD can manifest as one of three syndromes. The behavioural variant FTLD presents with prominent frontal features, with behavioural and psychiatric features at presentation, and is frequently misdiagnosed. The remaining two presentations (semantic dementia and progressive non-fluent aphasia) of FTLD are language-dominant disorders, and together are known as primary progressive aphasia. A rare subgroup of patients develop additional signs of weakness and wasting in bulbar and/or limb muscles in a pattern similar to that of amyotrophic lateral sclerosis (ALS). These cases have ubiquitin-positive pathology and are termed FTD-MND (frontotemporal dementia associated with MND). The EEG is usually normal in the early stages of FTLD, and CT or MRI scans show prominent frontotemporal atrophy.

No specific treatment has been found, and the disease progresses to death over 6–12 years.

FTLD is one of several neurodegenerative diseases associated with accumulation of tau. Other examples include corticobasal degeneration and progressive supranuclear palsy. These diseases are collectively known as the 'tauopathies'.

Vascular dementia

Cerebrovascular disease is a major cause of cognitive impairment in isolation or in combination with Alzheimer's disease. It is the second most common cause of dementia. Histopathologically, a spectrum of changes can be apparent; from large vessel atheromatous change to prominent small vessel disease and ischaemic changes including lacunar and micro-infarcts, leukoariosis, gliosis and demyelination.

Patients present in a variety of ways. The classical description is of 'multi-infarct dementia', which describes a stepwise deterioration due to recurrent strokes. A frontosubcortical pattern of presentation is common, reflecting the vulnerability of these structures to vascular damage. Patients present with executive and attentional impairment, behavioural change and cognitive slowing, with relative sparing of memory. Strategically localized single brain lesions may also profoundly affect specific cognitive functions (e.g. language or memory) without causing global dementia. Finally, vascular dementia can also present with gradual cognitive decline and no history of vascular episodes. This results from diffuse small vessel disease causing widespread white matter change. Patients present with marked slowness of thinking and memory retrieval, frontal deficits. Examination may reveal focal signs, brisk reflexes, parkinsonian signs, a pseudobulbar palsy or gait apraxia. This is called 'subcortical ischaemic leucoencephalopathy'.

Diagnosis

The diagnosis of multi-infarct dementia is made based on the history and the presence of multiple areas of large vessel infarction and/or prominent small vessel disease on CT or MRI. Patients often also have evidence of other vascular disease (e.g. ischaemic heart disease, peripheral vascular disease) or vascular risk factors.

Treatment

Primary prevention for patients at risk, to prevent the onset of multiple strokes (see Ch. 29). Secondary prevention of atherosclerosis in established cases with good control of hypertension, hyperlipidaemia and antiplatelet agents such as aspirin, and dipyridamole or clopidogrel in patients with a history of dyspepsia. Current NICE guidelines do not recommend the use of cholinesterase inhibitors in vascular dementia.

VASCULITIS

Vasculitis is an uncommon cause of dementia, but should be recognized as most cases are amenable to treatment. They include:

- polyarteritis nodosa
- primary granulomatous angiitis: isolated vasculitis of the central nervous system
- systemic lupus erythematosus
- giant-cell arteritis
- thrombotic microangiopathies.

DEMENTIA AS A PART OF OTHER DEGENERATIVE DISEASES

In the following conditions, dementia may be a prominent finding with other neurological features:

- Parkinson's disease (frontotemporal)
- Huntington's disease (frontal/subcortical)
- Progressive supranuclear palsy (frontal)
- Motor neuron disease (frontotemporal).

PSEUDODEMENTIA

Depression in the elderly can mimic the initial phases of dementia and is termed 'pseudodementia'. Pseudodementia can be successfully treated with antidepressant medications and counselling if necessary.

HINTS AND TIPS

It is vital to take a good social and psychiatric history in patients with dementia. The social circumstances surrounding a patient with dementia are critical for optimal management, e.g. familiar environments and routine. Remember that the carers also need social support. Even when depression is not the main cause of memory difficulties, its treatment can still lead to significant stabilization in the patient's symptoms.

Epilepsy 19

Objectives

- Describe the main types of seizure
- Describe the aetiological factors associated with epilepsy
- Understand which drugs are used in the common epilepsy syndromes and their side-effects
- Be able to manage status epilepticus
- Understand the issues relating to pregnancy and epilepsy

DEFINITIONS

- **Epileptic seizure:** a paroxysmal, synchronous and excessive discharge of neurons in the cerebral cortex manifesting as a stereotyped disturbance of consciousness, behaviour, emotion, motor function or sensation. An epileptic seizure typically has a sudden onset, lasts seconds to minutes and usually ceases spontaneously. They often recur.
- **Epilepsy:** the condition in which there is a propensity to have recurrent and unprovoked seizures. A single seizure is therefore not usually sufficient to make a diagnosis of epilepsy and seizures occurring solely in association with precipitants (e.g. fever in young children, metabolic disturbance, alcohol or drug abuse, acute head injury) are termed acute symptomatic or situation-related seizures, and are not considered as epilepsy.
- **Status epilepticus:** a state of continued or recurrent seizures, with failure to regain consciousness between seizures over 30 minutes. This is a medical emergency and has a mortality rate of 10–15%.
- **Prodrome:** premonitory changes in mood or behaviour; these may precede the attack by some hours.
- **Aura:** the subjective sensation or phenomenon that may precede and mark the onset of the epileptic seizure. It may localize the seizure origin within the brain.
- **Ictus:** the attack or seizure itself.
- **Postictal period:** the time after the ictus during which the patient may be drowsy, confused and disorientated. The patient may also have residual focal neurological signs, e.g. Todd's paralysis.

CLASSIFICATION OF SEIZURES

The International Classification of Epileptic Seizures (ICES) was proposed in 1981 to replace older classifications (Fig. 19.1). It is currently being revised and updated, but is still widely used.

EPIDEMIOLOGY

Between 3 and 5% of the population suffer one or two seizures during their lives. Recurrent seizures occur in 0.5% of the population and 90% of these cases are well controlled with drugs and have prolonged remissions.

Epilepsy more commonly presents during childhood or adolescence, but can occur at any age. Incidence rates vary with age, being between 20 and 70 cases per 100 000 persons a year; the prevalence rate ranges between 4 and 10 per 1000. There are two peaks in the incidence of grand mal seizures. The first occurs in children and adolescents, in whom usually no cause can be found. The second occurs in patients in their fifties and sixties, in whom the disease is probably caused by subcortical ischaemic changes secondary to hypertension.

AETIOLOGY

Epilepsy is a symptom of numerous disorders but in over 50% of patients with epilepsy, no apparent cause is found, in spite of full investigation.

Of the symptomatic causes in adults, vascular disease (especially stroke), alcohol abuse, cerebral tumours and head injury are the most common. With modern neuroimaging, structural causes of partial epilepsies such as hippocampal sclerosis and neuronal migrational defects have grown in importance.

Factors that may predispose to seizures are described below.

Family history

There is an increased liability to seizures in relatives of patients with epilepsy. This is especially true in the case of absence seizures, where up to 40% of cases have a family history. No single genetic trait can account for the vast heterogeneity of all epileptic syndromes. The

Fig. 19.1 International Classification of Epileptic Seizures

Partial seizures (seizures beginning focally)

Simple (consciousness not impaired)
With motor symptoms
With somatosensory or special sensory symptoms
e.g. taste/smell.
With autonomic symptoms
With psychological, e.g. 'jamais vu' or 'deja vu'
symptoms

Complex (with impairment of consciousness)
Beginning as a simple partial seizure and progressing
to a complex partial seizure
Impairment of consciousness at onset

Partial seizure becoming secondarily generalized

Generalized seizures

Absence seizure
Typical (petit mal)
Atypical

Others
Myoclonic seizure
Clonic seizure
Tonic seizure
Tonic–clonic seizure (grand mal)
Atonic seizure

Unclassified seizures

mechanism probably involves factors that alter membrane structure or function, which may lead to a lowered seizure threshold.

Antenatal and perinatal factors

Intrauterine infections such as rubella and toxoplasmosis, as well as maternal drug abuse and irradiation in early gestation, can produce brain damage and neonatal seizures. Perinatal trauma and anoxia, when sufficiently severe to cause brain injury, may also result in epilepsy.

Trauma and surgery

Severe closed or open head trauma is often followed by seizures. These can be within the first week ('early'), or may be delayed up to several months or years ('late'), when the likelihood of chronic epilepsy is greater. Surgery to the cerebral hemispheres is followed by seizures in about 10% of patients.

Metabolic causes

Many electrolyte disturbances can cause neuronal irritability and seizures such as hyponatraemia and hypernatraemia, hypocalcaemia, hypomagnesaemia and hypoglycaemia. Other metabolic causes include uraemia, hepatic failure, acute hypoxia and porphyria.

Chronic metabolic encephalopathies can produce permanent grey-matter injury.

Toxic causes

Drugs such as phenothiazines, monoamine oxidase inhibitors, tricyclic antidepressants, amphetamines, lidocaine (lignocaine) and nalidixic acid may provoke fits, either in overdose or at therapeutic levels in patients with a lowered seizure threshold.

Withdrawal of antiepileptic medication and benzodiazepines may also cause seizures, especially when it is done rapidly.

Chronic alcohol abuse is a very common cause of seizures. These may occur while drinking, during a withdrawal phase or secondary to hypoglycaemia or trauma.

Other toxic agents capable of causing seizures include carbon monoxide, lead and mercury.

Infectious and inflammatory causes

Seizures may be the presenting feature or part of the course of encephalitis, meningitis, cerebral abscess or neurosyphilis, and usually indicate a poorer prognosis in these conditions. High fevers secondary to noncerebral infections in children over 6 months and under 6 years of age are a common cause of generalized seizures ('febrile convulsion'). These are usually self-limiting and seizures do not tend to recur in adult life.

Vascular causes

Up to 15% of patients with cerebrovascular disease experience seizures, especially with large areas of infarction or haemorrhage. Less common vascular causes of seizures include cortical venous thrombosis and arteritis (e.g. polyarteritis nodosa) as well as vascular malformations.

Intracranial tumours

Sudden onset of seizures in adult life, especially if partial, should always raise the possibility of an intracranial tumour.

Hypoxia

Seizures can develop during or following respiratory or cardiac arrest secondary to anoxic encephalopathy.

Degenerative diseases

All patients with degenerative corticoneuronal diseases of the brain have an increased risk of seizures (e.g. Alzheimer's disease).

Photosensitivity

Some seizure types are precipitated by flashing lights, or flickering television or computer screens.

Sleep deprivation

Sleep deprivation often precipitates seizures in susceptible patients.

CLINICAL FEATURES

The diagnosis of epilepsy is primarily a clinical one. A detailed history is therefore essential and usually requires eyewitness reports, particularly when consciousness is lost during the event.

If an aura preceded the attack, the patient may be able to describe this, which may help localize the focus. The aura may not be remembered by the patient, especially if there is secondary generalization.

Partial seizures

Partial seizures arise from a localized area of cerebral cortex. The clinical manifestations of the seizure depends on where in the cortex the seizure arises (see Fig. 19.2), and how fast and far it spreads. Sixty per cent of partial seizures originate in the temporal lobes, and the remainder mostly originate from the frontal lobes. Seizures originating from the parietal or occipital regions are rare. Partial seizures can be subdivided into simple partial, complex partial and partial with secondary generalization.

Simple partial seizures

Simple partial seizures are seizures in which consciousness is not impaired, and in which the discharge remains localized. They are typically brief and involve focal symptoms. A structural brain lesion must be excluded (e.g. stroke, tumour or abscess).

Complex partial seizures

Complex partial seizures may have similar features to simple partial seizures, but by definition always involve impairment of consciousness. They usually originate in the temporal or frontal lobe and cause a disturbance of consciousness usually without loss of postural control,

Fig. 19.2 Common clinical features of seizures

Seizure	Clinical features
Temporal lobe seizures	• Aura – epigastric sensation, olfactory or gustatory hallucinations, autonomic symptoms (e.g. change in pulse, or blood pressure, facial flushing), affective symptoms (e.g. fear, depersonalization), déjà vu • Seizure – motor arrest and absence prominent, automatisms (e.g. lip smacking, chewing, fidgeting, walking), automatic speech (if non-dominant hemisphere onset), contralateral dystonia • Duration – Slow evolution over 1–2 minutes • Postictal – confusion common, may be secondary generalization, postictal dysphasia (if dominant hemisphere onset)
Frontal lobe seizures	• Aura – typically abrupt onset with variable aura – often indescribable, forced thinking, ideational or emotional manifestations • Seizure – vocalization/shrill cry, violent and bizarre automatisms, cycling movements of legs, ictal posturing and tonic spasms, version of head and eyes contralateral to side of seizure focus, fencing posture (extension and abduction of one arm with rotation of head to same side and flexion of the other arm), sexual automatisms with pelvic thrusting, obscene gestures and genital manipulation • Duration – typically very brief (∼30 seconds) • Postictal – confusion brief with rapid recovery
Parietal lobe seizures	• Somatosensory symptoms common – e.g. tingling, pain, numbness, prickling, vertigo, distortions of space • Automatisms and secondary generalization may occur
Occipital lobe seizures	• Visual hallucinations common – e.g. seeing flashing lights, or geometrical figures, sometimes complex hallucinations of objects/people if seizures arise from visual association cortex • Eyelids may flutter, occasional eye turning or rapid blinking • Automatisms and secondary generalization may occur

i.e. the patient remains standing. The actual attack varies between and within individuals. They can start as a simple partial seizure and then progress, or they can involve alteration of consciousness from the outset. Complex partial seizures typically last 2 to 3 minutes, but can continue for several hours as a part of 'non-convulsive status epilepticus'. Patients are typically amnesic.

Secondarily generalized seizures

These are partial seizures in which the epileptic discharge spreads to both cerebral hemispheres, resulting in a generalized (usually tonic–clonic) seizure. The spread of the seizure may be so rapid that no features of the localized onset are apparent.

Generalized seizures

Generalized seizures are characterized by the bilateral involvement of the cortex at the onset of the seizure. Patients lose consciousness at seizure onset, so there is usually no warning.

Generalized tonic–clonic seizures

These seizures typically have no warning, although in some epilepsies they may be preceded by increasing frequency of myoclonic jerks or absences. Tonic–clonic seizures start with a sudden loss of consciousness and fall to the ground. This is followed by the 'tonic' phase, which lasts for about 10 seconds, when the body is stiff, the elbows are flexed, and the legs extended. Breathing stops and the patient may turn cyanotic.

The tonic phase is followed by the 'clonic phase', which usually lasts for 1–2 minutes, and during which there is violent generalized rhythmical shaking. The eyes are open and roll back, the tongue may be bitten and there is a tachycardia. Bladder and bowel control may be lost. The frequency of the clonic movements gradually decreases and, eventually, ceases, marking the end of the seizure. Following a tonic–clonic seizure, the patient often cannot be roused for several minutes and awakes with confusion (postictal confusion), headache, myalgia and some retrograde amnesia. It is not unusual for patients to fall asleep after a convulsion, and this can sometimes be mistaken for unconsciousness.

Clonic seizures are similar to tonic–clonic seizures, but without an initial tonic phase.

Absence seizures

Typical absence seizures have an onset between 4 and 12 years of age. The attacks may occur several times a day, with a duration of 5–15 seconds. The patient suddenly stares vacantly. There may be eye blinking and myoclonic jerks. They are often diagnosed following complaints about an inattentive child with poor academic performance. Typical absence seizures are associated with a characteristic EEG pattern of three-per-second generalized spike-and-wave discharges. Atypical absence seizures are usually associated with more severe epilepsy syndromes such as Lennox–Gastaut syndrome, and the EEG usually shows less specific changes. The seizures themselves have a less abrupt onset/cessation, with more marked eyelid fluttering and myoclonic jerking.

Myoclonic seizures

Myoclonic seizures are abrupt, brief involuntary movements that can involve the whole body, or parts of it such as the arms or head. Not all myoclonus is the result of epilepsy; it is epileptic if it occurs in the context of a seizure disorder, and is cortical (rather than brainstem or spinal cord) in origin. The majority of myoclonic seizures occur in benign, idiopathic generalized epilepsies.

Atonic and tonic seizures

These are rare generalized seizures, and are often termed 'drop attacks'. They typically occur in severe epilepsy syndromes. Atonic seizures involve a sudden loss of tone in the postural muscles, causing a patient to fall. Tonic seizures involve a sudden increase in muscle tone, causing a patient to become rigid and fall.

HISTORY AND INVESTIGATIONS TO AID DIAGNOSIS

The diagnosis of a seizure is based on the clinical history. Additional information can be provided by brain imaging, the EEG or blood tests. The use of neuroimaging is more important in cases with a late onset (over the age of 25 years), that are partial, refractory to treatment, are associated with persisting abnormal clinical signs, or when the presentation is with status epilecticus.

Clinical features during an attack that support the diagnosis of a seizure include pupil dilatation, raised blood pressure and heart rate, extensor plantar responses, and central and peripheral cyanosis.

In generalized seizures, the pO_2 and pH are lowered, the creatine phosphokinase (CPK) or creatine kinase (CK) is elevated, and there is a marked elevation of serum prolactin.

The EEG is extremely useful if recorded during an attack and may show spike-and-wave activity. Interictal EEGs may show focal spikes or slow waves suggesting subclinical seizure activity, but can be normal in 50% of adults with epilepsy. In some cases, abnormal activity can be provoked by hyperventilation or photic stimulation (flashing light). This is especially true for absence seizures, in which there is the characteristic three-per-second spike-and-wave pattern in all leads. Prolonged EEG in the form of video telemetry or ambulatory EEG may increase the probability of recording ictal EEG.

HINTS AND TIPS

A normal EEG does not exclude epilepsy. Not all cortical spikes are recorded by scalp EEG, especially in the case of simple partial seizures. Conversely, an EEG with suggestive or definite epileptic features is very helpful in making a diagnosis of epilepsy.

Computed tomography (CT) or magnetic resonance imaging (MRI) may reveal structural lesions that have caused the seizures, especially if there is focal onset.

DIFFERENTIAL DIAGNOSES

It is important to distinguish epilepsy from other causes of transient focal dysfunction or loss of consciousness, as there are social and economic implications when a diagnosis of epilepsy is made, e.g. the patient is unable to drive or operate certain machinery.

The most common differentials of a convulsive seizure include:

1. syncope (vasovagal attacks, arrhythmias, carotid sinus hypersensitivity, postural hypotension): there is usually prodromal pallor, nausea, sweating and tends not to occur when recumbent (unless caused by arrhythmias). The patient is floppy during syncopal event, but rigid during a seizure. Palpitations may be experienced with arrhythmias. Urinary incontinence and jerking of limbs can occur in syncopal episodes, but the latter does not have the co-ordinated pattern of a tonic–clonic seizure.
2. non-epileptic or functional seizures, which are surprisingly common, especially in patients with known epilepsy. The following features help to differentiate a pseudoseizure from an epileptic seizure: more common in young women with a past psychiatric history; seizures tend to be refractory to all drugs; pupils, blood pressure, heart rate, pO_2, and pH may remain unchanged during seizure; plantar responses are flexor; serum prolactin levels are normal; the EEG shows no seizure activity during the episode and no postictal slowing.
3. transient ischaemic attacks (TIAs): these can include transient loss of consciousness – among other brainstem symptoms – when the posterior circulation is involved, but this is very uncommon and often over-diagnosed.

4. migraine: syncope can occur during migraine, causing confusion with epileptic seizures. In addition, migraine preceded by visual or sensory disturbances can be mistaken for partial epilepsies, as seizures are commonly followed by headache. However the progression of visual and sensory symptoms is usually much more rapid in epilepsy than migraine.
5. hypoglycaemia: this can cause behavioural disturbance and seizures.

DRUG TREATMENT

When to start drug treatment

Research shows that after one seizure only 30–60% of patients have a recurrence within 2 years. Moreover, if there is an identifiable provoking factor (e.g. alcohol) recurrence rates are lower. Recurrence rates rise to 80–90% following two or more seizures within 1 year. For this reason, antiepileptic treatment should typically be considered when two or more unprovoked seizures have occurred within a short period. However, in certain circumstances it may be prudent to start treatment after a single unprovoked seizure. This includes a seizure associated with a clearly abnormal EEG, seizures associated with a neurological deficit present since birth and seizures associated with a progressive neurological disorder.

What drugs to choose

Whenever possible, treatment should involve only one drug, to avoid interaction between the anticonvulsants and additive side-effects. Treatment is aimed at making the patient seizure-free whilst minimizing drug side-effects. Seizure freedom can be achieved with monotherapy in about 80% of patients with epilepsy.

The most common anticonvulsants in current clinical use are carbamazepine, sodium valproate, lamotrigine and phenytoin. Second-line drugs include clobazam, clonazepam, gabapentin, topiramate, levetiracetam, pregabalin, zonisamide, lacosamide, rufinamide, retigabine, oxcarbazepine and phenobarbital. NICE guidelines state that the first-line drugs for primary generalized epilepsy in adults are sodium valproate or lamotrigine, for absence epilepsy in children are ethosuximide or sodium valproate, and for partial seizures are carbamazepine or lamotrigine. Many patients still take phenobarbital and phenytoin for generalized seizures but these are less commonly prescribed because of their side-effect profile. Some patients may still be taking vigabatrin, but this is used rarely now because it can cause progressive and irreversible visual field defects.

If one anticonvulsant fails at the maximum tolerated dose, then it is substituted by another first-line drug. The first-line drugs are then tried in combination and finally second-line anticonvulsants are added.

Whichever drug is used, the dose should be built up slowly. Measurement of blood drug concentrations is important for phenytoin, as it displays zero-order kinetics and small increases in dose can cause it to reach toxic levels. For other drugs, therapeutic drug monitoring, if available, can be used to check compliance or to confirm clinically diagnosed toxicity. If the patient is seizure- and side-effect-free and has a slightly high serum anticonvulsant level then it is usually more appropriate not to change the drug dosage. Phenobarbital is still used in refractory epilepsy and status epilepticus, and levels should be monitored.

Pharmacokinetics of antiepileptic drugs

Phenytoin, phenobarbital, topiramate and carbamazepine are well known to induce enzymes within the liver that metabolize other drugs. This effect is particularly important when the patient is on the combined oral contraceptive pill, which can be rendered ineffective unless higher doses are used. Many of the antiepileptic drugs also block pathways within the liver for metabolism of drugs, e.g. sodium valproate prolongs the half-life of lamotrigine. Care must be taken when prescribing these drugs, especially in combination, to avoid toxic levels and other adverse reactions.

Adverse effects of antiepileptic drugs

All antiepileptic drugs can produce acute, dose-related, idiosyncratic or chronic toxicity and variable degrees of teratogenicity (damage to the developing foetus).

Acute toxicity

All anticonvulsants can cause drowsiness and slowed cognition, especially at higher doses. Some antiepileptic drugs cause a non-specific encephalopathy when blood levels are high. This is associated with sedation, nystagmus, ataxia, dysarthria and confusion. If any of these features is present, blood levels must be measured.

Idiosyncratic toxicity

Allergic skin reactions occur in up to 10% of patients on phenytoin and in up to 15% on carbamazepine. Lamotrigine can be associated with a particularly severe skin rash. These can be reduced by introducing these drugs slowly, at low doses and building up to therapeutic levels. Bone marrow aplasia is a rare idiosyncratic complication of carbamazepine.

Chronic toxicity

Chronic toxicity is especially associated with phenytoin and includes the development of coarsened facies, acne, hirsutism, gum hypertrophy and possibly peripheral neuropathy. All anticonvulsants appear to have some effect on cognitive function and can cause drowsiness. This is especially a problem with phenytoin. Carbamazepine and phenytoin can cause a sometimes-irreversible cerebellar ataxia in a dose-related manner. Generally, carbamazepine and sodium valproate have fewer chronic effects than phenytoin. Lamotrigine is being increasingly used for many types of epilepsy because of its low side-effect profile, to date. Levetiracetam is also being used more frequently because of a relatively lower incidence of side-effects and absence of effect on hepatic metabolism.

Teratogenicity and pregnancy

The background risk of major foetal malformations in the general population is 1–2%. This increases to 3% in patients who have epilepsy but do not take anticonvulsants, and to 4–9% in those patients who do take anticonvulsants. This risk increases in those with high plasma anticonvulsant concentrations, and is higher in those on polytherapy. Sodium valproate (particularly doses >800 mg) appears to have the highest individual risk of the anticonvulsants, and may also be associated with an increase in learning difficulties. The aim of drug treatment during pregnancy is to minimize drug exposure whilst maintaining seizure control, and safety of mother and foetus. In addition, NICE recommends that a 5 mg dose of folic acid should be taken prior to conception by women with epilepsy, and for the first trimester of pregnancy. The use of sodium valproate and carbamazepine, in particular in pregnancy, is associated with neural tube defects. Women on these drugs need early screening using ultrasound +/− amniocentesis (to test for alpha-fetoprotein) for early detection of neural tube defects.

Patients with epilepsy and on treatment who wish to become pregnant should seek specialist advice before conception and require regular follow-up by a neurologist during the pregnancy. The pharmacokinetics may markedly change during pregnancy, necessitating regular monitoring of seizures and serum drug concentrations. In the last month of pregnancy women should be given daily oral vitamin K if they are taking enzyme-inducing drugs, and at birth the baby should also receive intramuscular vitamin K. Breast-feeding is not contraindicated, except for women taking phenobarbital or ethosuximide which can be excreted in significant quantities in breast milk.

Withdrawal of antiepileptic drugs

In view of the many adverse reactions associated with anticonvulsants, a patient who has achieved remission for over 2 years should be considered for drug withdrawal. However, there is the risk of recurrence of seizures, especially in some forms of epilepsy, or in those taking more than one anticonvulsant or with abnormal EEGs. This has important consequences for driving, employment and self-esteem. Thus, the final decision to attempt withdrawal must be made by the patient and, if undertaken, must be carried out very slowly, with gradually decreasing doses.

STATUS EPILEPTICUS

Status epilepticus is defined as a seizure, or a series of seizures, that last more than 30 minutes without regaining consciousness. This definition is of little practical value as it can be applied to all seizure types, but convulsive status epilepticus is particularly important as it is associated with a mortality rate of up to 20%. For this reason, emergency treatment of convulsive seizures should begin if the seizure has lasted more than 5 minutes, or if repeated convulsions have occurred within an hour.

Patients with status epilepticus require immediate resuscitation. This involves establishing an airway and venous access, and administering oxygen. The circulation should be assessed and an infusion set up with normal saline.

Blood tests comprise blood gases, glucose, electrolytes, renal and liver function, and anticonvulsant levels.

HINTS AND TIPS

If hypoglycaemia is suspected in a patient with a possible history of alcohol abuse or malnutrition, then thiamine must be given with intravenous glucose, as glucose alone can precipitate Wernicke's encephalopathy.

Drug treatment

It is helpful to plan therapy in a series of progressive phases:

- Premonitory stage (0–10 minutes): rapid treatment may prevent the evolution to status. Lorazepam, diazepam, midazolam or paraldehyde can be used at this stage.
- Early status (10–30 minutes): a dose of fast-acting intravenous benzodiazepines such as lorazepam. This can be repeated once if seizures are not terminated. Repeated doses of benzodiazepines may lead to an accumulation and an increased risk of respiratory depression, especially with diazepam.

- Established status (30–60 minutes): phenobarbital or phenytoin is usually given at this stage with intravenous loading doses.
- Refractory status (after 60 minutes): by this stage, anaesthesia is required, with ventilation and intensive care treatment. The most common agents used are intravenous thiopental or propofol. EEG monitoring is very helpful to confirm when status has been aborted. In all cases, neuromuscular blockade should be avoided if possible, because if the seizures return, the patient's muscles will be paralysed and therefore the return of seizure activity may go unnoticed.

Once the patient is stable, further investigations may be necessary to elucidate the cause of the status epilepticus.

NEUROSURGICAL TREATMENT OF EPILEPSY

The indication for surgical treatment requires the accurate identification of a localized site of onset of seizures or the ability to disconnect epileptogenic zones and prevent spread as a palliative procedure. Patients should also have been shown to have epilepsy that is intractable (adequate trials of therapy with at least two first-line drugs) to medical therapy.

The majority of the procedures undertaken in centres worldwide involve some form of temporal lobe surgery. Less commonly, extratemporal cortical excisions, hemispherectomies and corpus callosotomies are carried out. Temporal lobe and extratemporal surgery can result in up to 80% and 40%, respectively, of patients becoming seizure-free in the first year after surgery.

MORTALITY OF EPILEPSY

Deaths directly related to epilepsy fall into several categories: status epilepticus; accidents during seizures or as a consequence of a seizure; sudden unexpected death in epilepsy (SUDEP). SUDEP is defined as a non-traumatic, unwitnessed death occurring in a patient with epilepsy who had previously been healthy, for which no cause is found even after a thorough post-mortem examination. There are many postulated mechanisms of death, including respiratory or cardiovascular arrest, but the underlying pathophysiology is still unknown. The annual mortality rate is 1 per 1000 epilepsy patients in the community, but this increases to 1 per 200 per year for those with refractory epilepsy, and is >1% for patients undergoing surgical evaluation.

It is important to be aware when seeing patients with epilepsy that fear, misunderstanding and the resulting social stigma surrounding epilepsy can result in social, and sometimes even legal, discrimination against those living with the condition.

DRIVING AND EPILEPSY

The DVLA can revoke a British driving licence in any individual felt to be unsafe to himself/herself and/or the public. Patients who have had one or more seizures need to contact the DVLA regarding the length of period they are not allowed to drive. As a guide, the following conditions need to apply before the patient can return to driving with or without treatment, though it should be noted that those drivers with group 2 licenses have more severe restrictions:

- Patients who have a diagnosis of epilepsy cannot drive for 1 year after a single seizure.
- Patients who have only nocturnal seizures may drive if they are seizure-free during the daytime for 3 years.
- For single seizures with a specific provocative cause (acute symptomatic seizure) that is unlikely to recur, the DVLA will deal with drivers on an individual basis.
- Following a single unprovoked epileptic seizure or isolated seizure, patients are barred from driving for 6 months, provided there is no history of epilepsy, previous solitary seizures, or a high risk of recurrence, in which case they are prevented from driving for 12 months.
- Patients who are driving and taking antiepileptic drugs but who wish to stop epileptic medication are recommended to stop driving during cessation and for 6 months following the last dose of their drug.

Headache and craniofacial pains

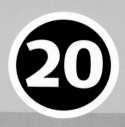

Objectives

* Understand the main headache syndromes and their management
* Describe the features that differentiate primary and secondary headaches
* Understand the types of brain shift that occur in raised intracranial pressure

Headache is one of the most common symptoms in medicine and may account for up to 40% of neurological consultations. The most important role of the general physician is in determining whether the patient has a primary or secondary headache. Primary headaches are those in which the headache and its features are the disease itself, and secondary headaches are those in which the headache is the result of another pathological process. Important examples of primary headache syndromes are migraine, tension-type headache and cluster headache. Important examples of secondary headaches are systemic infection, head injury, subarachnoid haemorrhage, vascular disorders and brain tumours (see Ch. 6).

TENSION-TYPE HEADACHE

Primary tension-type headache should only be diagnosed when it is completely featureless, with no nausea, vomiting, phonophobia, photophobia, osmophobia, throbbing or aggravation with movement. It is increasingly recognized that in many patients the development of persistent daily headache arises from a transformation of increasingly frequent migraine, rather than a primary tension headache syndrome, often in the context of overuse of analgesics. These patients have 'chronic migraine' and may respond to antimigrainous treatments.

The patient often complains of a diffuse, 'bandlike', dull headache, which may be accompanied by scalp tenderness and be aggravated by noise and light. The headache may last hours to days and occur infrequently or every day. There are no abnormal physical signs.

True episodic (headache on <15 days per month) tension-type headache should be managed with physical treatments (massage, relaxation therapy), and simple analgesics such as paracetamol, aspirin or other NSAIDs. When chronic (headache on >15 days per month), the only proven effective treatment is with amitriptyline. Chronic opiate and analgesic use should be avoided.

Paradoxically, these headaches can be exacerbated by analgesic overuse, including the chronic use of paracetamol and opiate based painkillers. In patients who probably have a mixture of analgesic and tension-type headache, the first aim should be to wean the patient off their opiate-based analgesia and concurrently commence a small dose of amitriptyline and restrict paracetamol or anti-inflammatories (e.g. aspirin, ibuprofen) for acute exacerbations of the headache.

MIGRAINE

Migraine is a common, often familial, condition characterized by an episodic unilateral throbbing headache typically lasting up to 4 to 72 hours. The patient often complains of photophobia, phonophobia and occasionally osmophobia, as well as nausea and sometimes vomiting. Patients with migraine often cannot bear to do anything apart from lying quietly in a dark room until their headache subsides. Exacerbation of pain by movement is a prominent feature of migraine. It is more common in young women and the headache is often preceded by a visual aura with fortification spectra or flashing lights or, less commonly, a sensory aura with numbness and tingling in the fingers and/or face.

The headache is thought to have a neurovascular basis and to be related to the release of vasoactive substances by the trigeminovascular system. The level of serum 5-hydroxytryptamine (5-HT) rises with the prodromal symptoms and falls during the headache. The headache may follow abnormal electrical activity within the cortex or 'spreading depression' and subsequent brainstem activation leads to alterations in cranial vascular tone.

There are various subdivisions of migraine, although migraine with aura (classical) and without aura (common) are the most frequently encountered forms.

Migraine with aura or 'classical migraine'

Patients with a classical migraine complain of an aura, which usually consists of moving white lights or spectra in the shape of fortifications ('fortification spectra'). Some patients experience a sensory aura which involves paraesthesias or numbness that spreads up a limb or part of the face. These precede the migrainous headache by up to 40 minutes and usually last about 20 minutes, rarely more than 60 minutes. The gradually spreading nature of the visual or sensory symptoms is important for making the diagnosis. The aura may extend into the headache phase.

Common migraine

There is no aura in common migraine but the headache is similar to classical migraine.

Basilar migraine

In basilar migraine, the brainstem aura causes symptoms that arise from dysfunction in the territory of the posterior cerebral circulation, which supplies the brainstem, cerebellum and most of the occipital cortices. The aura can consist of bilateral visual symptoms, ataxia, dysarthria, vertigo, limb paraesthesia and weakness. There may be loss of consciousness before, during or after the onset of headache, which often causes diagnostic confusion.

Hemiplegic migraine

Hemiplegic migraine is rare and causes lateralised weakness during the aura and headache, that can persist for days after the headache has settled. In some cases, there is an autosomal dominant transmission and in 50% of these, it is associated with defects in genes that encode calcium, sodium and potassium channels. Hemiplegic migraine must be differentiated from stroke or transient ischaemic attacks (TIAs). In a patient who presents for the first time with hemiplegia and headache it must be initially assumed that the patient has had a stroke or TIA unless there is a family history of hemiplegic migraine.

Management

The patient needs to be reassured that there are no secondary causes of the headache and that migraine is essentially an inherited tendency to headache caused by a patient's genes that cannot be cured, but can be modified and controlled. The avoidance of any precipitating lifestyle factors (e.g. particular food types, stress, sleep deprivation, dehydration, too much sleep) may be helpful. For patients using oral contraceptives/HRT and who have migraine with aura, there is an increased incidence of stroke. The risk is especially high in smokers with aura. In these patients the hormone treatment should be stopped.

During an attack

In the stepped model of migraine care, assuming there are no contraindications, patients use simple analgesia such as soluble aspirin 900 mg or paracetamol 1000 mg with an antiemetic (e.g. domperidone) to allow ingestion of the other drugs. Other NSAIDs can also be useful, but adequate doses must be given. Gastrointestinal side-effects such as dyspepsia may be limiting. Patients should avoid the regular use of codeine because of the risk of induction of a chronic 'analgesic' headache.

More severe, or refractory, attacks may be terminated by the use of 5-HT agonists (e.g. sumatriptan, naratriptan, zolmitriptan, rizatriptan, eletriptan). There are now preparations that can be given subcutaneously or nasally which bypass the need for gastric absorption. They may have different rapidity and duration of action, which should dictate choice in individual patients. Ergotamine is still used for acute attacks, but relatively infrequently because of liability to side-effects.

Prophylaxis

For frequent and severe attacks that occur more than twice per month, daily treatment for 6 months or more may be required to prevent headaches. Medications include:

- propranolol (beta-adrenergic receptor blocker)
- amitriptyline (tricyclic agent)
- pizotifen (5-HT antagonist)
- sodium valproate or topiramate (anticonvulsants)
- verapamil (calcium antagonist)
- methysergide (5-HT antagonist): rarely used now because it can cause retroperitoneal fibrosis.

HINTS AND TIPS

In patients with 'medication overuse' headache, preventative medications are unlikely to be effective until the regular analgesic use has been curtailed.

CLUSTER HEADACHE

Cluster headache is a rare, primary headache syndrome with a prevalence of approximately 0.1%. It occurs more commonly in men, with an onset in early middle life. Features of cluster headache comprise severe unilateral pain localized around the eye with ipsilateral autonomic features such as conjunctival injection, lacrimation, rhinorrhoea and sometimes a transient Horner's syndrome.

The headache and associated features last between 15 minutes and 3 hours, typically occurring one to eight times daily in clusters typically lasting 8 to 10 weeks at a time. Intervals between clusters may extend to several years. The onset of an attack typically has circadian periodicity, often being in the early hours of the morning, waking the patient from sleep. There may be migrainous features, but movement sensitivity is not typical and in fact patients with cluster headache often want to pace around, rather than lie still in bed. Patients with cluster headache should have brain neuroimaging as they can sometimes be associated with underlying pituitary pathology.

Treatment

Cluster headaches peak rapidly, and therefore the acute attack should be treated promptly. Many patients respond well to the inhalation of 100% oxygen at 10–15 L/min for 15–20 minutes. Sumatriptan injections, or sumatriptan/zolmitriptan nasal sprays are also effective, and rapid in their onset of action.

Specific preventative treatments for cluster headache depend on the length of a bout. The first-line agent for prolonged bouts is verapamil, often in high doses. Regular ECGs should be carried out as the dose is titrated upwards (especially above 240 mg) due to the risk of bradycardia and heart block. Other options include lithium, which requires careful monitoring of levels and topiramate. Limited courses of corticosteroids (e.g. 60 mg of prednisolone tapering over 10–20 days) can be useful in shorter bouts. Methysergide can be used for resistant cases, but this should be under hospital supervision because it can cause retroperitoneal fibrosis.

In patients with medically intractable, chronic (a bout of attacks lasting 1 year with <1 month remission) cluster headaches, neuromodulation may have a role to play, and include occipital nerve stimulation and deep brain stimulation.

OTHER NEUROLOGICAL CAUSES OF HEADACHE AND CRANIOFACIAL PAIN

Headache of raised intracranial pressure

The headache of raised intracranial pressure can be due to idiopathic intracranial hypertension or an intracranial tumour or a space-occupying lesion. It has certain characteristic features:

- There is a generalized ache
- It is aggravated by bending, coughing, or straining, which all raise intracranial pressure
- It is worse in the morning or after prolonged recumbency

- It may awaken the patient from sleep
- The severity gradually progresses.

It is often accompanied by:

- vomiting
- visual obscurations (transient loss of vision with sudden changes in intracranial pressure)
- progressive focal neurological signs
- papilloedema, enlarged blind spots and decrement in visual acuity
- risk of herniation: there is a risk that tonsillar herniation will occur in rapidly expanding or chronic untreated space-occupying lesions. When this happens, the cerebellar tonsils herniate through the foramen magnum and can result in brainstem compression and death, referred to as 'coning'. This usually occurs with expanding lesions in the posterior fossa (cerebellum and brainstem) or following untreated supratentorial herniation (Fig. 20.1). Supratentorial lesions usually cause lateral and central tentorial herniation initially. This is associated with a reduced level of consciousness, a third nerve palsy, especially loss of pupillary reflexes and pupillary dilatation, and ipsilateral hemiparesis due to pressure on the contralateral cerebral peduncle. If left untreated, transtentorial herniation will progress to tonsillar herniation.

Urgent imaging of the brain with computed tomography or magnetic resonance imaging is essential. Contrast may be required to visualize any lesions. See Chapter 30 for further management of intracranial masses.

> **HINTS AND TIPS**
>
> A worsening or a change in patients with a chronic primary headache disorder must be independently assessed, as these patients can develop a new pathology causing secondary headache in addition to their original condition.

Low pressure headache

This type of headache typically arises after a lumbar puncture. Patients report no pain whilst recumbent, but develop a headache when they sit or stand up. The headache may worsen as the day progresses. Symptoms improve within minutes with recumbency and typically worsen again within minutes to an hour on standing or with vigorous Valsalva (e.g. straining or coughing). The underlying cause can also include an epidural or a spontaneous CSF leak. MRI of the brain with contrast may show diffuse meningeal enhancement. Treatment options include bedrest,

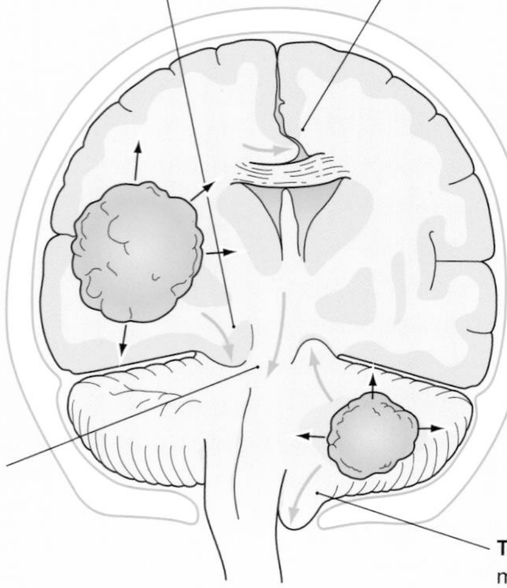

Brain shift — types

Tentorial herniation (lateral): a unilateral expanding mass causes tentorial (uncal) herniation as the medial edge of the temporal lobe herniates through the tentorial hiatus. As the intracranial pressure continues to rise, 'central' herniation follows

Subfalcine 'midline' shift: occurs early with unilateral space-occupying lesions. Seldom produces any clinical effect, although ipsilateral anterior cerebral artery occlusion has been recorded

Tentorial herniation (central): a midline lesion or diffuse swelling of the cerebral hemispheres result in a vertical displacement of the midbrain and diencephalon through the tentorial hiatus. Damage to these structures occurs either from mechanical distortion or from ischaemia secondary to stretching of the perforating vessels

Tonsillar herniation: a subtentorial expanding mass causes herniation of the cerebellar tonsils through the foramen magnum. A degree of *upward* herniation though the tentorial hiatus may also occur. Clinical effects are difficult to distinguish from effects of direct brainstem/midbrain compression

Fig. 20.1 Types of brain shift in a coronal section.

intravenous caffeine or autologous blood patches around the lumbar puncture site.

Other neurological causes of headache include:

- stroke, especially intracranial haemorrhage: see Chapter 29
- meningitis: see Chapter 31
- trigeminal and postherpetic neuralgia: see Chapter 22.

NON-NEUROLOGICAL CAUSES OF HEADACHE AND CRANIOFACIAL PAIN

Giant-cell arteritis (temporal arteritis)

Giant-cell arteritis is a granulomatous inflammation that usually affects the branches of the external carotid artery, including the palpable superficial temporal artery, in those over 60 years of age. The majority of patients experience pain over thickened, tender, often non-pulsatile, temporal arteries. The headache is accompanied by:

- a raised erythrocyte sedimentation rate (ESR): often highly elevated (60–100)
- visual loss (25% of untreated cases): amaurosis fugax (a TIA involving the retinal vessels) or permanent visual loss due to inflammation or occlusion of the posterior ciliary vessels. Once infarction has occurred in one eye, there is a severe risk that the second eye may also be affected without prompt treatment with steroids
- jaw claudication and scalp tenderness
- systemic features include proximal muscle pain in the form of polymyalgia rheumatica in up to 50% of cases, weight loss, fatigue
- rarer complications: brainstem ischaemia, cortical blindness, cranial nerve palsies, aortitis, involvement of coronary and mesenteric arteries.

Diagnosis

The diagnosis is made from the history and a raised ESR, and all cases should be confirmed by a biopsy of the temporal artery. At least 1 cm of the artery needs to be excised as the disease process may be patchy and missed by shorter biopsy samples.

Treatment

Treatment is with high-dose corticosteroids (e.g. prednisolone 60 mg per day). There is a risk of blindness if treatment is delayed and, therefore, the steroids should be started immediately and not be delayed until after the biopsy. The dose of steroids is gradually reduced as the ESR falls. It is usually possible to withdraw steroids slowly after several months to years.

Local causes

- Sinus disease
- Ocular-glaucoma, refraction errors
- Temporomandibular joint dysfunction
- Dental disease.

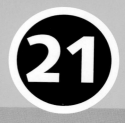
- Define akinetic–rigid syndrome
- Describe the main clinical features of Parkinson's disease
- Differentiate idiopathic Parkinson's disease from atypical parkinsonian syndromes
- Have an understanding of neuroleptic-induced movement disorders and restless legs syndrome

AKINETIC–RIGID SYNDROMES

The akinetic–rigid syndromes are defined by akinesia, which encompasses three main features: a poverty of movement (hypokinesia), a slowness of movement (bradykinesia) and fatiguing of repetitive movement. The definition also includes muscle stiffness with and a resistance to passive movement referred to as rigidity. These conditions are caused by neurodegeneration of, (or lesions) in, the basal ganglia and their connections and are also referred to as extrapyramidal syndromes. The basal ganglia consist of the caudate nucleus, globus pallidus, putamen, substantia nigra and subthalamic nucleus. The akinetic rigid syndromes can be divided into that which is the most common and typical, namely Parkinson's disease, and the atypical parkinsonian disorders of multiple system atrophy (MSA), progressive supranuclear palsy (PSP) and corticobasal degeneration (CBD).

Parkinson's disease

Parkinson's disease was first described by James Parkinson in 1817, who named it the 'shaking palsy'. It is the most common of all the akinetic–rigid syndromes with a prevalence of 170 per 100 000 of population in the UK. It is more common in men than in women, and the average age at disease onset is 60 years. It is a slowly progressive, degenerative disease involving the basal ganglia as well as other brain areas. It causes an akinetic–rigid syndrome, commonly associated with a rest tremor, that is later accompanied by a flexed posture, shuffling gait and impaired balance. The disease also manifests with a variety of non-motor symptoms, cognitive and psychiatric complications.

Pathology

There is progressive degeneration of cells within the pars compacta of the substantia nigra in the midbrain (Fig. 21.1). These neurons are dopaminergic. Eosinophilic intraneuronal inclusions called Lewy bodies can be found in the surviving neurons of the substantia nigra. These contain the protein alpha-synuclein, aggregated with abnormally phosphorylated neurofilaments and ubiquitin. The nigral cells projecting to the striatum are mostly affected – the 'nigrostriatal' pathway. This causes a loss of dopamine in the striatum. Pathological changes may also be seen in other non-dopaminergic brainstem nuclei such as locus ceruleus. The involvement of the non-dopaminergic system may account for the lack of response of some features of Parkinson's disease to dopamine replacement therapy, and the development of non-motor complications.

Aetiology

The cause of Parkinson's disease is unknown. Twin studies have provided conflicting information about the possible genetic component of Parkinson's disease. Recently, several family pedigrees have been described with familial Parkinson's disease. These include rare autosomal dominant gene mutations in alpha-synuclein and LRKK2, and autosomal recessive gene mutations in Parkin, PINK1 or DJ1 genes.

A consistent environmental factor has not been elucidated. Increased interest in exogenous toxins as a cause arose with the finding that drug addicts taking heroin contaminated with 1-methyl-4-phenyl-1,2,3, 6-tetrahydropyridine (MPTP) developed a similar condition, with selective destruction of the nigral cells and their striatal connections. There is also some evidence that pesticides and herbicides may increase the risk of developing Parkinson's disease.

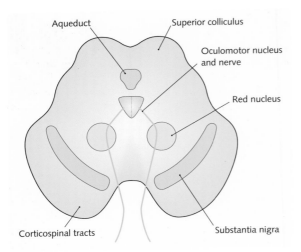

Fig. 21.1 Cross-section of the midbrain.

Fig. 21.2 The differences between spasticity and rigidity	
Spasticity	**Rigidity**
Lesion in upper motor neuron	Lesion in basal ganglia and connections
Increased tone more marked in flexors in arms and extensors in legs	Increased tone equal in flexors and extensors
Increased tone most apparent early during movement ('clasp-knife effect')	Increased tone apparent throughout range of movement (lead-pipe rigidity)
Reflexes brisk with extensor plantars	Normal reflexes with flexor plantars

Clinical features

Clinical features of Parkinson's disease comprise the classical triad of rest tremor, limb rigidity and not only bradykinesia but also akinesia, with progressive fatiguing of movements, in association with changes in posture and gait and a host of non-motor symptoms and cognitive decline.

An important and characteristic feature of Parkinson's disease is the striking asymmetry of the clinical signs. If a patient presents with symmetrical parkinsonian clinical signs, they are unlikely to have idiopathic Parkinson's disease.

Tremor

Tremor is the initial presenting symptoms in about 60% of patients with Parkinson's disease. This is a characteristic coarse resting tremor (4–7 Hz) of the hands and can affect any part of the body, including the chin, tongue and the legs. It can be exacerbated by emotion and distraction, e.g. walking or using the contralateral limbs. The rest tremor disappears in sleep. It is often 'pill-rolling' in nature on account of the thumb moving rhythmically backwards and forwards on the palmar surface of the fingers. The rest tremor may lessen or disappear during voluntary movement (e.g. when raising arms in front of body), but then reappears after a delay, in the new position ('re-emergent tremor').

Rigidity

There is stiffness of the limbs, which can be felt as resistance throughout passive movement of the arms and, equally, in the flexors and extensors. This is termed 'lead-pipe' rigidity. When combined with the tremor,

which can be subclinical, there is a jerky element ('cog-wheel' rigidity). The increase in tone can be felt most easily when the wrist is rotated in both clockwise and anticlockwise directions and can be made more apparent when the patient is asked to voluntarily move the opposite limb (synkinesis). The rigidity is usually asymmetrical in the limbs.

> **HINTS AND TIPS**
>
> Both rigidity and spasticity produce an increase in tone, but there are important differences (Fig. 21.2).

Bradykinesia, hypokinesia and akinesia

Akinesia is often the most disabling feature of Parkinson's disease. It is a grouping of symptoms that includes bradykinesia (slowness of movement with additional fatiguing and decrement of repetitive alternating movements) and hypokinesia (reduced amplitude of movements). Bradykinesia and hypokinesia affect not only the limbs but also the muscles of facial expression to give mask-like facies known as hypomimia and reduced blinking. The muscles of mastication, speech and voluntary swallowing, and some of the axial muscles, can also be involved. There is particular difficulty in initiating and terminating movements.

Speech is altered, producing a monotonous, hypophonic dysarthria, due to a combination of bradykinesia, rigidity and tremor. Power is usually preserved, although in advanced disease the slowness (bradykinesia) and rigidity make testing power difficult. Sensory examination is also normal, although patients can often describe discomfort and sensory abnormalities in the legs. Handwriting reduces in size and becomes spidery (micrographia).

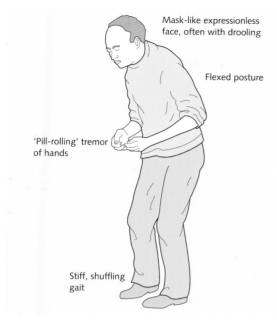

Mask-like expressionless
face, often with drooling

Flexed posture

'Pill-rolling' tremor
of hands

Stiff, shuffling
gait

Fig. 21.3 Parkinsonian posture.

Postural changes

The posture is characteristically stooped (Fig. 21.3), with a shuffling, flexed, festinant (steps that become increasingly fast) gait with poor asymmetrical arm swing. Falls are common later in the disease process, as the normal righting reflexes are affected. There may be difficulty initiating gait ('start hesitation'), and when the patient tries to turn either when walking or lying (e.g. in bed), there are great difficulties ('freezing') and the patient is said to move 'en bloc'.

Non-motor, cognitive and psychiatric features

Constipation is usual and urinary difficulties are common, especially in men. Depression is also common. Cognitive function is preserved in the early stages but dementia is a common complication later in the disease.

HINTS AND TIPS

Patients with Parkinson's disease often have additional non-motor symptoms which are equally important to manage. These may result directly from the disease or drug therapy. They include cognitive decline, depression, sensory complaints/pain, gastrointestinal complaints (e.g. weight loss and constipation), detrusor hyperreflexia (urinary urgency and frequency), erectile dysfunction in men, loss of libido, postural hypotension and intrusive REM sleep behavioural disorder.

Natural history

Parkinson's disease progresses over a period of years. The rate of progression is very variable, with the mildest forms running over several decades. The course is usually over 10–15 years with progressive immobility, falls and cognitive decline. The cumulative incidence of dementia approximates to 80%. Death is usually from bronchopneumonia.

Investigations

Parkinson's disease is a clinical diagnosis, and an MRI brain in uncomplicated disease is typically normal. A dopamine transporter (DaT) single-photon emission computed tomography (SPECT) scan typically shows decreased dopamine transporter binding in the basal ganglia. DaT scans should not be routinely used to confirm a diagnosis of Parkinson's disease, nor can they distinguish between Parkinson's disease, multiple system atrophy (MSA) and progressive supranuclear palsy (PSP). However a normal scan can be used to exclude Parkinson's disease. NICE therefore recommends its use where it is difficult to differentiate essential tremor from parkinsonism.

Treatment

The main aim of treatment is to restore the dopamine levels within the striatum. NICE guidelines highlight that it is not possible to pick a universal first-choice drug therapy for patients with early or late Parkinson's disease. Instead, a patient's clinical and lifestyle characteristics, together with their preference once fully informed about medication options, should be taken into consideration.

Levodopa (L-dopa)

L-dopa forms the mainstay of treatment for most patients with Parkinson's disease. It is given in a combined form with a peripheral decarboxylase inhibitor (benserazide – as Madopar; carbidopa – as Sinemet) to prevent the peripheral conversion of the inactive L-dopa to the active form, dopamine, reducing the peripheral side-effects of nausea, vomiting and hypotension. The conversion to dopamine still occurs within the CNS because benserazide and carbidopa can not cross the blood–brain barrier, but L-dopa can.

L-dopa improves bradykinesia and rigidity, but has a variable effect on tremor; however, the majority of patients with Parkinson's disease have a good response on treatment and this is often used as additional support for the diagnosis. As disease progresses, the duration of action of the medication decreases and marked fluctuations in motor symptoms occur with L-dopa-responsive phases called the 'on period', followed by 'off periods' where medication overtly wears off or does not take effect. As the disease progresses, motor fluctuations may become more severe and unpredictable. The 'on periods' can become associated with dyskinesias which are excessive choreiform movements caused by the use of L-dopa, which can be troubling, and the 'off periods' can become associated with sudden and unpredictable periods of immobility or other instances where the feet suddenly get stuck or frozen to the ground for seconds or minutes called 'freezing'. L-dopa may be held in reserve, to reduce the risk or delay L-dopa-induced dyskinesias, especially for those with an earlier age of onset of parkinsonism (55 years years or less), while other treatments are used. Other side-effects of L-dopa include drowsiness, postural hypotension, and psychiatric complications such as vivid dreams, nightmares, illusions, hallucinations and impulse control disorders.

Dopamine agonists

Dopamine agonists are analogues of dopamine and directly stimulate the dopamine receptors. The most effective anti-parkinsonian dopamine agonists stimulate D_2 receptors predominantly, but other types of dopamine receptor stimulation are probably important.

Dopamine agonists have varying selectivity and include bromocriptine, cabergoline, pergolide, ropinirole, pramipexole and apomorphine. Apomorphine is administered as individual subcutaneous injections or as a subcutaneous infusion and is usually reserved for patients at the end stages of the disease, particularly those with severe motor fluctuations or dyskinesias. The dopamine agonists are usually prescribed alone as the first-line treatment of Parkinson's disease, especially in younger patients, to delay the use of L-dopa, and therefore early and troublesome dyskinesias. They rarely produce the same dramatic motor response as L-dopa. Dopamine agonists share a similar side-effect profile to L-dopa, but may cause more marked nausea and vomiting, and in the elderly can have particularly severe psychiatric side-effects such that they are often avoided. Older agonists (pergolide, cabergoline, bromocriptine) are associated with a long-term risk of pleuro-pulmonary-retroperitoneal and cardiac valve fibrosis, and for this reason they are avoided.

Anticholinergic drugs

Anticholinergic drugs include benzhexol (trihexyphenidyl), benztropine and procyclidine, which are antimuscarinic agents that penetrate the central nervous system. They can be effective in reducing tremor, although not so effective for reducing rigidity and bradykinesia. Side-effects such as dry mouth, constipation, urinary retention, visual blurring, hallucinations, confusion and memory impairment often prevent their use, especially in the elderly. They are often reserved for younger patients who have an intrusive tremor. Amantadine is an antiviral agent, which has some dopamine reuptake

blocking and anticholinergic activity, and releases stored dopamine. It can be useful in the early stages of the disease, and for L-dopa-induced dyskinesias. Side-effects include ankle swelling, skin changes and confusion.

Monoamine oxidase B inhibitors

Selegiline and rasagiline are irreversible inhibitors of monoamine oxidase B (MAO-B), which act to block the degradation of dopamine in the CNS. Early use can delay the need for L-dopa, or prolong its duration of action.

COMT (catechol-*O*-methyltransferase) inhibitors

Dopamine is broken down peripherally by both dopa decarboxylase and by COMT. The rationale of these drugs is, therefore, to prevent the additional COMT-mediated breakdown and increase dopamine availability centrally. They are used in conjunction with L-dopa to reduce the L-dopa dose, and increase its duration of action. Entacapone is the most widely used drug in this group, while tolcapone is a second-line agent due to a risk of liver failure and rhabdomyolysis.

Management of hallucinations, psychosis and confusion

After excluding a superimposed infection or metabolic derangement, medication to treat parkinonsism can often be the cause of these symptoms and should be withdrawn in the following order: anticholinergics, dopamine agonists, MAO-BIs, COMPT-Is. If necessary the total L-dopa dose should also be reduced. If additional medication is needed, conventional neuroleptics should be avoided as they can worsen extrapyramidal features, in favour of atypical neuroleptics. Within this group, quetiapine, olanzapine and clozapine are the preferred options, although the latter will need regular blood monitoring.

Surgery

Functional stereotactic neurosurgery for Parkinson's disease is also included in the management of patients with complex disease. Deep brain stimulation of the subthalamic nucleus has a significant effect on underlying parkinsonism, including tremor and dyskinesias.

Differential diagnosis of Parkinson's disease

Parkinsonism refers to a syndrome where the clinical features resemble Parkinson's disease but have a different pathological basis. Hypothyroidism and depression may superficially mimic Parkinson's disease but will have no physical signs of parkinsonism.

Causes of parkinsonism include:

- medications: dopamine antagonists (e.g. phenothiazines, reserpine, haloperidol), lithium

- trauma: subdural haematomas, repetitive head injury, e.g. boxing
- cerebrovascular disease: lacunar infarcts of the basal ganglia and small vessel disease of the cerebral white matter
- hydrocephalus or tumour
- infections such as encephalitis lethargica and Japanese B encephalitis
- atypical parkinsonian disorders: multisystem atrophy, progressive supranuclear palsy and corticobasal degeneration (see below).

The atypical parkinsonian disorders

The atypical or 'Parkinson's plus' syndromes refers to other forms of parkinsonism that have clinical features that are not typical of Parkinsons's disease. These include symmetrical parkinsonism, little or no tremor and a poor or an absent response to L-dopa therapy. There are also additional neurological symptoms and signs.

Progressive supranuclear palsy

PSP is a rare condition with a mean age of onset of 63 years, and an average survival of 7 years. It is characterized by falls early on, symmetrical parkinsonism and a prominence of axial features with cognitive decline, dysarthria, dysphagia and a striking supranuclear gaze palsy that initially affects vertical gaze, but subsequently may affect all eye movements. The speed and range of voluntary eye movements are limited and can be overcome with the 'doll's head' or oculocephalic manoeuvre which demonstrates a full range of eye movements. The pathway from the cranial nerve nuclei responsible for ocular movements to the extraocular muscles is intact, and the pathology lies above the nucleus (i.e. supranuclear). There may be an astonished facial expression with overreaction and increased wrinkling of the frontalis muscle. There is usually a history of falls backwards early in the disease and PSP should be strongly considered in any patient with parkinsonian signs who suffers frequent falls within the first few years of onset. A pseudobulbar palsy develops insidiously with dysarthria, dysphagia and prominent emotional lability. Cognitive decline is common, particularly with frontal release signs and dysexecutive features. Pathological findings include neuronal loss, gliosis and aggregates of tau protein and neurofibrillary tangles in the brainstem, basal ganglia and cerebral cortex. The diagnosis is based on the clinical features and the MRI may identify atrophy of the midbrain (the 'hummingbird' sign) and superior cerebellar peduncles. There is usually little response to treatment with L-dopa, but amantadine may be useful.

Multisystem atrophy

MSA is a neurodegenerative disorder characterized by parkinsonism and cerebellar signs, or autonomic failure. It is rare, with a mean age of onset of 57 years, and an average survival of 7 years. Two forms are recognized; MSA-P and MSA-C. MSA-P is associated with asymmetrical parkinsonism that is poorly responsive to L-dopa and autonomic failure. The latter includes a postural drop in blood pressure, loss of sweating, urinary incontinence or retention and early erectile dysfunction.

In MSA-C, a cerebellar ataxia predominates with autonomic failure. Other features that occur in MSA and may help to differentiate it from other parkinsonian conditions include postural instability, orofacial dystonia and anterocollis, myoclonus that manifests as an irregular and jerky tremor of the upper limbs, pyramidal signs, abnormal respiratory patterns (e.g. stridor, gasps and sleep apnoea), and prominent emotional lability referred to as emotional incontinence. Cognitive decline is not a feature of MSA. The pathological hallmark of the disease is glial cytoplasmic inclusions that contain alpha-synuclein in the basal ganglia, cerebellum, pons/medulla and motor cortex. Cell loss and gliosis is also seen in Onuf's nucleus in the spinal cord which underlies the intrusive dysfunction of bladder and bowel. The diagnosis is a clinical one which can be supported by an MRI that may show degeneration of the middle cerebellar peduncles and pons ('hot-cross bun' sign). Abnormal autonomic function tests may also aid diagnosis. Treatment is essentially symptomatic, though amantadine and L-dopa should be trialled.

Corticobasal degeneration

CBD is a rare disorder that is characterized by strikingly unilateral involvement with rigidity and dystonia in an arm. There is no tremor, but other parkinsonian symptoms and signs are often prominent in addition to cognitive and visuospatial neglect, limb apraxia (inability to make purposeful movements) and myoclonus of the affected arm. Dysphasia and dysphagia may also occur. Patients also report 'alien limb' phenomenon where the arm appears to have a mind of its own and also appears alien. The arm may eventually become functionally useless. Initial symptoms typically begin at the age of 60 years. Eventually, both sides are affected as the disease progresses. Patients usually become bed-bound through immobility and die within 6–8 years. Treatment is mainly supportive and L-dopa has little or no effect. Post-mortem examination of the brain demonstrates tau inclusions.

Other parkinsonian syndromes

Medication-induced parkinsonism

Medications that have dopamine antagonist effects can cause a parkinsonian syndrome with bradykinesia and rigidity and tremor. The neuroleptics which include the phenothiazines (e.g. chlorpromazine), butyrophenones (e.g. haloperidol), thioxanthenes (e.g. flupentixol) and substituted benzamides (e.g. sulpiride) can commonly cause parkinsonian, or extrapyramidal side effects. These typically resolve after drug withdrawal, though some of the effects may be irreversible despite discontinuing the offending drug. Other commonly used dopamine receptor blocking drugs include prochlorperazine, metoclopramide and flunarizine, which are commonly used to treat vertigo, nausea and vomiting, and migraine.

Cerebrovascular disease

The pathological basis of cerebrovascular disease causing parkinsonism is usually multifocal small vessel disease, particularly subcortical ischaemia and lacunar infarcts. Patients often have a degree of cognitive impairment and pyramidal signs in the limbs with symmetrical bradykinesia and rigidity and little resting tremor. It typically affects the lower limbs and is sometimes called 'lower limb parkinsonism'. Patients typically have a small-stepped gait called 'marche a petit pas' with an upright stance (as compared with the stooped posture of Parkinson's disease) and an unsteady wide-based gait. Treatment is aimed at secondary prevention by treating underlying cardiovascular risk factors, especially hypertension.

Wilson's disease

Wilson's disease is an inherited autosomal recessive disorder of copper metabolism, resulting in low levels of the copper-binding protein caeruloplasmin. This causes elevated levels of free copper in the blood, which results in copper deposition in the brain, particularly in the basal ganglia, in the Descemet's membrane in the cornea (Kayser–Fleischer rings only seen on slit lamp examination of the eyes) and in the liver, which causes cirrhosis. Patients typically present in their teens or early adult life with atypical parkinsonism, tremor, dystonia, cerebellar signs and cognitive decline. Patients can also present with prominent psychiatric symptoms, including a personality change, emotional lability and psychosis. It is uncommon for neurological manifestations to occur after the age of 40 years. The diagnosis is made by identifying low levels of caeruloplasmin with high free copper in the urine and serum after a penicillamine challenge. An MRI brain may show cortical atrophy or signal change in the putamen and a liver biopsy can provide a tissue diagnosis. Genetic testing is not practical due to the large number of mutations that have been found. The disease is treated with copper-binding agents such as penicillamine, trientine or tetrathiomolybdate and the neurological damage may be partly reversible.

NEUROLEPTIC-INDUCED MOVEMENT DISORDERS

Dopamine blocking drugs used to treat psychiatric illness or as antiemetics or vestibular sedatives can cause a variety of movement disorders.

Acute dystonic reactions

Dystonia develops in 2–5% of patients on neuroleptics or antiemetics (metoclopramide and prochlorperazine). This reaction is unpredictable and can occur even after single doses of the medication. The range of dystonias includes torticollis, oculogyric crisis and trismus. They respond rapidly to intravenous injection of an anticholinergic drug (e.g. procyclidine or benztropine). Some patients on neuroleptics who develop these reactions are also treated or cotreated with an oral anticholinergic.

Medication-induced parkinsonism

See above.

Akathisia

Akathisia is a restless, repetitive and irresistible need to move, usually caused by neuroleptics. It may cease with drug withdrawal or be treated with a benzodiazepine or propranolol.

Tardive dyskinesia

Tardive dyskinesia is a movement disorder that develops after chronic exposure to neuroleptics. It can be irreversible and may worsen when the offending medication is stopped. Involuntary movements affect the face, mouth and tongue (orobuccolingual movements) causing lip smacking, grimacing and dystonic grimacing. It can be avoided by using newer atypical neuroleptics. It is thought to be due to drug-induced supersensitivity of the dopamine receptors.

Neuroleptic malignant syndrome

Occasionally, dopamine receptor blocking drugs can cause this syndrome, which manifests with extreme rigidity, fluctuating conscious level, fever, autonomic disturbance and elevated serum creatine kinase. The drug in question should be withdrawn and the patient treated with a dopamine agonist/levodopa and dantrolene.

RESTLESS LEGS SYNDROME

This is a common syndrome that can be familial or sporadic. It can be associated with iron deficiency, anaemia, pregnancy, peripheral neuropathy or uraemia. Patients complain of an unpleasant sensation in their legs and an irresistible urge to move their legs, which is worst at night when they are resting or inactive. Symptoms are relieved by movement, and can be treated with dopaminergic medication.

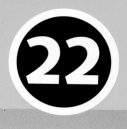
- Define the 12 cranial nerves and their functions
- Describe the most common pathologies affecting the cranial nerves
- Be able to infer the location of a lesion from the associated clinical symptoms and signs

The most common cranial nerve lesions and the symptoms and signs associated with them are summarized in Figure 22.1.

OLFACTORY NERVE (FIRST, I)

The most common causes of either hyposmia (diminished sense of smell) or anosmia (absent sense of smell) are nasal and sinus disease, often in association with smoking. Head injury can also cause anosmia secondary to trauma to the cribriform plate, severing the delicate olfactory sensory axons that pass through it. A tumour or other space-occupying lesion of the frontal lobe may occasionally cause anosmia by compression of the olfactory bulb and tract (e.g. meningioma of the olfactory groove). Neurodegenerative disorders such as Alzheimer's and Parkinson's disease can also cause a diminished sense of smell.

OPTIC NERVE (SECOND, II)

Visual field defects

Lesions at various points in the visual pathway cause characteristic patterns of visual field loss (see Ch. 8).

Papilloedema

Papilloedema refers to swelling, with elevation, of the optic disc, and is a term that should strictly only be used to refer to elevation of the optic disc caused by raised intracranial pressure. Initially, there is redness of the disc, with blurring of the margins and loss of retinal venous pulsation. Then there is loss of the physiological cup and the disc becomes engorged. In severe papilloedema, there may be retinal haemorrhages around the disc. It is typically bilateral. The causes of papilloedema are shown in Figure 22.2.

On clinical examination of papilloedema there is an enlarged blind spot, but usually no loss of visual acuity or visual disturbance unless the disc swelling is caused by local inflammation or infiltration of the optic nerve head, or acute ischaemia of the optic nerve. If papilloedema is severe, prolonged and untreated, there is often constriction of the visual fields and blindness due to infarction secondary to pressure on the blood vessels that supply the optic nerve. There may be transient visual obscurations, that is, transient loss of vision lasting a few seconds, and precipitated by measures that produce a transient rise in intracranial pressure such as coughing, bending and straining.

Optic neuritis

Optic neuritis describes acute inflammation of the optic nerve, and if the nerve head is involved, causing it to swell, it is termed papillitis. The most common cause of this is multiple sclerosis, though there are many other causes (Fig. 22.3).

In contrast to papilloedema, in optic neuritis there is early severe visual loss, especially to colour, but also to acuity, and there is often a central or paracentral scotoma (visual field defect). There may be an afferent pupillary defect. There is also often pain in or behind the affected eye, unlike in papilloedema. Anterior optic neuritis may cause swelling of the optic disc, but often the inflammatory process is in the posterior part of the nerve and is named 'retrobulbar neuritis'. The optic disc will be normal on ophthalmoscopy in retrobulbar neuritis. When optic neuritis is caused by multiple sclerosis, the prognosis for recovery of vision is very good. There is usually gradual improvement in vision over a few days, weeks or months, and patients often return to near-normal visual acuity. However, there is often a relative loss of colour vision and the visual evoked potentials show delay in conduction of signals from the eye to the occipital cortex. This and other causes of optic neuritis may result in permanent visual loss.

Fig. 22.1 Summary of the cranial nerves and the clinical features resulting from lesions of individual nerves

Cranial nerve number	Cranial nerve name	Symptoms and signs caused by lesions
1	Olfactory nerve	• Loss of smell/taste
2	Optic nerve	• Papilloedema/ papillitis • Visual field defect
3	Oculomotor nerve	• Ophthalmoplegia with diplopia • Pupillary dysfunction • Ptosis • Divergent strabismus
4	Trochlear nerve	• Diplopia (superior oblique palsy)
5	Trigeminal nerve	• Loss of sensation to the face • Weakness of muscles of mastication • Loss of corneal reflex
6	Abducens nerve	• Diplopia (lateral rectus palsy) • Convergent strabismus
7	Facial nerve	• Weakness of muscles of facial expression • Loss of taste (anterior two-thirds of the tongue) • Hyperacusis • Loss of tears
8	Vestibulocochlear nerve	• Loss of hearing and imbalance
9	Glossopharyngeal nerve	• Loss of taste (posterior one-third of the tongue) • Difficulties swallowing (motor and sensory loss) • Carotid sinus dysfunction
10	Vagus nerve	• Weakness of palate, vocal cords with swallowing difficulties
11	Accessory nerve	• Weakness of shrugging shoulders and head turning
12	Hypoglossal nerve	• Weakness of tongue movement

Fig. 22.2 Causes of papilloedema

• Raised intracranial pressure:
  • mass lesions – tumours, abscesses, haematomas
  • cerebral oedema – trauma, infarcts
  • increased CSF production – e.g. choroid plexus papilloma
  • decreased CSF absorption – e.g. arachnoid granulation post meningitis
  • obstructive hydrocephalus
  • obstruction of venous outflow – e.g. venous sinus thrombosis
  • idiopathic intracranial hypertension
• Raised optic nerve head due to medical causes – includes anaemia, hyperviscosity, diabetes, malignant hypertension
• Raised optic nerve head due to acute papillitis (Fig. 22.3)

Fig. 22.3 Causes of optic neuritis/neuropathy

• Inflammation (optic neuritis), e.g. multiple sclerosis, sarcoidosis, Behçet's
• Optic nerve compression, e.g. local fracture or cerebral tumour, aneurysm
• Infiltration, e.g. glioma, lymphoma
• Ischaemic, e.g. anterior ischaemic optic neuropathy (AION), including temporal arteritis
• Metabolic, e.g. vitamin B_{12} deficiency
• Toxins and drugs, e.g. tobacco – alcohol amblyopia, methanol, ethambutol
• Hereditary, e.g. Leber's optic neuropathy (mitochondrial cytopathy) Friedreich's ataxia
• Infective, e.g. direct spread from paranasal sinuses or orbital cellulitis, syphilis, Lyme disease, EBV
• Trauma

Optic atrophy

Optic atrophy is usually seen on ophthalmoscopy as a pale featureless disc and it may follow many different pathological processes, including any of the causes of optic neuropathy in Figure 22.3. It represents the end stage of damage to the optic nerve and patient's vision can be very poor (e.g. Leber's optic neuropathy) or near normal (e.g. multiple sclerosis).

OCULOMOTOR (THIRD, III), TROCHLEAR (FOURTH, IV) AND ABDUCENS NERVES (SIXTH, VI)

The oculomotor, trochlear and abducens nerves are considered together because they innervate the muscles responsible for movement of the eye. Lesions of these nerves cause the clinical sign of ophthalmoplegia,

Fig. 22.4 Conditions causing combined ocular palsies

Brainstem lesions	Multiple sclerosis Encephalitis Tumour, especially glioma
Multiple cranial neuropathies	Basal meningitis (TB, sarcoid, neoplastic, syphilis) Tumours (meningioma, lymphoma, chordoma) Cavernous sinus thrombosis
Neuromuscular disorders	Myasthenia gravis Botulinum toxin injection
Ocular muscle disorders	Thyroid eye disease Orbital myositis Infiltration, e.g. lymphoma Rare ocular myopathies Local trauma

Fig. 22.5 Causes of trigeminal nerve palsy according to site

Brainstem (nuclei and connections)	Multiple sclerosis Infarction Brainstem gliomas Syringobulbia
Cerebellopontine angle	Acoustic neuroma Meningioma
Cavernous sinus	Internal carotid aneurysm Meningioma Cavernous sinus thrombosis Carotico-cavernous fistula Extension of pituitary tumour
Gasserian (trigeminal) ganglion	Herpes zoster (shingles) Neoplastic infiltration Idiopathic trigeminal neuropathy (associated with connective tissue diseases including Sjögren's, rheumatoid arthritis, systemic lupus erythematosus, and systemic sclerosis)

which is weakness or paralysis of these muscles or dysfunction of the cranial nerve innervating these muscles, and the symptom of double vision or 'diplopia'. The causes and features of isolated ocular nerve palsies are considered in detail in Chapter 9.

Combined ocular palsies

Many conditions can cause combinations of third, fourth and sixth nerve palsies. Some of the more common causes are listed in Figure 22.4, including conditions that are not neuropathies but which produce similar clinical pictures.

TRIGEMINAL NERVE (FIFTH, V)

The sensory fibres of the trigeminal (fifth) nerve supply sensation to the face, including the cornea. The motor fibres supply the muscles of mastication. The sensory fibres are divided into three branches:

- Ophthalmic (V_1): which also supplies the cornea and is the afferent part of the corneal reflex
- Maxillary (V_2)
- Mandibular (V_3).

A lesion of the trigeminal nerve involving all segments will cause unilateral touch, pain and temperature sensory loss to the face, tongue and buccal mucosa, with reduction in the corneal reflex on the affected side. There will also be deviation of the jaw towards the side of the lesion when the mouth is opened if the motor component is involved.

The causes of a trigeminal nerve palsy are listed according to anatomical site in Figure 22.5.

Trigeminal neuralgia ('tic douloureux')

Trigeminal neuralgia is uncommon in young adults and mostly presents in those over the age of 75 years. There is a female:male ratio of about 2:1. It consists of sudden and severe paroxysms of electric-shock-like or shooting pain, usually in the V_2 and V_3 divisions of the trigeminal nerve, occurring up to several times per minute, and these may last from a few seconds up to 2 minutes. Often there may be brief, pain-free refractory periods where futher pain does not occur or cannot be triggered. The paroxysms of pain are usually stereotyped and can be triggered by certain stimuli (e.g. washing the face, shaving, cold wind or eating), or by touching a particular position on the face. It is unilateral in over 95% of cases, and may persist for days to months, but with a tendency for periods of remission to become shorter over time. The pain can be so severe as to cause the patient severe distress to the point of precipitating a reactive depressive illness. Idiopathic trigeminal neuralgia is not associated with any physical signs such as trigeminal sensory loss. Symptomatic trigeminal neuralgia refers to that caused by compression or infiltration of the trigeminal root by pathology such as a tumour or an arteriovenous malformation. In these cases the pain is not paroxysmal and there may be signs of trigeminal sensory loss. Multiple sclerosis can also cause trigeminal neuralgia from inflammation in the brainstem or secondary atrophic areas in the trigeminal root.

Patients should be investigated with MRI to exclude secondary causes. Medical treatment usually consists of carbamazepine, which acts as a membrane stabilizer and therefore reduces the frequency of spontaneous nerve impulses within the nerve. Alternatives with less evidence for their efficacy include gabapentin and lamotrigine. If symptoms are refractory to these medications, then surgical intervention may be required. Older surgical techniques such as obliteration of the trigeminal ganglion and root with a sclerosant or radiofrequency thermocoagulation of the ganglion are less popular now. Microvascular decompression is the surgical treatment of choice and aims to separate the nerve root from the vessel causing partial compression.

Postherpetic neuralgia

Herpes zoster (shingles) most commonly affects the dermatomes of the ophthalmic division of the trigeminal nerve and mid-thoracic sensory roots. The maxillary and mandibular trigeminal divisions may also be affected, although not typically in isolation. Pre-eruptive pain in these areas is common, and may last for several days before the rash of acute herpes zoster appears. The resolution of the vesicular eruptions may subsequently be followed by pain within the distribution of the affected divisions.

FACIAL NERVE (SEVENTH, VII)

The muscles of the upper part of the face have bilateral innervation from the motor cortex. An upper motor neuron lesion (i.e. above the level of the facial nucleus in the pons), such as a stroke or tumour, will cause contralateral weakness of the lower half of the face and spare eye closure and forehead movement. Weakness unilaterally of all the facial muscles (upper and lower face) is caused by a lower motor neuron lesion, i.e. facial nucleus or facial nerve.

The facial nerve carries mainly motor fibres supplying the muscles of facial expression. It also has a sensory component, subserving taste from the anterior two-thirds of the tongue, and a parasympathetic component to the lacrimal, submaxillary and submandibular glands (lacrimation and some of salivation). The most common cause of facial weakness is a supranuclear lesion (e.g. in the cerebral hemisphere), such as stroke or tumour, causing an upper motor neuron type of weakness.

The causes of lower motor neuron-type facial weakness are listed anatomically in Figure 22.6.

Bell's palsy

Bell's palsy is a common condition that presents with an acute lower motor neuron facial palsy, which is usually unilateral. It has an annual incidence of 20 per 100 000,

Fig. 22.6 Causes of facial weakness (lower motor neuron) according to site

Pons – there may be associated sixth nerve lesions (lateral rectus palsy), lesions of the parapontine reticular formation (failure of conjugate gaze towards the lesion) and lesions of the corticospinal tracts (contralateral hemiparesis)	• Demyelination – multiple sclerosis • Vascular lesions • Pontine tumours, e.g. glioma • Motor neuron disease
Cerebellopontine angle	• Acoustic neuroma • Meningioma • Basal meningitis (TB, sarcoid, syphilis, Lyme disease, neoplastic)
Within the petrous temporal bone	• Bell's palsy • Middle ear infection • Trauma • Herpes zoster (Ramsay Hunt syndrome) • Tumours, e.g. glomus tumour
Within the face – the branches emerge from the stylomastoid foramen and pierce the parotid gland to supply the muscles of facial expression	• Parotid gland tumours • Mumps • Sarcoidosis • Guillain–Barré syndrome • Mononeuritis multiplex
Other causes of facial weakness – often bilateral	Neuromuscular junction • Myasthenia gravis Myopathies • Myotonic dystrophy • Facio-scapulo-humeral muscular dystrophy

and though all age groups can be affected, it is most common in those aged 30 to 50 years. The exact cause and site of the pathology is uncertain. It may be related to inflammation of the facial nerve within the petrous temporal bone, and herpes viruses have been implicated in some studies. Bell's palsy may be preceded by a history of aching around the ear in the 24 hours before onset. The palsy is usually complete within a few hours. There should be no sensory loss in the face, though patients may complain of 'numbness' of the affected side. Depending on the location of the lesion (see Ch. 10), there may be other associated features. A lesion below the geniculate ganglion but above the chorda tympani may be associated with disturbed taste on the ipsilateral anterior part of the tongue. Patients may also notice hyperacusis as the stapedius muscle is supplied by a branch of the facial nerve proximal to the chorda tympani. If herpes zoster infection is responsible (Ramsay Hunt syndrome), herpetic vesicles on the pinna, or external auditory canal, will be seen. In these patients the eighth cranial nerve may also be affected, causing vertigo, deafness and tinnitus.

The prognosis is usually extremely good, with 80% of patients making a full recovery within 2–8 weeks. If recovery is delayed, the ultimate degree of recovery is often incomplete and may be accompanied by synkinesis or 'crocodile tears' due to aberrant reinnervation.

The use of a short course of high-dose steroids within the first week may speed the recovery. Treatment with aciclovir in Bell's palsy does take place but conclusive evidence is lacking, though it should be used in Ramsay Hunt syndrome. Eye care is important in those patients with incomplete lid closure, and includes regular lubrication and an eye patch to prevent corneal abrasions. Surgery may be required if there is incomplete recovery of facial movements.

Fig. 22.7	Neurological causes of deafness and vertigo
Brainstem	Demyelination (multiple sclerosis) Infarction (vertigo lasts minutes)
Eighth nerve	Acoustic schwannoma (rarely causes vertigo – more commonly deafness and ataxia) Basal meningitis Trauma
End-organ disease	Trauma Degenerative syndromes Vascular, including vasculitis Ménière's syndrome (vertigo lasts hours) Infection (herpes zoster, mumps, etc.) Benign positional vertigo (mainly vertigo rather than deafness and vertigo lasts seconds) Vestibular neuronitis (mainly vertigo rather than deafness and vertigo lasts days)

HINTS AND TIPS

Acoustic schwannomas are tumours of the eighth cranial nerve and often spare the motor fibres of the seventh nerve. Unfortunately, surgical removal of the tumour often involves sacrificing the seventh nerve and patients are then left with severe facial weakness postoperatively.

VESTIBULOCOCHLEAR NERVE (EIGHTH, VIII)

The vestibulocochlear (eighth) nerve has two components, the vestibular and cochlear components, which are responsible for hearing and balance, respectively. Lesions cause deafness, tinnitus, loss of balance, vertigo with or without vomiting, and the clinical sign of horizontal gaze-evoked jerky or rotary nystagmus.

Causes of deafness and vertigo are listed in Figure 22.7.

Cerebellopontine angle lesions

The most common lesions in the cerebellopontine angle are an acoustic schwannoma of the vestibular part of the eighth cranial nerve or a meningioma. Other causes include metastases and other primary tumours. Bilateral acoustic neuromas are diagnostic of neurofibromatosis type 2.

There is often additional involvement of the fifth and seventh cranial nerves, cerebellar connections, and sometimes the sixth nerve, because of their close proximity to each other as they leave the pons (see Ch. 30). This results in the clinical picture of unilateral progressive sensorineural deafness, occasional tinnitus, vertigo with or without nystagmus, loss of facial sensation including the corneal reflex, lower motor neuron pattern weakness of the muscles of facial expression (which suggests a malignant cause as benign lesions usually spare the seventh nerve in the early stages), cerebellar ataxia and sometimes diplopia due to damage to the sixth nerve.

To make the diagnosis requires magnetic resonance imaging focused on the internal auditory meatus and brainstem. The treatment is surgical for large tumours and radiotherapy for smaller tumours.

Ménière's disease

Ménière's disease tends to affect the 30-to-50-year-old age group. It can be unilateral involvement, but in up to 50% it can be bilateral. Excessive fluid in the vestibular system, caused by failure to reabsorb endolymph, causes recurrent episodes of disabling vertigo, transient sensorineural deafness, tinnitus and a feeling of pressure in the ears. The vertigo can last from 30 minutes to hours, during which the patient will be very unsteady and may have nystagmus with fast phase away from the affected ear. Even afterwards there may be a sense of imbalance. Ultimately, the vertigo diminishes but deafness often becomes permanent. In some cases the condition may remit at an earlier stage. Treatment is with episodic use of vestibular sedatives (e.g. cinnarizine, cyclizine, or prochlorperazine) and vestibular rehabilitation exercises. Thiazide diuretics and a low-salt diet may also reduce the excess of endolymphatic fluid that contributes to the symptoms.

Benign paroxysmal positional vertigo

Benign paroxysmal positional vertigo comprises transient vertigo lasting typically less than 30 seconds and is precipitated by head movements, usually due to particulate material in the posterior semicircular canal. Other forms of positional vertigo can occur following viral infection, trauma or age-related degenerative change in the labyrinth. Although the vertigo is brief, many patients can feel unsteady for hours to days. In benign positional vertigo, symptoms can be reproduced using Hallpike's manoeuvre, which involves tilting the patient backwards from a sitting position and turning the patient's head suddenly to one side when they are horizontal (see Ch. 11). Treatment is usually with specific repositioning manoeuvres, e.g. Epley's, or a programme of vestibular exercises. Central lesions can also cause positional vertigo, but on assessing patients with the Hallpike manoeuvre, there is no latent period, the nystagmus lasts longer and may be variable, and does not fatigue. Patients are not so symptomatic with centrally driven vertigo, and there are often other signs of brainstem or cerebellar disease.

Acute vestibular failure

Patients presenting with acute unilateral vestibular failure primarily have symptoms of severe vertigo, nausea and vomiting without cochlear symptoms (hearing loss, tinnitus). On examination there may be nystagmus present with the fast phase away from the affected ear and caloric testing may show ipsilateral canal paresis. Bedrest, antiemetics and vestibular sedatives are the main modes of treatment in the acute setting, and often symptoms will settle after 2–3 weeks. Causes can be uncertain but commonly include viral infections, where the term vestibular neuronitis or viral labyrinthitis may be used. It is important to be able to differentiate vestibular neuronitis from an acute vestibular syndrome arising from an inferior cerebellar/brainstem stroke. In the latter, in addition to the above symptoms, ataxia may also be prominent. Patients also tend to have vascular risk factors, and there may be other signs of brainstem dysfunction such as diplopia, dysarthria, dysphagia and sensory-motor deficits. The nystagmus may also be more complex with vertical or torsional components. Clearly, these patients needs to be scanned with MRI to look for evidence of infarction.

LOWER CRANIAL NERVES (GLOSSOPHARYNGEAL, VAGUS, ACCESSORY AND HYPOGLOSSAL)

Isolated palsies of the lower cranial nerves are rare. Combined palsies, especially involving the ninth, tenth and twelfth nerves, produce 'bulbar palsies' and are found with:

- brainstem infarcts
- motor neuron disease
- tumours: brainstem, nasopharyngeal carcinoma, glomus tumour
- polyneuropathy, e.g. Guillain–Barré syndrome
- myasthenia gravis
- polymyositis
- trauma, especially to the base of skull.

Jugular foramen syndrome

Cranial nerves IX, X and XI pass through the skull base in the jugular foramen. Pathology in this location, such as tumour, carcinomatous infiltration, granuloma or chronic meningitis, can therefore cause a combination of lower cranial nerve palsies which sometimes includes the hypoglossal nerve. If there is involvement of the brainstem, there may be an associated Horner's syndrome and long tract signs. These patients need imaging with MRI and CT, and treatment of the underlying cause of their presentation.

Diseases affecting the spinal cord (myelopathy)

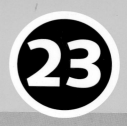

● Objectives

- Understand the anatomy of the spinal cord and be able to sketch a cross-section of the cord showing the central grey matter and major surrounding tracts
- Describe the syndromes of motor, sensory and sphincter dysfunction that arises from a spinal cord lesion
- Understand the clinical features arising from spinal cord compression, transverse myelitis, metabolic cord disease, intrinsic cord lesions or complete transection of the spinal cord
- Understand the causes of mixed upper and lower motor neuron signs in the limbs

ANATOMY

The spinal cord extends from the top of the C1 vertebra to the bottom of the body of the L1 or L2 vertebra in adults. There is an expansion in the diameter of the cord in the cervical and lumbar regions due to increased numbers of anterior horn motor cells to the arms and legs. The lower end of the spinal cord is known as the conus medullaris (Fig. 23.1). The spinal cord is continuous with the medulla oblongata superiorly, and inferiorly with the cauda equina and filum terminale. This is a thin connective tissue filament that descends from the conus medullaris with the spinal nerve roots. Thus, pathology at T12 and L1 affects the lumbar cord, at L2 affects the conus medullaris, and lesions below L2 involve the cauda equina and represent injuries to the spinal roots, rather than the spinal cord.

The spinal cord, cauda equina and filum terminale, down to the S2 level, is surrounded by a thick covering of dura mater, which is separated from the fine arachnoid mater by the potential subdural space. The arachnoid mater is separated from the pia mater, which invests the spinal cord and nerve roots, by the subarachnoid space.

A representative part of the spinal cord in cross-section is shown in Figure 23.2. It contains the central grey matter, consisting of neuronal cell bodies and the peripheral white matter, which contains the ascending and descending axonal pathways. The ascending pathways relay sensory information from the periphery to the brain, brainstem and cerebellum, and the descending pathways relay motor instructions from the brain. There are three main white matter tracts. The two main ascending tracts are the spinothalamic tract and dorsal columns and the main descending pathway is the lateral corticospinal tract (see Fig. 23.2 and Ch. 16).

Most of the main sensory and motor pathways cross to the contralateral side during their course in the CNS. It is important to know these sites of decussation because clinically different syndromes result from interruption of the pathways at various levels.

MAJOR PATHWAYS WITHIN THE SPINAL CORD

Pain and temperature

The dorsal nerve roots subserving pain and temperature enter the spinal cord and the fibres synapse within the dorsal horn. The second-order neurons immediately cross over to the opposite side of the cord and join the spinothalamic tract, which ascends to the thalamus. This pathway runs anterolaterally in the spinal cord (see Fig. 23.2).

A lesion of the spinothalamic tract on one side will result in loss of pain and temperature below the level of the lesion on the contralateral side.

Proprioception (joint-position sense) and vibration

Fibres carrying information regarding proprioception and vibration enter the spinal cord in the dorsal root and do not synapse but join the ipsilateral dorsal (posterior) columns. The posterior columns lie posteromedially in the spinal cord and ascend to synapse in nuclei at the lower end of the medulla (see Fig. 23.2 and Ch. 16). The second-order neurons cross over in the medulla to form the medial lemniscus, which ascends to the thalamus.

A lesion of the dorsal columns on one side will result in loss of proprioception and vibration below the level of the lesion on the ipsilateral side.

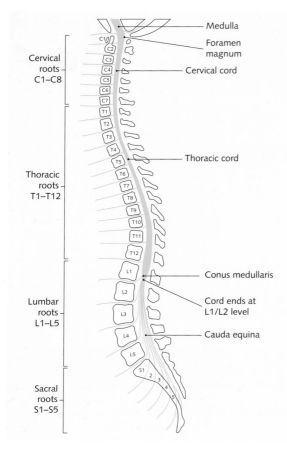

Cervical roots C1–C8

Medulla

Foramen magnum

Cervical cord

Thoracic roots T1–T12

Thoracic cord

Lumbar roots L1–L5

Conus medullaris

Cord ends at L1/L2 level

Cauda equina

Sacral roots S1–S5

Fig. 23.1 Anatomy of the spinal cord.

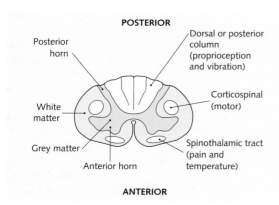

POSTERIOR

Posterior horn

Dorsal or posterior column (proprioception and vibration)

Corticospinal (motor)

White matter

Grey matter

Spinothalamic tract (pain and temperature)

Anterior horn

ANTERIOR

Fig. 23.2 A cross-section of the spinal cord, showing the positions of the major pathways.

Motor pathways

The corticospinal tracts begin in the motor area of the cerebral cortex as upper motor neurons and their axons descend ipsilaterally through the corona radiata and the internal capsule. The axons then cross in the medulla as the 'pyramidal decussation' and descend laterally in the spinal cord (see Fig. 23.2). The axons in the tracts enter the anterior horn of the spinal cord (see Ch. 15) and synapse on the lower motor neuron cell body or 'anterior horn cell'. Weakness can therefore be caused by lesions of either the upper motor neuron (UMN) or the lower motor neuron (LMN) (see Ch. 15). These two types of weakness have distinct clinical signs and symptoms that usually allow them to be differentiated and therefore enable gross anatomical localization of the lesion.

A lesion of the corticospinal tract on one side of the spinal cord will cause an ipsilateral upper motor neuron defect (spastic hemi- or monoparesis, clonus, brisk reflexes, and an extensor plantar response).

The clinical syndromes of spinal cord disease

There are three main motor syndromes associated with spinal cord disease:

- Paraparesis (UMN involvement of legs only)
- Tetraparesis (UMN involvement of all four limbs)
- Brown–Séquard syndrome (unilateral lesion causing UMN involvement of one side).

These three patterns of weakness are often associated with sensory signs. They may develop rapidly or slowly, and over days to months to years, depending on the cause. Any lesion involving the spinal cord results in a syndrome called a 'myelopathy'. If the lesion damages the anterior horn cells as well as the corticospinal tracts then the patient will have UMN signs below the level of the lesion and LMN signs at and about the level of the lesion. If a myelopathy occurs together with a radiculopathy (i.e. root involvement), then the condition is called a 'myeloradiculopathy'. For example, the most common cause of compression of the cervical spinal cord is due to 'wear and tear' osteoarthritis and degenerative changes within the cervical vertebrae or 'cervical spondylosis'. This leads to damage to the corticospinal tracts in the cervical cord, resulting in UMN signs in the legs (paraparesis) and sensory loss below the level of the lesion (sensory level) (i.e. 'myelopathy'), as well as LMN signs in the arms due to damage of spinal roots at the level of the spondylotic lesion, i.e. 'radiculopathy'.

Paraparesis (spastic paraparesis or paraplegia)

Paraparesis indicates bilateral upper motor neuron damage involving the axons that innervate the legs from both corticospinal tracts. The clinical signs include increased tone with spasticity, pyramidal distribution of weakness, increased reflexes with clonus and extensor plantar

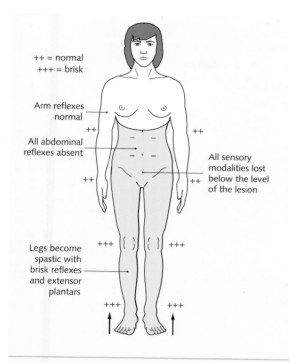

++ = normal
+++ = brisk

Arm reflexes
normal

All abdominal
reflexes absent

All sensory
modalities lost
below the level
of the lesion

Legs become
spastic with
brisk reflexes
and extensor
plantars

–, Absent reflex; +, Reduced reflex; ++, Normal
+++, Pathologically brisk reflex; ↑, Extensor plantar

Fig. 23.3   Clinical signs of cord compression caused by a lesion of the thoracic cord at the T7 level.

responses. The abdominal and cremasteric reflexes or 'cutaneous reflexes' may be absent (Fig. 23.3). There is often also involvement of the two sensory pathways from the level below the lesion. This is called a 'sensory level'. Sphincter dysfunction is also typical of spinal cord disease and occurs early with intrinsic spinal cord lesions and later in the course of extrinsic spinal cord lesions.

Tetraparesis (spastic tetraparesis, tetraplegia, quadriparesis and quadriplegia)

Spastic tetraparesis produces the same clinical picture as paraparesis but involves both arms and legs; it is usually caused by a lesion in the high cervical cord, but is occasionally due to brainstem or bilateral cortical damage.

Brown–Séquard syndrome (unilateral cord lesion)

Brown–Séquard syndrome is rare in its pure form but partial forms are more common.

The pure Brown–Séquard clinical picture (Fig. 23.4) consists of:

- ipsilateral spastic leg and sometimes arm if the lesion is above C5, with brisk reflexes and an extensor plantar response
- ipsilateral loss of joint-position sense and vibration (dorsal columns)
- contralateral loss of pain and temperature (spinothalamic tracts cross at their level of entry).

The sensory level is often a few segments lower than the level of the lesion because pain fibres ascend a few spinal segments before entering the dorsal horn to synapse then cross (see Ch. 16).

There are other less common clinical syndromes affecting the spinal cord which will be discussed below.

CAUSES OF SPINAL CORD DISEASE

Transection of the cord

Spinal cord transection is usually the result of trauma following anterior dislocation of one vertebra on another. The forces required to do this often result in associated fractures. It causes loss of all motor, sensory and autonomic function, including the sphincters, below the level of the lesion either immediately, if the transection is complete, or within hours if the damage is partial, but later results in secondary oedema causing involvement of the whole spinal cord at the level of the partial lesion.

With any severe, acute spinal cord lesion there are usually two clinical stages:

- **Spinal shock**: initially, there is loss of all reflex activity below the level of the lesion, with flaccid limbs, atonic bladder with overflow incontinence, atonic bowel, gastric dilatation and loss of genital reflexes and vasomotor control.
- **Heightened reflex activity**: this occurs after about 1–2 weeks and is associated with spasticity of the limbs, brisk reflexes and extensor plantar responses. Patients develop a spastic bladder (small capacity with urgency, frequency and automatic emptying) and hyperactive autonomic function (sweating and vasomotor changes).

HINTS AND TIPS

The supply to the diaphragm is via the phrenic nerve (C3, C4 and C5) and therefore any cord lesion above C3 may cause neuromuscular respiratory failure.

Fig. 23.4 Clinical signs of a Brown–Séquard lesion at level C7 on the left.

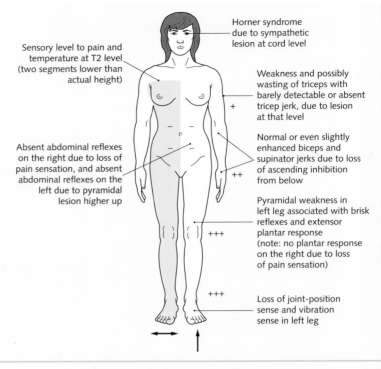

Horner syndrome due to sympathetic lesion at cord level

Sensory level to pain and temperature at T2 level (two segments lower than actual height)

Weakness and possibly wasting of triceps with barely detectable or absent tricep jerk, due to lesion at that level

Absent abdominal reflexes on the right due to loss of pain sensation, and absent abdominal reflexes on the left due to pyramidal lesion higher up

Normal or even slightly enhanced biceps and supinator jerks due to loss of ascending inhibition from below

Pyramidal weakness in left leg associated with brisk reflexes and extensor plantar response (note: no plantar response on the right due to loss of pain sensation)

Loss of joint-position sense and vibration sense in left leg

–, Absent reflex; +, Reduced reflex; ++, Normal
+++, Pathologically brisk reflex; ↑, Extensor plantar

Bilateral upper motor neuron signs in the legs (with or without arm involvement) with no cranial nerve signs usually indicate spinal cord pathology. The lesion must be above the body of L1, because the spinal cord ends at this level and lesions below this level involve the cauda equina and so cause lower motor neuron signs.

Differential diagnosis

In the absence of trauma, similar symptoms and signs of a very severe cord lesion should make one consider the following:

- Ischaemic infarction of the cord: occlusion of a major segmental artery, dissecting aortic aneurysm, vasculitis or anterior spinal artery thrombosis
- Haemorrhage into the spinal cord from an arteriovenous malformation, epidural or subdural haemorrhage
- Acute or subacute necrotizing or demyelinating myelopathy
- Epidural abscess
- Acute vertebral collapse – usually associated with neoplastic disease of the vertebrae.

Treatment

Complete transection of the spinal cord has a very poor neurological outcome. It is more usual for incomplete cord transection to occur. In this scenario, it is vital to treat any spinal fracture and instability with orthopaedic or neurosurgical input as this may prevent secondary damage to the intact cord from the spinal injury. The reduction of spinal cord oedema with immediate administration of high-dose corticosteroids may help.

Spinal cord compression

The clinical picture is determined by the site of compression or inflammation. Pain is the most common presenting symptom, followed by limb weakness, sensory loss and sphincter disturbance. Rarely, cord compression can present with ataxic symptoms, without pain. Lesions affecting the cord below T1 will not involve the arms, whereas lesions between C5 and T1 cause LMN and sometimes UMN signs in the arms, and UMN signs in the legs. Lesions above C5 cause UMN signs in the arms and legs. Compressive lesions may spare sphincter function until the patient has severe disease. Therefore, any patient with sphincter involvement needs urgent investigation.

Causes

- Trauma (see above)
- Degenerative disease – spondylotic/disc disease and spinal canal stenosis
- Tumours: metastatic or myeloma
- Infective lesions: epidural abscess, tuberculoma, HIV, HTLV-1, granuloma
- Epidural haemorrhage.

Degenerative disease – spondylotic/disc disease and spinal canal stenosis

Spondylosis is the term for degenerative changes within the spine that occur during ageing or secondary to trauma or rheumatological disease. The degenerative process starts with dehydration and disintegration of the nucleus pulposus, leading to a reduction in disc height and tears in the annulus fibrosus. This then causes loading and hypertrophy of the facet joints, bulging of the discs and ligamentum flavum hypertrophy, all of which contributes to narrowing of the spinal canal. Clinically the degenerative processes manifest in two ways, disc protrusion and spinal canal stenosis.

Damaged discs usually protrude laterally and cause compression of the nerve roots, resulting in a lower motor neuron lesion. The most common pathologies involve the most mobile parts of the spine which are the C5/C6 and C6/C7 discs, causing C6 and C7 radiculopathies (damage to the spinal segmental nerves) in the upper limbs, and L4/L5 and L5/S1 discs, involving the L5 and S1 spinal nerves in the lower limbs. However, discs can protrude centrally and posteriorly. This results in cord compression when it occurs above the level L1 and causes a spastic paraparesis (usually a low cervical or thoracic disc) or tetraparesis (high cervical disc), with variable sensory loss and sphincter dysfunction. If central disc protrusion occurs below the L1 vertebral level, the cauda equina will be affected and the patient will have a lower motor neuron syndrome affecting the legs and bladder (see Fig. 23.5).

In the cervical/thoracic spine, canal stenosis will cause compression of the spinal cord, while in the lumbar spine, canal stenosis will cause compression of the cauda equina. Canal stenosis can manifest in several ways: as a radiculopathy, cervical spondylotic myelopathy or neurogenic claudication. Localized areas of narrowing may cause compression of an individual nerve root, causing a painful radiculopathy. This is typically shooting in nature and referred into the dermatome of the affected root. The distribution of any neurological deficits (motor or sensory) will also be determined by the root affected. In the cervical spine, canal stenosis may cause compression of the spinal cord, causing a cervical spondylotic myelopathy. This may present clinically with a stepwise

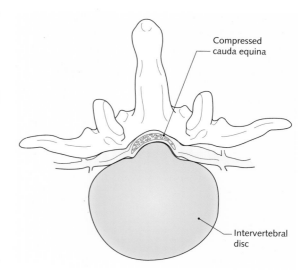

Fig. 23.5 Central disc protrusion compressing cauda equina below L1.

neurological deterioration. Initially, symptoms may begin in the legs with unsteadiness and difficulty walking, and there may be only mild signs in the arms. In the lumbar spine, canal stenosis may lead to compression of the cauda equina and may cause neurogenic claudication. This manifests as neurological symptoms of calf pain, weakness and sensory disturbance that worsen with walking, standing or maintaining certain postures, but ease with bending forwards, sitting or lying which enlarges the diameter of the spinal canal.

Treatment for degenerative spinal disease may be conservative (analgesia, anti-inflammatories, exercise and physiotherapy), or surgical when there is neurological compromise.

> **HINTS AND TIPS**
>
> It is important to remember that cervical cord compression can lead to a neurological deficit being confined to the legs, with only mild and subtle signs in the arms. Therefore, when requesting imaging studies for someone with symptoms and signs in the legs, the cervical spine should be assessed as well as the thoracic and lumbar spine.

Spinal cord tumours

Spinal cord tumours can be:

- **intramedullary** (within the substance of the spinal cord): these are usually malignant, e.g. glioma – ependymoma or astrocytoma causing an intrinsic cord lesion

- **intradural but extramedullary**, i.e. on the surface of the cord arising from the meninges (meningioma) or spinal root (schwannoma or neurofibroma), but within the dural sac. These are usually benign and present with spinal cord compression and back pain
- **extradural** (in the epidural space or within/between vertebrae): these are usually manifestations of multi-focal systemic neoplasia, e.g. metastatic carcinoma, lymphoma, myeloma, or can be other mass lesions, e.g. abscess, lipoma. Extradural tumours typically present with vertebral collapse or spinal cord compression.

Infective lesions

- Epidural abscess
- Tuberculoma
- HIV
- HTLV-1.

Infections in the spinal column occur in the facet joints (septic arthritis), the intervertebral disc (discitis) or within the vertebral bodies (osteomyelitis). Infections in the epidural space give rise to epidural abscesses, and are most often caused by *Staphylococcus aureus*. The organism usually reaches the cord via the bloodstream, but may spread directly from skin/soft tissue infections, or sites of invasive procedures or spinal surgery. Damage occurs through direct compression of nerve tissue or blood supply, thrombosis of veins, focal vasculitis or inflammation. The classic clinical triad consists of fever, spinal pain and neurological deficits. Diagnosis is made with magnetic resonance imaging (MRI) and lumbar puncture. Treatment is with appropriate antibiotics and surgical drainage. The treatment of the underlying source of infection is also important.

Tuberculomas are a frequent cause of cord compression in areas where tuberculosis (TB) is common (e.g. India, Pakistan, Africa, and in any areas populated from these countries of origin). It often occurs in the absence of pulmonary disease. Infection typically starts in a disc space, before spreading to form an epidural or paravertebral abscess. There may be destruction of vertebral bodies and spread of infection along the extradural space. This results in cord compression and paraparesis or 'Pott's paraplegia'. The clinical signs of TB meningitis may coexist. Diagnosis requires a high index of suspicion. The tuberculoma can be picked up on MRI, and *Mycobacterium tuberculosis* may be seen or grown from samples of cerebrospinal fluid. Treatment is with antituberculous therapy, as guided by the local microbiology sensitivities, but triple and often quadruple therapy is often needed. This is continued for at least 9 months and may be used in conjunction with the judicious use of corticosteroids for coexisting oedema.

Immunocompromised HIV patients carry an increased risk of pyogenic spinal infections, including *Staphylococcus aureus* and tuberculosis. In addition, they have a risk of opportunistic infections and, therefore, there should be a low threshold for investigating patients with HIV presenting with back pain, particularly those with a low CD4 count or high viral load. Patients with HIV are also at risk of developing spinal cord disease as a result of demyelination or vacuolar myelopathy.

Human T-cell lymphocytic virus type 1 (HTLV-1) also causes a progressive myelopathy primarily of the thoracic cord, which is otherwise known as tropical spastic paraparesis. Patients from tropical regions develop a progressive spastic paraparesis and urinary disturbance with sparing of the posterior columns.

Epidural haemorrhage and haematoma

Epidural or extradural haemorrhage and haematoma are rare sequelae of anticoagulant therapy, bleeding diatheses and trauma, including lumbar puncture. They often result in a rapidly progressive cord or cauda equina lesion, associated with severe pain. Treatment is surgical decompression, and management of any underlying disorder.

> **COMMUNICATION**
>
> Patients frequently do not clinically improve after decompression for cervical spondylosis, although myelopathic pain usually decreases with time. The main aim of decompression is to prevent progression of disease. This needs to be highlighted when discussing possible cervical decompressive surgery with patients.

Vascular cord lesions

Anterior spinal artery occlusion

Infarction of the spinal cord is rare in comparison with that of the brain. The blood supply of the spinal cord is predominantly from a single anterior and two posterior spinal arteries. The anterior artery supplies the anterior two-thirds of the spinal cord. It arises from the vertebral arteries in the neck, and is supported by radicular branches from the aorta. Anterior spinal artery occlusion is caused by thrombus or embolism, and the risk factors for these are identical to those for cerebral infarcts. Spinal cord infarction can also occur in the context of severe systemic hypotension or cardiac arrest. In an anterior spinal infarct, onset of symptoms is sudden and associated with back pain. Symptoms include paralysis, loss of bladder function and loss of pain and temperature below the level of the lesion. Position and vibration sense are spared. In the acute stage the weakness may be flaccid due to spinal shock, but this may progress to spasticity over time. The mid to lower thoracic region is the most vulnerable to ischaemia.

Dural ateriovenous fistulas

These are rare acquired lesions most typically seen in men over the age of 50 years. They exist on the dural surface and often affect the lower part of the spinal cord, including the conus medullaris. The most common presentation is of a progressive, stepwise myeloradiculopathy (or conus syndrome), probably related to venous hypertension. There is gradual loss of lower limb function with combined upper and lower motor neuron signs, and mixed cord and root sensory loss with saddle anaesthesia and bowel and bladder sphincter dysfunction. Some patients can also present with neurogenic claudication. The diagnosis is typically established with MRI/MRA and spinal angiography, and treatment involves endovascular embolization or surgical occlusion.

Intramedullary spinal arteriovenous malformations

These are congenital abnormalities consisting of arterial feeding vessels which drain into dilated, tortuous veins which are under high pressure. They can remain asymptomatic, but can present in patients in their 20s. Presentation can be with sudden loss of neurological function (associated with pain) below the level of the lesion as a result of haemorrhage or infarction. Patients can also present with stepwise neurological symptoms due to the mass effect of the lesion or due to spinal cord ischaemia resulting from vascular steal or venous hypertension. MRI/MRA can be used to diagnose these lesions, and they can be treated with endovascular occlusion or surgical resection.

Cavernous haemangiomas

These are capillary malformations that can occur within the spinal cord and in approximately one-third of cases are familial, and may be multiple. The whole spine and brain should, therefore, be imaged to exclude multiple lesions. Bleeding can occur from them, causing gradual loss of cord function distal to the lesion. The diagnosis is based on MRI alone, as angiography is unhelpful, and treatment is surgical.

Transverse myelitis

Transverse myelitis is a broad term used to describe segmental inflammation of the cord with resultant paraparesis (or tetraparesis), arising from a wide range of diseases. Most cases are idiopathic, but probably arise from an autoimmune process triggered by a preceding infection. Associations with transverse myelitis include:

- multiple sclerosis (MS) and, rarely, neuromyelitis optica
- viral infection – either as a result of direct virus infection or postviral demyelination, e.g. Epstein–Barr virus, varicella zoster, CMV, HSV, hepatitis C. It

should be noted that some viruses (e.g. enteroviruses such as poliovirus) selectively invade the anterior horn cells to produce asymmetrical flaccid weakness with absent reflexes and no sensory signs
- parasitic infection (e.g. schistosomiasis)
- sarcoidosis
- connective tissue diseases, e.g. systemic lupus erythematosus, Sjögren's, scleroderma, antiphospholipid syndrome, rheumatoid arthritis.

The inflammation of transverse myelitis is typically restricted to one or two segments and symptoms usually develop over several hours. Typically, the inflammation is bilateral with variable loss of distal motor, sensory and sphincter function, though unilateral syndromes have also been described. Almost all patients get leg weakness to varying degrees and arm weakness if the lesion is in the cervical cord. In addition to decreased sensation, pain and tingling are common and back and radicular pain may occur. The diagnosis is based on the clinical picture, MRI spine and CSF results. Treatment depends on the underlying cause but may include steroids.

Metabolic and toxic cord disease

Subacute combined degeneration of the cord

Subacute combined degeneration of the cord (SCDC) is the most important example of metabolic disease affecting the spinal cord and is caused by deficiency of vitamin B_{12}. The deficiency may result from nutritional deficiency (especially in vegans), pernicious anaemia, gastrectomy or disease of the terminal ileum (e.g. Crohn's disease, 'blind-loop' syndrome). Up to 25% of patients with neurological damage caused by vitamin B_{12} deficiency do not have haematological abnormalities (i.e. macrocytic megaloblastic anaemia). The deficiency causes a dorsal spinal cord syndrome; there is degeneration of the dorsal and lateral white matter of the spinal cord, producing a slowly progressive weakness, sensory ataxia and paraesthesias, and, ultimately, spasticity, paraplegia and incontinence. Other causes of a dorsal cord syndrome include multiple sclerosis, syphilis (tabes dorsalis), Friedreich's ataxia, vascular malformation, epidural and intradural extramedullary tumours, and cervical spondylotic myelopathy.

Treatment is with vitamin B_{12}, but this may not significantly improve the spinal cord damage. The condition can be made dramatically worse by giving folic acid without vitamin B_{12}.

Vitamin B_{12} deficiency can also cause damage to the peripheral nerves. The resulting syndrome is of a peripheral neuropathy, with a sensory ataxia due to loss of joint-position sense, and a spastic paraparesis. The full clinical picture of an upper motor neuron lesion in the legs is modified by the peripheral neuropathy (i.e. there is usually loss of ankle jerks but the plantar responses are usually extensor). Patients can also develop optic atrophy and a mild dementia.

Copper deficiency myeloneuropathy

A syndrome similar to the subacute combined degeneration of vitamin B_{12} deficiency can occur with acquired copper deficiency, which may be the result of gastrointestinal surgery, excessive zinc ingestion, or a primary disorder.

Intrinsic cord lesions

The signs of an intrinsic cord lesion are usually caused by MS. Much rarer causes include an intrinsic tumour or a syrinx (syringomyelia).

Syringomyelia and syringobulbia

Syringomyelia (relatively common) and syringobulbia (very rare) are caused by a fluid-filled cavity (syrinx) within the spinal cord and brainstem, respectively.

The cavitation of the cervical cord is associated, in the majority of cases, with a congenital abnormality of the foramen magnum, which is usually an Arnold–Chiari malformation. This causes the cerebellar tonsils to lie in the posterior foramen magnum and potentially they can compress the brainstem. A syrinx can also arise due to an intrinsic tumour or following traumatic or infectious, or inflammatory pathology. Most lesions are between C2 and T9, though they can extend upwards or downwards.

Clinically, there is an evolving picture as the expanding cavity damages the various neurons and pathways (Fig. 23.6). The signs can be unilateral, especially at

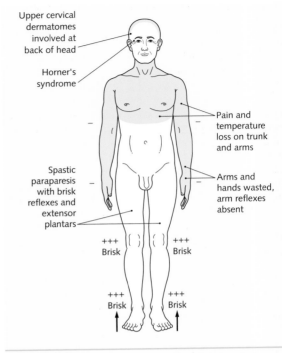

−, Absent reflex; ++, Normal; +++ Brisk; ↑, Extensor plantar

Fig. 23.6 The evolving pattern of an intrinsic cord lesion at T1. This pattern may be seen with syringomyelia and intrinsic cord tumours, e.g. glioma, ependymoma and astrocytoma.

presentation, but are ultimately bilateral, though there may be asymmetry:
- Pain in the upper limbs is often an early feature, which may be exacerbated by coughing or straining if associated with an Arnold–Chiari malformation.
- Dissociated spinothalamic sensory loss (i.e. loss of crossing pain and temperature fibres, but preservation of vibration and joint position pathways) in a 'cape-like' or 'suspended' distribution (i.e. the dermatomes above and below the level of the syrinx are spared). In advanced cases the impairment of pain sensation may lead to the development of neuropathic or Charcot joints in the hand, elbow or shoulder.
- There is unilateral or bilateral Horner's syndrome (meiosis, ptosis and anhydrosis) due to damage to sympathetic fibres within the spinal cord down to T1.
- There is wasting and weakness of the small muscles of the hand due to damage of the anterior horn cells at the level of T1 (a common site for a syrinx).
- Spastic paraparesis develops only after the cavity is markedly distended and compresses on the corticospinal tracts.

- Ultimately, the posterior columns may also become affected.

  With syringobulbia, there is also:

- bilateral wasting and weakness of the tongue
- hearing loss
- vestibular involvement with nystagmus
- facial sensory loss.

  Treatment of a syrinx associated with a Chiari malformation is surgical decompression of the foramen magnum.

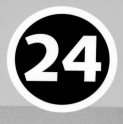
- Define 'upper motor neuron', 'lower motor neuron' and 'motor unit'
- Describe the types of motor neuron disease (MND)
- Understand how to diagnose MND
- Understand the management of MND

The motor neuron cell bodies within the primary motor cortex (pre-central gyrus of the frontal cortex) and their axons, which descend down to synapse with the motor nuclei of the cranial nerves and the anterior horn cells, are called the upper motor neurons (UMNs); the cell body of the anterior horn cell and its axon that projects to muscle via the nerve roots, plexus and peripheral nerves is the lower motor neuron (LMN) (see Ch. 15). Features of UMN and LMN defects are listed in Figure 24.1. Each LMN extends peripherally to innervate a variable number of skeletal muscle fibres (from 20 to over 1000). The motor neuron, and the muscle fibres it supplies, is known as a 'motor unit'.

TYPES AND CLINICAL FEATURES OF MOTOR NEURON DISEASE

Motor neuron disease (MND) is a disease in which there is progressive degeneration of motor neurons in the motor cortex and in the anterior horns of the spinal cord. There is also degeneration of the cells within the somatic motor nuclei of the cranial nerves within the brainstem. There is usually relentless progression of the disease to death within 1–5 years.

MND encompasses a number of conditions that affect motor neurons. These include: amyotrophic lateral sclerosis (ALS), progressive bulbar palsy (PBP), primary lateral sclerosis (PLS) and primary muscular atrophy (PMA). These categories do not represent distinct aetiological or pathological mechanisms, and often with disease progression the clinical features of all the groups merge. Originally MND was thought to affect only motor neurons, but it is now increasingly recognized that other systems, including cognitive centres, cerebellar, and extrapyramidal pathways, as well as the sensory system, can be affected. MND may, therefore, be

better thought of as a multisystem disease, with a relative preponderance for motor neurons.

Amyotrophic lateral sclerosis

Amyotrophic lateral sclerosis (ALS) is often used synonymously with MND in the USA and in Europe. It has an incidence of 2 per 100 000 per year, affects males more than females (M:F = 2:1), a mean age of onset of 60 years, and a mean duration of survival of 3 years. In the UK, it is used to represent a particular form of MND with a mixture of UMN and LMN signs in the limbs, head, neck and bulbar region (Fig. 24.2). Degeneration of the UMNs gives rise to increased tone, pyramidal distribution weakness and brisk reflexes with extensor plantars. LMN involvement may give rise to muscle cramps, fasciculations, including of the tongue, wasting and weakness. All these features may occur in combination within a body region.

Onset of disease tends to be focal, distal and asymmetrical, and progresses in a segmental fashion from one limb to another. A small proportion of patients may present with symmetrical, proximal flaccid weakness of the arms, with sparing elsewhere, though as the disease progresses UMN signs will develop. This is known as the 'flail arm variant' of MND.

In addition to motor features, it is now also increasingly recognized that up 50% patients with MND may also have cognitive impairment, with up to 10% fulfilling the diagnostic criteria for frontotemporal dementia (FTD). Thus, MND and FTD may represent two ends of a disease continuum.

Progressive muscular atrophy

Progressive muscular atrophy (PMA) is associated with LMN signs (wasting, weakness and fasciculations, although tendon reflexes are usually preserved), which often begin asymmetrically in the small muscles of the hands or feet and spread. This form often progresses to include UMN signs with time.

Fig. 24.1 Features of upper and lower motor neuron lesions

Upper motor neuron	Lower motor neuron
Spastic paralysis	Flaccid paralysis
No wasting	Muscle wasting
No fasciculations	Fasciculations present
Brisk reflexes	Reduced or absent reflexes
Clonus	No clonus
Extensor plantar response (Babinski)	Plantar response flexor or absent

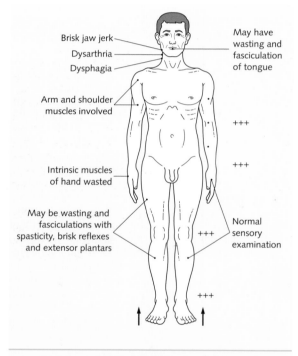

Brisk jaw jerk
Dysarthria
Dysphagia

May have wasting and fasciculation of tongue

Arm and shoulder muscles involved

+++

+++

Intrinsic muscles of hand wasted

May be wasting and fasciculations with spasticity, brisk reflexes and extensor plantars

+++

Normal sensory examination

+++

++, Normal; +++, Pathologically brisk reflex; ↑, Extensor plantar

Fig. 24.2 Clinical findings in a patient with classic amyotrophic lateral sclerosis with a mixture of upper and lower motor neuron signs. There is often a mixed bulbar and pseudobulbar picture, e.g. wasted, fasciculating tongue with a spastic palate, which may remain isolated or be the presenting feature of amyotrophic lateral sclerosis.

Progressive bulbar and pseudobulbar palsy

'Bulbar' refers to the lower brainstem motor nuclei. 'Bulbar' palsy usually refers to involvement of the LMN with prominent fasciculations in the tongue, often with wasting, in addition to a weak palate with nasal regurgitation and a nasal voice. 'Pseudobulbar' palsy involves the UMN bilaterally and leads to a spastic dysarthria ('Donald Duck' voice), dysphagia, hypersalivation, laryngospasm and emotional lability ('pseudobulbar affect'). Approximately 25% of MND patients may present with bulbar onset, with symptoms and signs restricted to the tongue and muscles innervated by the lower cranial nerves. Most of these patients will go on to develop classical ALS/MND. Those whose disease remains restricted to the bulbar region tend to have a worse prognosis, due an increased risk of aspiration. These patients often lose the ability to speak also, due to lack of movement of the tongue, palate and mouth.

Primary lateral sclerosis

A small number of patients (typically 1 to 5%) may present solely with UMN signs, typically initially in the legs before progressing to involve the arms and bulbar muscles. This variant is known as primary lateral sclerosis, and the diagnosis can only be made once other conditions are excluded, and the signs have remained solely UMN for at least 3 years. Unlike the other variants, these patients tend to have a slower progression and better prognosis.

Eye movements and sphincter involvement are never affected in MND and their abnormality virtually excludes the diagnosis. Respiratory muscles may be involved and occasionally patients present with type 2 respiratory failure from the onset. Patients may complain of sensory symptoms, including pain in the limbs, but have no sensory signs. They may also experience troublesome cramps, especially at night.

PATHOGENESIS

The majority of cases of MND are sporadic with no family history. Familial cases account for between 5 and 10% of patients. The most common familial form is due to abnormal expression of the superoxide dismutase-1 gene (SOD-1) found on chromosome 21, which typically causes autosomal dominant ALS. Our understanding of the genetic basis of this condition has recently expanded, with the discovery that in both familial and sporadic ALS, ubiquitin-positive neuronal cytoplasmic inclusions within the motor neurons are present, and these contain the nuclear protein TDP-43. This protein is also found in ubiquitin-positive frontotemporal lobe dementia. The pathological overlap between these two conditions mirrors the clinical overlap described above, and a number of genetic mutations are now being identified that are thought to play a role in this overlap, the most recent and important being the gene C9orf72 on chromosome 9.

DIFFERENTIAL DIAGNOSIS

The differential diagnosis depends on the mode of presentation.

Amyotrophic lateral sclerosis

Differential diagnoses for ALS include conditions that present with a mixture of UMN and LMN signs:

- Cervical spondylotic radiculomyelopathy: combination of spinal cord compression (UMN), spinal root compression and anterior horn cell loss (LMN)
- Spinal tumours: can cause LMN signs at the level of the pathology and also UMN signs below the level of the lesion
- Spinal conus medullaris lesions: can present with a mixture of UMN and LMN features
- Hyperthyroidism: wasted, fasciculating muscles secondary to a myopathy with brisk reflexes.

Progressive muscular atrophy

Differential diagnoses for PMA include conditions with LMN signs only:

- Spinal muscular atrophy: a heterogeneous hereditary condition with anterior horn cell loss
- Inclusion body myositis: a common cause of myopathy in older patients (see Ch. 28)
- Poliomyelitis (new onset is rare in the UK)
- Postpolio syndrome: progressive weakness and wasting 30–40 years after having had polio, which usually affects limbs involved in the initial disease. The exact cause is uncertain, but it does not involve reactivation of the poliomyelitis virus
- Multifocal motor neuropathy with conduction block: autoimmune condition with high levels of anti-GM1 antibody. This is treatable with intravenous immunoglobulin and immunosuppression
- Lead neuropathy.

Pseudobulbar/bulbar palsy

Differential diagnoses for pseudobulbar palsy include conditions that cause bilateral UMN lesions:

- Cerebrovascular disease can cause a pseudobulbar palsy as well as UMN signs in the limbs
- Multiple sclerosis usually gives a pseudobulbar picture, but this is often in association with cerebellar features, optic atrophy and other brainstem syndromes
- Kennedy's disease (spinal bulbar muscular atrophy): an X-linked recessive hereditary condition giving rise to a slowly progressive lower motor neuron syndrome with predominant bulbar and facial muscle involvement as well as axial and limb weakness. Patients may also have sensory symptoms, and gynaecomastia and testicular atrophy.

Differential diagnosis for bulbar palsy (i.e. an LMN syndrome with no UMN features), include:

- myasthenia gravis
- multiple lower cranial nerve lesions caused by infiltrating skull base tumours, e.g. nasopharyngeal carcinoma and glomus tumours
- rare neuropathies presenting with bulbar weakness, e.g. rare cases of Guillain–Barré or diphtheria.

DIAGNOSIS

The diagnosis is made clinically and this is supported by electromyography (EMG), which shows the presence of denervation (fibrillation potentials and positive sharp waves) in the muscles supplied by more than one spinal region. The presence of EMG changes in the tongue in association with changes in the limbs is often helpful in confirming the diagnosis. Nerve conduction studies may show a reduction in motor nerve conduction amplitudes (see Ch. 3). Prolonged central motor conduction times (CMCTs) may be useful for detecting clinically silent UMN lesions.

Other conditions must be excluded if suspected. This may require MRI of the brain and spinal cord in order to exclude skull base lesions, and cervical myeloradiculopathies, which may present with mixed UMN and LMN features.

TREATMENT

There is no cure for MND. The diagnosis should be carefully and fully discussed with the patient and carers. Ideally, counselling and multidisciplinary support should be available.

Drug treatment

Riluzole, a glutamate receptor antagonist, has been shown to increase survival by 2–3 months, but it has no effect on disability; it is now recommended by National Institute for Clinical Excellence (NICE) in those patients with probable or definite ALS. Liver enzymes should be checked regularly while a patient is taking it.

Symptomatic treatment

Symptomatic treatment is of paramount importance in MND and includes:

- speech therapy and communication aids
- treatment to reduce or thicken secretions for sialorrhoea caused by dysphagia and weak facial muscles
- altered food consistency for safe swallowing and, ultimately in some cases, a percutaneous endoscopic gastrostomy (PEG) or radiologically inserted gastrostomy (RIG)
- baclofen or tizanidine for spasticity
- appropriate management of pain, cramps and affective symptoms
- physiotherapy, splints, walking aids and wheelchairs
- adaptations to allow patients to stay at home
- full palliative care in the terminal stages
- patients often have nocturnal hypoventilation due to neuromuscular respiratory weakness. This can often be helped with non-invasive respiratory support (NIPPV, CPAP), and there are clear guidelines to their use outlined by NICE.

HINTS AND TIPS

Some groups of motor neurons are spared in MND. These include motor nerves from the oculomotor nuclei responsible for eye movements, and those from Olaf's nucleus in the sacral spinal cord and important for bladder and bowel control. Sensory signs also do not occur in pure MND, though up to one-quarter of patients may complain of mild sensory symptoms.

COMMUNICATION

When assessing a patient for possible MND, specific enquiries should be made about breathing difficulties. Often patients may present with subtle features of respiratory muscle/diaphragm weakness and central hypoventilation. These include symptoms such as orthopnoea, morning headaches, daytime somnolence and fatigue.

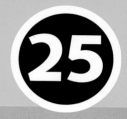

Radiculopathy and plexopathy 25

● **Objectives**

- Understand the anatomy of the spinal nerve roots
- Describe the clinical features associated with radiculopathy
- Understand the difference in the clinical features between a central and lateral lumbar and cervical disc protrusion
- Describe the common causes of plexopathy

ANATOMY

Thirty paired spinal nerve roots provide the means of entry and exit of information from the CNS. The dorsal root contains the sensory (afferent) fibres arising from sensory receptors in the periphery, as well as a collection of sensory cell bodies, termed the dorsal root ganglion (Fig. 25.1). The ventral (anterior) root contains the motor (efferent) fibres derived from the anterior horn cell bodies in the anterior horn of the spinal cord grey matter (see Fig. 25.1). The dorsal and ventral spinal roots lie within the spinal subarachnoid space and come together at the intervertebral foramen to become a mixed sensorimotor nerve called the spinal root.

The spinal roots are named by the vertebral level at which they emerge from the spinal cord. In the cervical region, the roots exit above each vertebral body and there are therefore eight cervical roots (C1–C8), even though there are only seven cervical vertebrae. By contrast, at all other levels the roots emerge below the respective vertebral body (i.e. T1–T12, L1–L5) (see Fig. 25.1).

After emerging from the intervertebral foramina, the spinal roots pass into the brachial plexus to supply the upper limb or into the lumbosacral plexus to supply the lower limb. In the thoracic region, they form the intercostal nerves, which supply sensation and motor activity to the chest and upper abdominal wall.

The brachial plexus lies in the posterior triangle of the neck, between scalenius anterior and scalenius medius, and is derived from the C5–T1 spinal roots. At the root of the neck, the plexus lies behind the clavicle. The plexus gives off several motor branches before forming the 'cords' and ultimately becomes the median (C6, C7, C8, T1), ulnar (C8, T1) and radial nerves (C5, C6, C7, C8, T1) (see Ch. 15).

The lumbosacral plexus is subdivided into the lumbar plexus (T12–L5) and the sacral plexus (L4–S3) (see Ch. 15). The lumbar plexus is located in the psoas muscle and forms the femoral nerve (L2, L3, L4), which supplies the anterior thigh muscles and knee extensors. The sacral plexus is on the posterior wall of the pelvis and forms the sciatic nerve (L4, L5, S1, S2, S3), which supplies the hip extensors and knee flexors. The sciatic nerve consists of two parts: those nerves that will form the common peroneal nerve (L4, L5, S1, S2 posterior divisions) and the tibial nerve (L4, L5, S1, S2 anterior divisions), which supplies the ankle invertors and plantar flexors. The common peroneal nerve further divides into the superficial peroneal nerve, which supplies the ankle evertors, and the deep peroneal nerve, which supplies the toe and ankle dorsiflexors.

When a spinal nerve root is damaged, the patient is said to have a 'radiculopathy' and when a plexus is damaged, the patient is said to have a 'plexopathy'.

RADICULOPATHY (SPINAL NERVE ROOT LESIONS)

Nerve roots may be affected by pathology, causing symptoms and signs referred to that root. Causes of radiculopathy include:

- cervical and lumbar spondylosis (degenerative changes including disc prolapse and osteophytes – see Ch. 23)
- trauma
- tumours, e.g. neurofibroma, neuroma, lymphoma, metastases
- herpes zoster virus (shingles)
- meningeal inflammation and infiltration
- diabetes
- arachnoiditis, e.g. chemical or infections, such as TB.

The most common cause is degenerative changes affecting the cervical and lumbar regions.

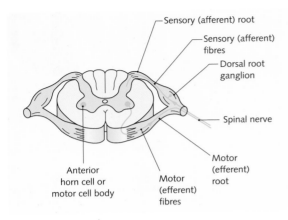

Fig. 25.1 Anatomy of spinal roots.

Clinical features

- Pain: severe, sharp, shooting and/or burning pain radiating into the cutaneous distribution (dermatome) or muscle group (myotome) supplied by the root. It can be aggravated by movement, straining or coughing. Pain may also arise from the soft tissues and joints
- Neurological signs: lower motor neuron signs, i.e. wasting with or without fasciculations, flaccid weakness and reduced/absent reflexes in the affected myotome and sensory impairment in the affected dermatome.

Specific radiculopathies

Lateral cervical disc protrusion

Lateral disc protrusion in the cervical region often causes severe pain in the upper limb. A C6/C7 disc protrusion causing a C7 radiculopathy is the most common lesion followed by a C5/C6 disc lesion affecting C6. T1 radiculopathy is rarely caused by spondylotic disease and, if present, should be investigated promptly.

In cervical radiculopathies, there is root pain that radiates into the affected dermatome (into the middle finger with a C7 lesion). Subsequently, there is wasting and weakness of the muscles innervated by the root (triceps, and wrist and finger extensors in a C7 lesion), and the reflexes involved in this root will be lost (triceps jerk in a C7 lesion). If the compression is severe the nerve root may infarct, leading to loss of pain, but the motor features will remain.

Lesions can be visualized on magnetic resonance imaging (MRI) or myelography with computed tomography (CT). Most cases in which pain is the only symptom recover with rest, the aid of a neck collar, and analgesia as the disc prolapse resolves spontaneously. When recovery is delayed, and especially if motor neurological signs exist or there is severe intractable pain, surgical spinal root decompression may be performed.

In some cases, the patient may have a central and a lateral disc protrusion, in which case the patient may have cervical cord compression with upper motor neuron signs in the legs and a sensory level as well as the radiculopathy at the level of the lesion, and disturbed bladder and bowel function. In older patients, cervical spondylotic changes themselves (see Ch. 23) can compress the nerve roots, spinal cord or both, causing a spondylotic radiculomyeloathy.

Lateral lumbar disc protrusion

The most common lesion in the lumbar region causes compression of L5 and S1 roots due to lateral prolapse of L4/L5 and L5/S1 discs, respectively (Fig. 25.2). This results in low back pain and 'sciatica', which is pain radiating down the buttock and back of the leg to the foot (and does not refer to disease of the sciatic nerve). Mechanical pain alone without a radiculopathy only causes pain to radiate as far down as the knee. If the pain is particularly severe or there are atypical features, consider rarer causes such as tumours, neoplastic, infectious or inflammatory infiltration, structural causes or, very rarely, diabetic infarction.

In sciatica there is limitation of straight-leg-raising in the affected leg due to pain referred in a sciatic distribution. This is caused by root tension that stretches the affected root. This pain may be aggravated by dorsiflexion of the foot. There may be weakness of extension of the great toe (L5) or of plantar flexion (S1). The reflexes may be lost (ankle jerk in an S1 root lesion, or, rarely,

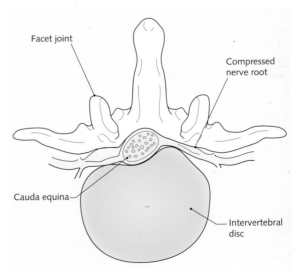

Fig. 25.2 Lateral disc protrusion in the lumbosacral region.

the knee jerk in an L3/L4 lesion). Sensory loss may be found in the affected dermatome.

Investigations include MRI or myelography if MRI is not available. Most cases of disc protrusion resolve with rest and analgesia, but decompressive surgery may be required.

Central lumbar disc protrusion

The spinal cord ends at L1/L2. A central disc protrusion below this level will result in a polyradiculopathy and not a myelopathy. Multiple nerve roots (cauda equina) may be involved and will cause lower back pain with radiation down the legs, lower motor neuron weakness of the legs and feet, sacral numbness, retention of urine, bowel dysfunction and impotence.

The onset may be acute, causing a flaccid paraparesis, or chronic, producing symptoms similar to intermittent claudication caused by vascular insufficiency; this is called 'neurogenic claudication'. A patient with back pain who develops retention of urine should be suspected of having a central lumbar disc protrusion. Urgent imaging and decompression should follow.

HINTS AND TIPS

It is a common mistake to assume that a central lumbar disc protrusion causes spinal cord compression. The spinal cord ends at L1/2 and, therefore, the more common central disc protrusions (L4/5 or L5/S1) cause damage to the cauda equina, which is the loose bundle of nerve roots descending through the lumbosacral canal. The resulting syndrome is, therefore, a lumbosacral polyradiculopathy, i.e. pure LMN weakness with sensory loss in a dermatomal pattern (perineum and backs of legs) with severe sphincter dysfunction and reflex loss. Any patient presenting with lumbosacral root symptoms should be questioned about bowel and bladder function, and erectile dysfunction in the male. Furthermore, these patients should have a rectal (and pelvic where appropriate) examination to exclude palpable masses, and their sacral dermatomes and anal sphincter tone should be assessed.

PLEXOPATHIES

Disease of the brachial and lumbosacral plexuses is relatively uncommon. Several specific conditions affect the plexuses. The clinical features of a plexopathy will reflect motor and sensory findings extending over more territory than that of a single nerve root or peripheral nerve.

Brachial plexopathies

Causes of brachial plexopathies include:

- trauma
- neuralgic amyotrophy
- malignant infiltration
- radiotherapy
- compression, e.g. thoracic outlet syndrome (cervical rib or fibrous band).

Trauma

Trauma is the most common cause of a brachial plexus lesion and, in severe cases, early referral to a specialist unit with experience in the surgical repair of plexus injuries is advised as some recovery of function can be obtained even with complete disruption:

- Upper plexus lesion (C5, C6): upper plexus injury is usually caused by falling on the shoulder or traction on the neck and shoulder at birth ('Erb's palsy'). It is associated with the characteristic posture of a 'waiter's tip' with the arm internally rotated, extended, and slightly adducted with loss of shoulder abduction and elbow flexion. Sensory loss occurs in the outer aspect of the shoulder, arm, forearm and thumb in the C5, C6 dermatomes.
- Lower plexus lesion (C8, T1): lower plexus injury is usually caused by forced abduction of the arm, which may occur at birth ('Klumpke's palsy') and following trauma in later life, e.g. motorcycle accidents. There is characteristically a 'clawed hand' with loss of function of the intrinsic muscles of the hand and long flexors and extensors of the fingers as well as loss of sensation in C8 and T1 dermatomes and a Horner's syndrome.

Neuralgic amyotrophy (acute brachial neuropathy, brachial neuritis)

Neuralgic amyotrophy is a condition in which severe pain in the muscles of the shoulder is followed 2–7 days later, as the pain resolves, by rapid wasting and weakness in the proximal, more commonly than distal, muscles of the arm. It may occur bilaterally and tendon reflexes may be lost in the affected limb. Sensory findings are usually minor. It may follow an infection, inoculation or surgery, but most often a precipitating cause is not found. It is thought to be caused by an inflammatory process affecting the nerve roots and plexus, often causing demyelination and subsequent axonal degeneration. Recovery is gradual over many months, but may not be complete. Recurrent episodes can occur. A very similar process can affect the lumbosacral plexus.

Episodic painful brachial neuropathy may be a presenting symptom of hereditary neuropathy with liability to pressure palsies (HNPP). HNPP shows autosomal dominant inheritance and is characterized by episodes of mononeuropathy at vulnerable sites of nerve compression. A more generalized peripheral neuropathy may be evident upon clinical examination. Mildly reduced nerve conduction velocities are usually associated with a deletion of the PMP22 gene on chromosome 17. The same gene can be affected by different mutations and cause Charcot–Marie–Tooth disease type 1.

Malignant infiltration

Invasion of the brachial plexus usually occurs in association with metastatic or locally invasive breast carcinoma and can occur many years after the initial tumour was diagnosed and treated. There is usually severe and intractable pain in the arm.

Pancoast tumour

An apical lung tumour (usually squamous cell carcinoma) can involve the brachial plexus by affecting C8/T1-derived roots.

Clinically, the patient has:

- severe pain in the arm
- ipsilateral weak and wasted hand
- sensory loss (C8, T1)
- Horner's syndrome.

Radiotherapy-induced plexopathy

Irradiation of the brachial plexus following breast carcinoma can lead to damage of the brachial plexus, especially the lower parts. The onset is usually delayed between 5 and 30 months and can be difficult to differentiate from metastatic breast cancer clinically and radiologically.

Compression

Cervical rib (thoracic outlet syndrome)

A fibrous band or cervical rib extending from the tip of the transverse process of C7 to the first rib can stretch the lower part of the brachial plexus (C8, T1). There is pain along the ulnar border of the forearm and sensory loss initially in the distribution of T1, with wasting of the abductor pollicis brevis more than the interossei or hypothenar muscles (Gilliatt-Sumner hand). There might also be a Horner's syndrome. Patients often complain of pain in the shoulder and numbness in the forearm especially on carrying heavy objects.

Some patients also develop a vascular syndrome if there is compression of the subclavian artery or vein by a cervical rib or fibrous band. This will be associated with vascular symptoms, such as an audible bruit in the supraclavicular fossa, unilateral Raynaud's phenomenon, pallor of the limb on elevation and loss of the radial pulse on abduction and external rotation of the shoulder. This is known as Adson's sign.

The vascular and neurological syndromes rarely coexist. Treatment is surgical decompression.

Lumbosacral plexus

Symptoms of a lumbosacral plexus lesion may be unilateral or bilateral. Diabetic 'amyotrophy' and malignant infiltration in the pelvis are the most common causes. Weakness, reflex change and sensory loss depend on the location and extent of plexus damage. In general, the following features are found:

- Upper plexus lesion: weakness of hip flexion and adduction, with anterior leg sensory loss.
- Lower plexus lesion: weakness of the posterior thigh (hamstrings) and foot muscles, with posterior leg sensory loss.

Diabetic amyotrophy

Diabetic amyotrophy is usually seen in older men with mild-to-moderate diabetes and may be associated with periods of poor glycaemic control. The site of the pathology may be in the lumbosacral plexus or in the roots and may have an inflammatory aetiology. Patients present with painful wasting – usually strikingly asymmetrical – of the quadriceps and psoas muscles. There is loss of the knee jerks and extreme tenderness in the affected area. There is usually minimal sensory loss. It resolves with careful control of blood glucose over many months.

Other causes of a lumbosacral plexopathy:

- **Infiltration by neoplasia**, e.g. prostate, ovarian and cervical, can infiltrate or metastasize to the lumbosacral plexus. This is usually associated with severe pain in the pelvis or/and legs
- **Radiotherapy**
- **Trauma** following abdominal or pelvic surgery, e.g. hysterectomy
- **Compression** from an abdominal aortic aneurysm or retroperitoneal haematoma.

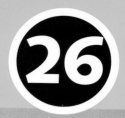
Objectives

- Understand the types of peripheral nerves
- Define mononeuropathy, polyneuropathy and multifocal neuropathy
- Describe the symptoms and signs associated with damage to peripheral motor nerves as well as large and small sensory fibres
- Understand how to investigate peripheral neuropathy
- Describe common mononeuropathies and polyneuropathies

ANATOMY

Peripheral nerves are made up of numerous axons bound together by three types of connective tissue – endoneurium, perineurium and epineurium (Fig. 26.1). The vasa nervorum located in the epineurium provides the blood supply.

Peripheral nerve trunks contain myelinated and unmyelinated fibres. Myelin is a protein–lipid complex that forms an insulating layer around some axons, resulting in increased rates of conduction in these fibres.

All peripheral nerves have a cellular sheath, the Schwann cell, but only in some does the membrane of the cell 'spiral' around the axon, forming the multi-layered myelin sheath.

Schwann cells of myelinated nerves are separated by nodes of Ranvier. At these points, the axons are not surrounded by myelin. During conduction, impulses jump from one node to the next, which is called saltatory conduction. Conduction in unmyelinated nerves is slower and dependent on the diameter of the axon.

Within the peripheral nerve, the axons vary structurally and this is related to function. Three distinct types of fibre can be distinguished (Fig. 26.2). All are myelinated, apart from the C fibres, which carry impulses from painful stimuli.

The function of peripheral nerves can be disrupted by damage to the cell body, the axon, the myelin sheath, the connective tissue or the blood supply.

Two basic pathological processes occur:

1. **Wallerian degeneration:** the axon and myelin sheath degenerates distal to injury to the axon. The process occurs within 7–10 days of the injury and the degenerating portion of the nerve is electrically inexcitable. Regeneration can occur because the basement membrane of the Schwann cell survives and acts as a skeleton along which the axon regrows up to a rate of about 1 mm per day

2. **Demyelination:** segmental destruction of the myelin sheath occurs mostly without axonal damage although prolonged demyelination may cause secondary axonal damage. The primary lesion affects the Schwann cell and causes marked slowing of conduction or conduction block. Local demyelination is caused by pressure, e.g. entrapment neuropathies or by inflammation, e.g. Guillain–Barré syndrome.

DEFINITIONS OF NEUROPATHIES

- **Neuropathy:** a pathological process that affects a peripheral nerve or nerves and may involve axonal degeneration (Wallerian degeneration) or demyelination, as discussed above
- **Mononeuropathy:** focal involvement of a single nerve is affected, e.g. the median nerve in carpal tunnel syndrome. If multiple single nerves are affected either simultaneously or sequentially in an asymmetrical pattern, it is termed **multifocal neuropathy** or mononeuritis multiplex. With time the pattern may become more symmetrical in appearance and, therefore, difficult to distinguish from a polyneuropathy
- **Polyneuropathy:** a diffuse disease process affecting many nerves that is usually distal and symmetrical with some proximal progression. In certain disease processes there may be a more proximal involvement initially, e.g. demyelinating neuropathies. However, it is most commonly axonal and, therefore, length-related, affecting the longest axons first, i.e. the feet, and gradually involves shorter axons in the legs and hands. Depending on the underlying cause, it can be acute, subacute or chronic. It may be progressive, relapsing or transient, and can be motor, sensory, autonomic or mixed (sensorimotor ± autonomic).

Fig. 26.1 Transverse section of a peripheral nerve.

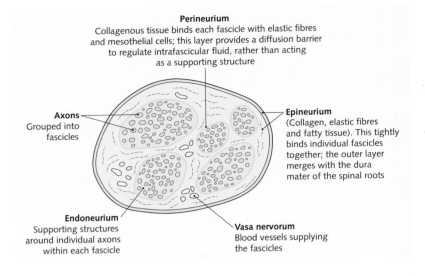

Perineurium
Collagenous tissue binds each fascicle with elastic fibres and mesothelial cells; this layer provides a diffusion barrier to regulate intrafascicular fluid, rather than acting as a supporting structure

Axons
Grouped into fascicles

Epineurium
(Collagen, elastic fibres and fatty tissue). This tightly binds individual fascicles together; the outer layer merges with the dura mater of the spinal roots

Endoneurium
Supporting structures around individual axons within each fascicle

Vasa nervorum
Blood vessels supplying the fascicles

Fig. 26.2 Fibre types in peripheral nerve

Fibre type	Fibre diameter (μm)	Velocity (m/s)	Function/nerve type
Type A (myelinated); Group I	12–20	90	Vibration and position sense alpha motor neurons
Group II	6–12	50	Touch and pressure afferents
Group III	1–6	30	Gamma afferents
Type B (myelinated)	2–6	10	Autonomic preganglionic
Type C (unmyelinated)	<1	2	Pain and temperature afferents autonomic postganglionic

SYMPTOMS OF NEUROPATHY

Sensory symptoms and signs

Negative symptoms (loss of sensation)

Large myelinated fibre disease causes loss of touch, vibration and joint-position sense (proprioception), leading to:

- difficulty discriminating textures
- feet and hands feeling like 'cotton wool'
- gait unsteady through loss of position sense, especially at night when vision cannot compensate.

Small unmyelinated fibre disease causes loss of pain and temperature appreciation, leading to:

- painless burns and trauma
- damage to joints (Charcot's joint), resulting in painless deformity.

Positive symptoms

Large myelinated fibre disease can cause paraesthesia ('pins and needles'). Small unmyelinated fibre disease produces painful positive symptoms:

- Burning sensations
- Dysaesthesia: pain on gentle touch
- Hyperalgesia: lowered threshold to pain
- Hyperpathia: pain threshold is elevated, but pain is excessively felt
- Lightning pains: sudden, very severe, shooting pains, which usually suggest a diagnosis of tabes dorsalis (tertiary syphilis)
- Allodynia: when non-painful stimuli are perceived as painful.

Sensory examination

Functions of large myelinated sensory fibres include:

- light touch
- two-point discrimination
- vibration sense
- joint-position sense.

Functions of small unmyelinated and thinly myelinated sensory fibres include:

- temperature perception
- pain perception.

- flaccid weakness of muscles
- depressed or absent tendon reflexes.

Skeletal symptoms

When a neuropathy is present during early development, skeletal deformities may be seen. These include clawing of the toes, pes cavus and kyphoscoliosis.

When joint-position sense is lost, gait may be abnormal due to 'sensory ataxia' and Romberg's test is positive (loss of joint-position sense is compensated for by vision; therefore, when the eyes are closed, the stance becomes unsteady, whereas it is steady when the eyes are open). Romberg's test is not a test of cerebellar dysfunction.

Sensory examination should include the search for neuropathic burns, trauma, ulcers on the heels and between the toes and Charcot joints. There might also be trophic changes within the skin due to loss of sensory and autonomic fibres. These changes include loss of hairs, oedema, purple discoloration and shiny featureless skin (see Ch. 2).

Autonomic symptoms

Autonomic symptoms and signs include postural hypotension, impotence, constipation, diarrhoea, loss of bladder control, abnormal sweating and blurring of vision. In any assessment of a neuropathy, it is important to check pupillary responses and to check for postural hypotension.

Motor symptoms

Weakness is usually the main presenting feature. This is usually distal (e.g. difficulty clearing the kerb when walking or unable to open jars) but some neuropathies can be proximal (e.g. difficulty climbing stairs or combing hair).

Patients may also complain of cramps and twitching of muscles (fasciculations), although these symptoms are more commonly due to diseases affecting the anterior horn cell (e.g. motor neuron disease).

Motor examination

The classic features of a lower motor neuron abnormality include:

- distal wasting of muscles: distal wasting can also occur with generalized weight loss, but weakness is rare, although the muscles may fatigue easily in this context
- fasciculations

INVESTIGATION OF PERIPHERAL NEUROPATHY

In up to 30% of cases, the cause of a neuropathy may not be identified. The following investigations may be helpful in the diagnosis:

- **Blood tests:** routine blood tests to exclude certain causes of peripheral neuropathy should include full blood count (FBC), erythrocyte sedimentation rate (ESR), C-reactive protein (CRP), urea and electrolytes (U&E, especially renal function tests), liver function tests, glucose, autoantibodies, vitamin B_{12} and serum protein electrophoresis
- **Nerve conduction studies:** these can differentiate axonal degeneration (reduced amplitude of electrical impulse) from demyelination (reduced conduction velocity) and can characterize whether sensory and/or motor fibres are involved. They can also localize the sites of abnormality, e.g. in entrapment neuropathies
- **Electromyography (EMG):** use of a fine needle inserted into the muscle can discern whether complete or partial denervation is present and whether reinnervation is occurring. This can help in localization, depending on the distribution of muscles affected
- **Nerve biopsy:** the sural nerve is the most commonly biopsied because it is purely sensory and the small resulting clinical deficit is therefore trivial. Pathological information can be gained from light and electron microscopy. Nerve biopsies can be useful to confirm the presence of vasculitis or other inflammatory infiltration, when the cause of a progressive neuropathy has not been revealed by other investigations. In addition small punch biopsies are being increasingly used to help diagnose small-fibre neuropathies
- **Cerebrospinal fluid (CSF) examination:** this may be helpful, for example, in inflammatory demyelinating neuropathies such as Guillain–Barré syndrome or chronic inflammatory demyelinating polyradiculoneuropathy, when the protein content is usually raised, without inflammatory cells.

SPECIFIC NEUROPATHIES

Mononeuropathies

Peripheral nerve compression and entrapment neuropathies

Nerves can be damaged by compression either acutely (e.g. by a tourniquet or a tight-fitting cast over the leg) or chronically (e.g. carpal tunnel syndrome). This usually causes localized demyelination, although, if prolonged, it may lead to axonal degeneration.

Acute compression tends to affect nerves that lie superficially to the skin (e.g. the common peroneal nerve at the fibular head by prolonged knee crossing or a tight-fitting plaster cast, or the radial nerve as it passes around the humerus, causing 'Saturday-night palsy').

Chronic compression causes 'entrapment neuropathies', which occur when the nerve passes through tight anatomical spaces (e.g. the median nerve in the carpal tunnel). A history of recurrent compressive neuropathic lesions should raise the possibility of an underlying hereditary neuropathy with a liability to pressure palsies.

The most common nerves to be involved by compression are described below.

Carpal tunnel syndrome

The median nerve is supplied from the C6, C7, C8 and T1 nerve roots. The median nerve may become compressed in the fibro-osseous carpal tunnel at the wrist, in which case the C8/T1 small muscles of the hand are affected. Carpal tunnel syndrome is usually idiopathic but can be associated with:

- hypothyroidism
- pregnancy

- diabetes mellitus
- rheumatoid arthritis
- acromegaly.

It presents with tingling, pain and numbness in the hand, which tends to wake the patient from sleep or in the morning. The pain may extend up the arm to the shoulder and be relieved by shaking of the arm and hand. In some cases there is weakness of the thenar muscles (1st lumbrical, opponens pollicis, abductor pollicis brevis and flexor pollicis brevis), especially abductor pollicis brevis. Sensory loss affects the palm and the lateral three-and-a-half digits. If it is long-standing and severe, there may be wasting of abductor pollicis brevis. Tinel's sign may be present – tapping on the carpal tunnel reproduces tingling and pain. In Phalen's test, forced wrist flexion may provoke similar sensory symptoms.

Diagnosis is clinical and by electrophysiology, confirming slowing of the impulse across the wrist with a reduced amplitude in some cases. Surgical decompression is the definitive procedure, although splints and steroid injections into the carpal tunnel may provide temporary relief (Fig. 26.3).

Ulnar nerve compression

The ulnar nerve arises from the roots of C8 to T1. Ulnar nerve compression is less common than carpal tunnel syndrome. Entrapment typically occurs at the elbow, where the nerve is compressed within the olecranon groove within the cubital tunnel, which lies behind the medial epicondyle. It can follow fracture of the ulna or prolonged/recurrent pressure at this site. The ulnar nerve may be compressed at other sites within the cubital tunnel, such as between the two heads of flexor carpi ulnaris.

In an ulnar neuropathy a patient may complain of tingling or numbness affecting the little finger, part of the ring finger and, sometimes, the ulnar side of the hand distal to the wrist. If sensory loss extends to the medial

Fig. 26.3 Carpal tunnel syndrome – in more proximal median nerve lesions sensory loss may also be apparent in the palm.

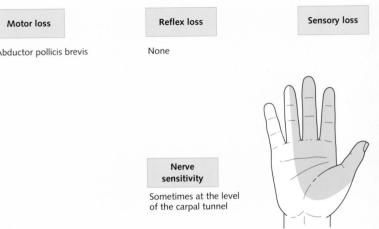

Motor loss
Abductor pollicis brevis

Reflex loss
None

Sensory loss

Nerve sensitivity
Sometimes at the level of the carpal tunnel

side of the forearm, this indicates a more proximal lesion, such as a brachial plexus or C8 root lesion. In severe cases there may be wasting of the hypothenar muscles and weakness of ulnar-innervated muscles of the forearm and hand. The patient may develop an 'ulnar claw hand' due to involvement of the medial two lumbricals, especially when the nerve is affected at the wrist, leaving the long ulnar flexors unopposed. Weakness of the adductor pollicis (which adducts the thumb), abductor digiti minimi (which abducts the little finger) and the interossei (which abduct and adduct the fingers) muscles may be present.

Electrophysiology localizes the lesion. Surgical decompression or anterior transposition can be performed, but results from the latter procedure are generally poor and it is seldom performed in modern practice.

A more distal ulnar compression neuropathy can occur in the deep motor branch as it passes across the palm. This is due to regular pressure from tools, e.g. screwdrivers, crutches or cycle handlebars (Fig. 26.4). The deep palmar branch is purely motor and, therefore, damage will cause wasting and weakness of the interossei muscles and adductor pollicis, but sensation will be spared. The hypothenar muscles are also typically spared.

Radial nerve compression
The radial nerve is supplied by C6, C7 and C8 roots. It supplies the triceps, brachioradialis, supinator, wrist and finger extensors, and long thumb abductor. Radial nerve compression occurs when the radial nerve is compressed against the humerus, e.g. when the arm is draped over the back of a chair for several hours ('Saturday-night palsy'), and results in wrist drop and weakness of finger extension and brachioradialis. Sensation is lost in the region of the 'anatomical snuffbox' on the dorsum of the hand over the base and shafts of the first two metacarpals. Recovery is usually spontaneous, but may take up to 3 months (Fig. 26.5). More proximal lesions can cause impaired sensation on the posterolateral aspect of the forearm.

Common peroneal nerve palsy
The common peroneal nerve is supplied by L4, L5, S1 and S2 nerve roots. It has two branches: the superficial branch supplies the ankle evertors, and skin on the lateral side of the lower leg. The deep branch supplies the toe and ankle dorsiflexors, and a small area of skin on the dorsum of the foot between the first and second toes. Common peroneal nerve palsy occurs when the nerve is compressed at the fibular head and can result from prolonged squatting or leg crossing, wearing a tight plaster cast, prolonged bedrest or coma. It results in a foot drop and weakness of eversion and dorsiflexion, with sensory loss on the anterolateral border of the shin and dorsum of the foot. Recovery is usual, but not invariable, within a few months (Fig. 26.6).

Lateral cutaneous nerve of the thigh (meralgia paraesthetica)
The sensory lateral cutaneous nerve of the thigh is supplied by L2 and L3 roots. This nerve may be compressed beneath the inguinal ligament, which causes burning, tingling and numbness on the anterolateral surface of the thigh. There is no weakness or reflex change. It usually occurs in overweight patients and weight loss may help (Fig. 26.7).

Multifocal neuropathy (mononeuritis multiplex)
Certain systemic illnesses are associated with multiple mononeuropathies. They can be caused by preferential sites of entrapment but also by a focal pathological

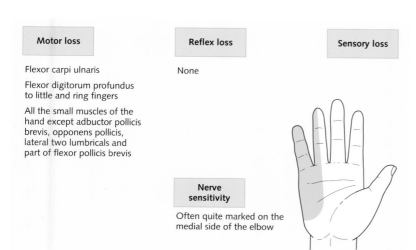

Fig. 26.4 Ulnar nerve compression.

Motor loss	Reflex loss	Sensory loss
Flexor carpi ulnaris	None	
Flexor digitorum profundus to little and ring fingers		
All the small muscles of the hand except adbuctor pollicis brevis, opponens pollicis, lateral two lumbricals and part of flexor pollicis brevis		

Nerve sensitivity

Often quite marked on the medial side of the elbow

Fig. 26.5 Radial nerve compression.

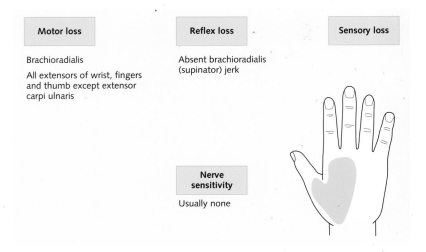

Motor loss	Reflex loss	Sensory loss
Brachioradialis	Absent brachioradialis (supinator) jerk	
All extensors of wrist, fingers and thumb except extensor carpi ulnaris		

Nerve sensitivity

Usually none

Fig. 26.6 Common peroneal nerve palsy.

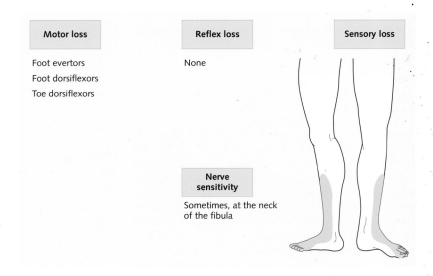

Motor loss	Reflex loss	Sensory loss
Foot evertors	None	
Foot dorsiflexors		
Toe dorsiflexors		

Nerve sensitivity

Sometimes, at the neck of the fibula

process in a nerve(s) (e.g. infarction in diabetes). These include:

- diabetes mellitus
- connective tissue disease, e.g. polyarteritis nodosa, systemic lupus erythematosus (SLE), rheumatoid arthritis – the pathology is usually a small vessel vasculitis
- sarcoidosis
- amyloidosis
- neurofibromatosis
- HIV
- leprosy.

HINTS AND TIPS

Small vessel vasculitic neuropathy can occur in isolation or in association with other connective tissue diseases, e.g. SLE, rheumatoid arthritis. Characteristically, it is associated with severe pain in the affected nerves and multiple mononeuropathy. It often affects muscle as well and, therefore, a combined biopsy of both muscle and nerve is often performed if the diagnosis is suspected. It is an important cause not to miss as a delay in diagnosis and treatment can lead to severe neurological deficits.

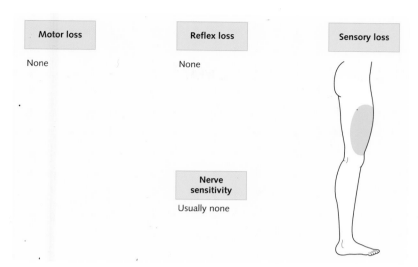

Motor loss

None

Reflex loss

None

Nerve sensitivity

Usually none

Sensory loss

Fig. 26.7 Meralgia paraesthetica.

Polyneuropathies

Polyneuropathies can be classified according to their mode of onset, functional or pathological type, distribution or causation. The classification used below is based on causation.

Polyneuropathies associated with systemic disease

A wide range of systemic diseases can affect the peripheral nerve. The following represent a small selection of the most common conditions.

Diabetic neuropathy

The neuropathies found in diabetes mellitus are often related to poor glycaemic control. The exact cause of the nerve damage is uncertain, but may relate to sorbitol accumulation or to vascular disease in both large and small vessels.

A number of different types of neuropathy complicate diabetes:

- distal symmetrical polyneuropathy: most commonly sensory, but may be sensorimotor and have autonomic features. Improving glycaemic control has been demonstrated to reduce the risk of developing peripheral neuropathy
- a painful small fibre neuropathy affecting the feet is common in diabetes and may often be the presenting feature of the disease
- proximal asymmetrical motor neuropathy: a lumbosacral radiculoplexus neuropathy, also known as 'diabetic amyotrophy', acutely painful and occurs in older men. There is lumbar or proximal leg pain from the outset, followed by asymmetric proximal leg weakness and wasting

- autonomic neuropathy: with gastroparesis and resultant diarrhoea, arrhythmias and postural hypotension. This neuropathy is also length-dependent and loss of sweating in the feet may be an early feature
- mononeuropathies can be single or multiple, especially entrapment
- cranial nerve lesions: especially isolated third (usually pupil sparing) and sixth nerve palsies
- mononeuritis multiplex.

Renal disease

Chronic renal failure produces a progressive sensorimotor neuropathy. The response to dialysis is variable, but the neuropathy usually improves after renal transplantation.

Paraneoplastic polyneuropathy

Malignant disease, especially small-cell carcinoma of the bronchus, can produce a pure sensory neuropathy affecting the large fibres, leading to a sensory ataxic neuropathy. This is also known as a sensory neuronopathy and is often associated with antineuronal antibodies, such as anti-Hu antibodies. The neuropathy may predate the appearance of the malignancy by months or years.

Haematological malignancies such as multiple myeloma and other monoclonal gammopathies characteristically produce peripheral neuropathies that resemble chronic inflammatory demyelinating polyradiculoneuropathy (CIDP) or vasculitic neuropathies.

Connective tissue diseases and vasculitides

Connective tissue diseases and vasculitides classically produce a very painful mononeuritis multiplex, although individual diseases may produce a symmetrical sensorimotor neuropathy (especially SLE), entrapment neuropathy (rheumatoid arthritis) or trigeminal neuropathy (Sjögren's syndrome). With progression, mononeuritis multiplex can resemble a polyneuropathy with a 'glove-and-stocking' distribution. Factors suggestive of vasculitic aetiology include subacute onset, asymmetrical distribution, pain, leg involvement and systemic symptoms. Treatment is with steroids and immunosuppressants.

Porphyria

Acute intermittent porphyria produces a predominantly axonal motor neuropathy/polyradiculopathy in addition to abdominal pain, psychosis and seizures. The onset is usually acute or subacute, similar to Guillain–Barré syndrome, and often presents with asymmetrical proximal weakness. Like Guillain–Barré syndrome, respiratory, facial, ocular, bulbar and autonomic function can be affected.

Amyloidosis

Amyloid is deposited around the vessels in the nerve, causing distortion. The neuropathy is characterized by predominantly sensory, painful, dysaesthetic features. Autonomic features are common.

Neuropathies caused by drugs and toxins

Drugs

A wide variety of drugs are known to cause a peripheral neuropathy. Most produce a chronic, progressive, sensorimotor polyneuropathy and are generally reversible. Examples of the most common include:

- sensory axonal neuropathy: chloramphenicol, isoniazid (by affecting pyridoxine metabolism), phenytoin, Taxol
- motor axonal neuropathy: amphotericin, dapsone, gold
- sensorimotor axonal neuropathy: chlorambucil, cisplatin, disulfiram, nitrofurantoin, vincristine
- sensorimotor demyelinating neuropathy: amiodarone.

Toxins

A wide variety of metals and industrial toxins have been shown to cause polyneuropathy. Peripheral nerve involvement is often accompanied by other systemic features. For example:

- lead causes a motor neuropathy
- arsenic and thallium cause a painful peripheral sensory neuropathy
- acrylamide, trichloroethylene and fat-soluble hydrocarbons, e.g. as in glue sniffing, cause a progressive polyneuropathy.

Alcoholic neuropathy

Alcohol is the most common toxin associated with peripheral neuropathy. Alcoholic neuropathy is one of the most common forms of peripheral neuropathy

(up to 30% of all cases of neuropathy) and is primarily axonal.

It progresses slowly, with distal sensory loss, paraesthesia and burning pains. Distal muscle weakness may occur and spread proximally, with muscle cramps and gait disturbance.

The cause may be primarily due to alcohol toxicity, but also due to a secondary deficiency of vitamins, particularly in thiamine and other B vitamins, as well as often having an inadequate general dietary intake.

Abstinence from alcohol, supplementation of thiamine and a balanced diet constitute the principal therapy. The painful symptoms may be eased with the use of neuropathic pain medications, such as antidepressants (e.g. amitriptyline or duloxetine) or antiepileptics (e.g. gabapentin or pregabalin).

Inflammatory demyelinating neuropathies

The group 'inflammatory demyelinating neuropathies' includes an acute neuropathy (Guillain–Barré syndrome) and a chronic neuropathy, CIDP.

Guillain–Barré syndrome (postinfective polyneuropathy)

Guillain–Barré syndrome is also called acute inflammatory demyelinating polyradiculoneuropathy (AIDP). It occurs worldwide, with an annual rate of 1.5 cases per 100 000.

It often follows 1–3 weeks after a respiratory infection or diarrhoea, which may have been mild. *Campylobacter jejuni* has been particularly implicated as a cause of the diarrhoea and is associated with a more severe form. It may also follow other infections such as HIV seroconversion or following vaccines.

The classic presentation is with distal paraesthesia, often with little sensory loss, and weakness tends to occur proximally, distally spreading proximally or generalized. The symptoms ascend up the lower limbs and body over days to weeks. Facial weakness is present in 50% of cases, and is often asymmetrical. Ophthalmoparesis occurs in 15% of patients with typical Guillain–Barré syndrome. In patients with cranial nerve involvement, bulbar weakness, or neck and proximal arm weakness, there is a significant risk of intercostal muscle and diaphragmatic weakness leading to respiratory failure. If the vital capacity drops to 1 litre or below, artificial ventilation is often necessary. Autonomic dysfunction may also occur in 60% of patients, and causes arrhythmias, urinary retention and constipation. Clinically, symptoms usually reach their peak within 6 weeks of the onset of symptoms.

A proximal variant of Guillain–Barré syndrome exists, involving ocular muscles and associated with areflexia and ataxia (Miller–Fisher syndrome).

Diagnosis is usually clinical, supported by slowed conduction velocities on nerve conduction studies and a raised CSF protein with a normal cell count or mild lymphocytosis. Both these investigations may be normal early in the disease. Patients with Miller–Fisher variant have anti-GQ1b ganglioside antibodies.

Differential diagnoses include other paralytic illnesses, such as poliomyelitis, myasthenia gravis, botulism and primary muscle disease.

Patients with Guillain–Barré syndrome should have adequate monitoring of cardiac and respiratory function. They should have continuous heart monitoring, and regular vital capacity and oxygen saturation assessments. The use of intravenous immunoglobulin has been shown to produce significant improvement in the course of the disease and is equivalent to the more invasive plasmapheresis. Corticosteroids and immunosuppressive agents have not been successful in acute Guillain–Barré syndrome. Careful management of the paralysed patient, and ventilation as indicated, are also essential. Recovery, although gradual over many months, is usual in 80% of patients. Approximately 10–15% patients may have a prolonged stay on an intensive care unit, with a recovery period extending up to 2 years. A mortality rate of 5% is associated with inadequate ventilatory support, complications of immobility (aspiration, pulmonary embolism) and arrhythmias. By definition, the symptoms and signs cease to progress after 8 weeks or the disease becomes termed CIDP.

HINTS AND TIPS

In the differential diagnosis of Guillain–Barré syndrome the following atypical features suggest an alternative diagnosis:

- Significant asymmetry – vasculitis
- Marked CSF lymphocytosis – HIV, Lyme disease, polio
- Sensory level – spinal cord syndrome
- Marked bladder or bowel dysfunction – spinal cord syndrome.

Chronic inflammatory demyelinating polyradiculoneuropathy

CIDP represents an often milder syndrome that is related to Guillain–Barré syndrome, but has a more protracted clinical course. The clinical, diagnostic features and pathology are similar to those of Guillain–Barré syndrome, though it is rarely associated with preceding infection. It is usually a symmetrical, progressive, polyradiculoneuropathy with symptoms of weakness, sensory loss and paraesthesia. The weakness can be both proximal and distal, and though neck weakness is common, facial weakness is rare. The sensory loss is typically 'glove-and-stocking' like in nature, with marked large-fibre loss leading to a sensory ataxia. CSF protein is elevated with a normal cell count. NCS show demyelination.

Drug treatment includes corticosteroids, with or without other immunosuppressive agents such as azathioprine or cyclophosphamide, or recurrent intravenous immunoglobulin infusions/plasmapheresis.

Multifocal motor neuropathy

This is an uncommon disorder, but an important differential for the lower motor neuron variant of motor neuron disease. It is characterized by progressive, asymmetrical weakness without sensory involvement. Cranial nerve and respiratory involvement are rare, and nerve conduction studies show multifocal conduction block. There are usually high levels of anti-GM1 ganglioside antibodies. It is potentially treatable with IVIG.

Neuropathies caused by nutritional deficiencies

Thiamine (vitamin B₁) deficiency (beriberi)

Thiamine deficiency is strongly implicated in the causation of alcoholic neuropathy. In addition to the peripheral neuropathy, deficiency can cause Wernicke–Korsakoff syndrome (see Ch. 34).

Pyridoxine (vitamin B₆) deficiency

Pyridoxine deficiency causes a mainly sensory neuropathy. It may be precipitated by isoniazid therapy for tuberculosis, and pyridoxine is, therefore, given in association with this drug.

Vitamin B₁₂ deficiency

Peripheral neuropathy can occur in association with subacute combined degeneration of the cord (spastic paraparesis, loss of proprioception, paraesthesia); vitamin B₁₂ deficiency is also linked to optic neuropathies and dementia. Treatment involves intramuscular replacement injections (see Ch. 23).

Vitamin E deficiency

Vitamin E deficiency occurs in the context of fat malabsorption. The onset of neurological symptoms takes many years. It involves a large-fibre sensory neuropathy with spinocerebellar degeneration.

Neuropathies caused by infection

In the Western world the most relevant infections that can cause a peripheral neuropathy are HIV and Lyme disease, and worldwide diphtheria and leprosy are also important. HIV can cause a variety of peripheral nerve syndromes, either directly or indirectly through immune suppression and co-morbid infections, or the side-effects of medications. Lyme disease can cause a cranial neuropathy, radiculopathy or an asymmetric peripheral neuropathy.

Hereditary neuropathies

The field of hereditary neuropathies is a complex one, with clinically and genetically heterogeneous conditions. This section will consider the group of conditions known as the hereditary motor sensory neuropathies (HMSN), also known as Charcot–Marie–Tooth (CMT) disease. Other, less common types of hereditary neuropathy are not discussed..

With the advent of molecular genetic studies, the original classification system for HMSN is undergoing modification. Categories are as follows:

- CMT type I: most common form, autosomal dominant demyelinating neuropathy with hypertrophy of nerves ('onion-bulb' formation on electron microscopy); onset at age between 5 and 15 years
- CMT type II: mostly autosomal dominant inheritance, axonal neuropathy; onset 10 and 20 years
- CMT type III (Dejerine–Sottas disease): autosomal dominant or recessive demyelinating neuropathy, variant of type I but more severe with earlier onset, gross hypertrophy of peripheral nerves and often the CSF protein is raised due to hypertrophied nerve roots
- X-linked CMT: the second most common form, and clinically similar to CMTI though there is no male-to-male transmission, demyelinating in males and axonal in females.
- Complex forms of HMSN: additional features such as optic atrophy, retinitis pigmentosa, deafness and spastic paraparesis can coexist.

General characteristics of hereditary motor sensory neuropathies

All forms of HMSN are characterized by distal wasting of the lower limbs, which progresses, often over many years, and may involve the upper limbs.

When the wasting in the legs is severe, they resemble 'inverted champagne bottles' (Fig. 26.8A). The wasting is accompanied by reduced or absent reflexes and a variable loss of sensation.

Pes cavus (loss of lateral arch) with clawing of the toes is almost invariable and reflects early onset of disease (Fig. 26.8B). These features may be the only signs in mild cases. Clawing of the hands may also be seen. One-third of patients may have a postural tremor and half have palpable thickening of peripheral nerves. Sensory features are not as marked as the motor features.

The age of onset varies from childhood to middle age. There is variability within subgroups and within families.

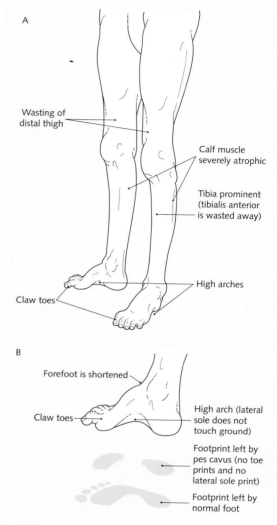

Fig. 26.8 'Inverted-champagne-bottle' legs of hereditary motor sensory neuropathy.

Critical illness polyneuropathy

This is an axonal sensorimotor polyneuropathy that can occur in patients who are critically ill on intensive care units with multiorgan failure and infection. It can cause significant problems in weaning from artificial ventilation and its pathogenesis is unknown. In some patients the weakness is muscular: that is, they have a critical illness myopathy.

The causes of peripheral neuropathies are summarized in Figure 26.9.

Fig. 26.9 Summary of causes of peripheral neuropathies

Inflammatory	Guillain–Barré syndrome Chronic inflammatory demyelinating polyradiculoneuropathy (CIDP) Multifocal motor neuropathy with conduction block
Metabolic	Diabetes Renal disease Porphyria
Nutritional deficiencies	Vitamin B_1 Vitamin B_6 Vitamin B_{12} Vitamin E
Toxic	Drugs: isoniazid, vincristine, nitrofurantoin Alcohol Lead
Vasculitis/connective tissue disease	Primary vasculitis – e.g. polyarteritis nodosa, Wegener's granulomatosis, Churg–Strauss syndrome, microscopic polyangiitis Secondary vasculitis – e.g. connective tissue disorders (rheumatoid arthritis, systemic lupus erythematosus, Sjögren's syndrome), drugs, viral infections (hepatitis C, HIV, CMV), malignancy
Malignancy (paraneoplastic)	Bronchus Breast, ovarian, uterus Haematological malignancies including monoclonal paraprotein of unknown significance (MGUS)
Infection	HIV Lyme disease Leprosy
Hereditary	CMT syndromes
Trauma	Often mononeuropathies or multiple mononeuropathies – crush, section, avulsion
Miscellaneous	Critical illness neuropathy

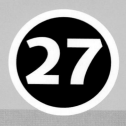
- Understand the anatomy and neurophysiology of the neuromuscular junction
- Describe the clinical features of myasthenia gravis
- Understand the investigations and management of myasthenia gravis

The normal anatomy and physiology of the neuromuscular junction are outlined in Figure 27.1. A normal electrical impulse passes down motor nerves towards skeletal muscle. Each motor axon divides up into a number of terminal branches just before it reaches the muscle. Each one of these branches ends at the presynaptic nerve terminal. The electrical impulse causes calcium to flood into the terminal and acetylcholine-containing vesicles to fuse with the nerve membrane, thereby releasing acetylcholine into the synaptic cleft. The acetylcholine crosses the synaptic cleft and binds to acetylcholine receptors on the postsynaptic muscle end-plate membrane. This results in depolarization of the muscle fibre and subsequent contraction of the muscle. The acetylcholine is then broken down by acetylcholinesterase, which is bound to the basement membrane in the synaptic folds.

Two main diseases of neuromuscular transmission will be discussed in this chapter – myasthenia gravis and Lambert–Eaton myasthenic syndrome (LEMS).

MYASTHENIA GRAVIS

Myasthenia gravis is an acquired, organ-specific autoimmune disorder, of unknown cause, in which antibodies are directed against the postsynaptic acetylcholine receptor. This results in weakness and fatigability of skeletal muscle groups. The most commonly affected muscles are the proximal limbs, the ocular and bulbar muscles.

There is often an associated abnormality of the thymus in patients with myasthenia gravis. Thymic hyperplasia is found in 70% of patients below the age of 40 years. In 10% of all patients with myasthenia gravis, a benign thymic tumour (thymoma) is found. The incidence of thymomas increases with age. In patients with thymoma, antibodies to striated muscle may also be found.

There appear to be two distinct groups of patients who develop myasthenia gravis, split by age and sex:

- Young women (20–35 years), who tend to have an acute, severely fluctuating, more generalized condition, with increased association with HLA-B8 and HLA-DR3.
- Older men (60–75 years), who tend to have a more oculobulbar presentation.

There is some crossover between the groups, and myasthenia gravis is seen in young men and older women, but less frequently.

Clinical features

The clinical features of myasthenia gravis are listed in Figure 27.2. The most important characteristic of myasthenia gravis is fatigability. All the features listed may present with fluctuating weakness, which is worse after exercise and at the end of the day. Ptosis and ophthalmoplegia are the presenting features in 50% of patients.

Fatigability of the levator palpebrae superioris can be demonstrated by asking a patient to look downwards for a period, before then instructing them to look up. In this situation the eyelid may twitch ('Cogan's lid twitch') as elevation is initially normal, before fatigue occurs due to myasthenia. Alternatively, the affected muscles can be exercised by making a patient, in whom ptosis is sometimes apparent, look upwards for 1–2 minutes. The ptosis will become more severe and the eyes may drift to the primary position. Similar manoeuvres can be carried out for the proximal limb muscles by testing power before and after repeated contractions such as shoulder abduction.

Limb reflexes are normal or hyperactive but fatigue on repeated testing. Muscle wasting is rare, occurring at a late stage in only a minority of more severe cases. It is rarely as severe as in disorders affecting the motor cell body or nerve. Sensory examination is normal.

Fig. 27.1 The neuromuscular junction. Antibodies directed against acetylcholine receptors cause myasthenia gravis, whereas antibodies against the presynaptic voltage-gated calcium channels cause Lambert–Eaton myasthenic syndrome.

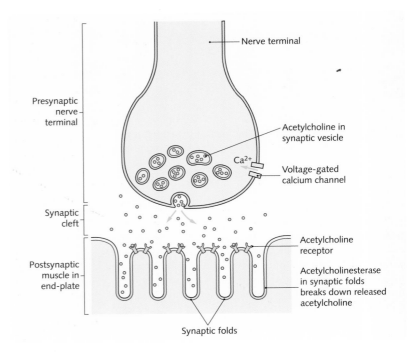

Nerve terminal

Presynaptic nerve terminal

Acetylcholine in synaptic vesicle

Ca²⁺

Voltage-gated calcium channel

Synaptic cleft

Postsynaptic muscle in end-plate

Acetylcholine receptor

Acetylcholinesterase in synaptic folds breaks down released acetylcholine

Synaptic folds

Fig. 27.2 Symptoms of myasthenia gravis – all these features show fatigability

Ocular	Ptosis Diplopia
Other cranial muscles	Weak face and jaw Dysarthria Dysphonia Dysphagia
Limb weakness	Usually proximal – shoulder and hips
Neck weakness	Neck flexion and extension – patients can present with difficulty lifting head up
Respiratory muscle weakness	Shortness of breath

HINTS AND TIPS

Any young woman with a complex ophthalmoplegia is likely to have myasthenia, MS or thyroid eye disease. With bilateral ptosis in addition to ophthalmoplegia, myasthenia is probable and, very rarely, ocular myopathies. In thyroid eye disease there will typically be proptosis, not ptosis, and in MS usually other brainstem symptoms or signs.

Investigations

Tensilon (edrophonium) test

Edrophonium is a fast-acting anticholinesterase (i.e. it antagonizes the action of acetylcholinesterase and thus prevents the breakdown of acetylcholine). This enables more acetylcholine to stimulate the reduced numbers of acetylcholine receptors. When edrophonium is given as an intravenous bolus, usually with atropine to prevent cardiac side-effects, ptosis, diplopia and proximal limb fatigability improves within seconds and for only 2–3 minutes. This can be used as a diagnostic test for myasthenia gravis, although many neurologists are now relying on the other tests available and reserving this test if the others are negative and the clinical suspicion is high.

Serum acetylcholine receptor and MUSK antibodies

The highly specific acetylcholine receptor (AChR) antibody is present in the serum of up to 85% of patients with generalized myasthenia gravis. About 50% of patients with ocular myasthenia gravis have the antibody. About 50% of patients who are seronegative for AChR test positive for muscle-specific kinase antibodies (anti-MUSK).

Electromyography

There are two classic electromyographic findings in myasthenia gravis:

- A decrement in amplitude (progressive 'fatigue') of the compound muscle action potential following repetitive stimulation.
- Increased jitter using a single-fibre electrode.

Thymus imaging

It is essential to image the chest with computed tomography or magnetic resonance imaging for the presence of thymic hyperplasia or tumour, as removal of a hyperplastic thymus may improve the condition in some patients and removal of thymomas prevents malignant transformation.

Autoantibodies

Other autoantibodies may be present, especially those against striated muscle and thyroid which are associated with thymomas.

Spirometry

The patient's vital capacity (VC) needs to be checked. AVC falling below 1.5 litres requires transfer of the patient to ITU/HDU before frank ventilatory failure occurs.

HINTS AND TIPS

Any known myasthenic with new-onset bulbar dysfunction should have their VC carefully monitored. There can often be very few other features of myasthenia at the start of a relapse and neuromuscular respiratory weakness can be missed. Patients may complain that their breathing is difficult lying flat but this is not invariable.

Management

The illness may have a protracted and fluctuating course. Acute exacerbations may be unpredictable or may follow infections or treatment with certain drugs. It is important to recognize respiratory involvemeant, as assisted ventilation may be required. However, patients may remit permanently, especially after thymectomy or with immunosuppressive treatment.

Oral acetylcholinesterases

Pyridostigmine is the most widely used drug; it has a time of onset of less than 60 minutes, and a duration of action of about 3–5 hours. The patient's response will determine the dosage required.

Overdosage causes a cholinergic crisis with severe weakness, which may be difficult to differentiate from the myasthenic weakness. Colic and diarrhoea may also occur.

Acetylcholinesterases are excellent symptomatic drugs but do not alter the natural history of the disease.

Thymectomy

In patients with thymic hyperplasia, thymectomy, for unknown reasons, improves the prognosis of the disease, especially in those under 40 years of age and in those who have had the disease for less than 10 years.

In patients with a thymoma, surgery is essential to remove a potentially malignant tumour but this rarely results in improvement of the myasthenia.

Immunosuppression

Corticosteroids provide the mainstay of immunosuppressive treatment. An excellent response is seen in 70% of patients but the dose must be increased slowly, preferably in hospital, as there is often a temporary exacerbation of symptoms before the therapeutic effect.

Plasmapheresis or intravenous immunoglobulin may sometimes be used during an acute exacerbation or when there is respiratory involvement. The effects are usually short-lived and therefore must be repeated if required.

Azathioprine is most commonly used as a steroid-sparing agent, though many other immunosuppressants are also used, e.g. methotrexate, ciclosporin and mycophenolate.

LAMBERT–EATON MYASTHENIC SYNDROME

Lambert–Eaton myasthenic syndrome (LEMS) is a rare condition associated with antibodies that are directed against the presynaptic voltage-gated calcium channels at the neuromuscular junction. This results in a failure of acetylcholine release from the presynaptic nerve terminal. In many cases, it is a non-metastatic manifestation of malignancy, especially small-cell carcinoma of the lung.

LEMS is characterized by weakness of the proximal limb muscles, especially in the lower limbs. Ocular and other cranial muscles are typically spared. There may be fatigability but, characteristically, there is a paradoxical initial improvement in power after exercise, followed by sustained weakness. Reflexes are usually absent, but then return following use of the muscle ('post-tetanic potentiation'). Autonomic involvement is especially common in cases associated with an underlying malignancy.

The diagnosis can be confirmed electromyographically by an 'incremental' increase of the compound muscle action potential after repetitive stimulation (the opposite to myasthenia gravis). AChR antibodies and edrophonium testing are negative. Voltage-gated calcium channel antibodies are usually positive. A search should be made for malignancy, especially small-cell carcinoma of the lung, although the tumour may not be found initially, only to appear several years later or to be seen only on positron emission tomography (PET) scanning.

Guanethidine hydrochloride and 4-aminopyridine (4-AP) may enhance acetylcholine release. Intravenous immunoglobulin and plasmapheresis may also help. The prognosis for those with a primary lung tumour is usually poor.

OTHER MYASTHENIC SYNDROMES

Even rarer myasthenic syndromes include:

- congenital myasthenia gravis: patients develop weakness as newborns often due to mutations within the apparatus that allows release of acetylcholine from the presynaptic terminal

- neonatal myasthenia gravis: this is caused by transfer of antibodies to the acetylcholine receptor across the placenta to the baby and usually resolves after delivery
- penicillamine-induced myasthenia.

BOTULINUM TOXIN

Clostridium botulinum is a bacterium that can make a preformed toxin, which, when ingested, can cause food poisoning. It is a very rare condition and the toxin can damage the neuromuscular junction, resulting in a paralytic condition resembling severe, acute myasthenia gravis, often with pupillary changes. However, this very powerful neuromuscular-blocking toxin is used routinely in neurological practice, in small, localized, subcutaneously injected doses, to treat unwanted muscular activity. The indications include cervical dystonia, blepharospasm and severe limb spasticity following stroke or multiple sclerosis.

Disorders of skeletal muscle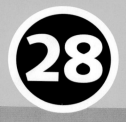

● **Objectives**

- Understand the basic anatomy of skeletal muscle
- Describe the features in the history which help diagnose a muscle disorder
- Understand the tests used to investigate muscle disease
- Understand the main clinical features of hereditary and inflammatory myopathies
- Describe the myopathies associated with systemic disease

ANATOMY

Skeletal muscle is made up of large numbers of multinu-cleated muscle fibres, which have an outer membrane (sarcolemma) and cytoplasm (sarcoplasm) and in which lie the contractile components of the muscle (myofibrils). The fibres are separated by connective tissue (endomysium) and arranged in bundles (fasciculi). Each fasciculus has a connective tissue sheath (perimysium). The muscle is made up of a number of fasciculi bound together and surrounded by a connective tissue sheath (epimysium) (Fig. 28.1).

There are two broad types of muscle fibre, which are functionally different:

1. Type I: rich in myoglobulin, with low metabolism (aerobic) and rich in sarcoplasm
2. Type II: low in myoglobin, with high metabolism (aerobic or anaerobic) and little sarcoplasm.

CLINICAL FEATURES OF MUSCLE DISEASE (MYOPATHY)

Muscle has rather uniform structure and function and thus diseases of muscles from a variety of causes can produce similar clinical features. The general features of muscle disease will, therefore, be summarized prior to discussion of the most common and important specific diseases.

Weakness

Myopathies are characterized by weakness of muscles and the distribution is usually proximal. Each muscle disease exhibits a particular pattern of involvement (e.g. proximal limb, facial and dysphagia), which is an important diagnostic clue. Proximal muscle wasting and weakness is common in inflammatory myopathies. In one of the hereditary forms, facio-scapulo-humeral dystrophy, muscle wasting and weakness is often asymmetrical and can affect the face, proximal upper limbs and distal lower limbs. Inclusion body myositis on the other hand causes focal wasting and weakness in the flexor compartment of the forearm and thighs in an asymmetrical pattern. Careful examination of all muscle groups is important to classify a myopathy and to differentiate it from a lower motor neuron (LMN) disorder or a disorder of the central nervous system.

Changes in muscle tone

There may be a loss of tone (hypotonia) secondary to disease of muscle, although this sign can be difficult to differentiate from normal tone.

Changes in muscle bulk

Wasting of the affected muscles is distinctive in contrast to the distal wasting of most neuropathies.

Enlargement of muscle may be the result of over-activity or an early sign in certain dystrophies, caused by infiltration of fat, exacerbating the weakness (pseudohypertrophy).

Changes in reflexes

These are usually preserved in muscle disorders, at least until wasting and weakness is severe, which helps to distinguish myopathies from LMN syndromes.

Changes in muscle contractility

Myotonia – persistence of contraction, often for several seconds, during attempted relaxation – is found in myotonic dystrophy, paramyotonia congenita,

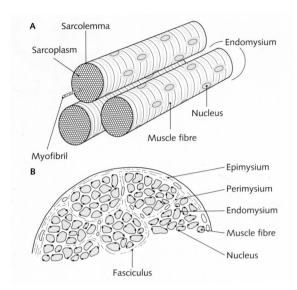

Fig. 28.1 Normal skeletal muscle morphology: (A) longitudinal muscle fibres; (B) cross-section of muscle.

hyperkalaemic periodic paralysis and congenital myotonia. On electromyography (EMG), the characteristic findings consist of rhythmic discharges. This phenomenon may also be elicited by a sharp tap on the muscle belly (percussion myotonia). Myotonia must be differentiated from fasciculations (muscle twitching) and myokymia (rippling of the muscle), which are typically due to denervation of muscle. Contractures indicate long-standing muscle weakness and can be seen in several dystrophies.

Pain

Pain is a rare complaint in primary muscle disease except in deficiencies of certain enzymes of the carbohydrate or lipid pathways or in severe inflammatory myopathy (e.g. polymyositis, vasculitis). It is important to ask about a change in the colour of urine, as this may indicate myoglobinuria secondary to rhabdomyolysis, which can occur in some metabolic disorders.

COMMUNICATION

The pattern of wasting and weakness of muscles in muscle disease and presenting symptoms:

• Proximal weakness – difficulty standing up from chairs, getting out of bed, climbing stairs, hanging clothes on the washing line and storing items in overhead cupboards
• Distal weakness – difficulty with writing, doing up buttons, opening bottles and tripping over feet/toes

---

• Facial weakness – expressionless/myopathic facies, drooling and difficulty whistling
• Eyes – ptosis, diplopia and ophthalmoplegia (rare)
• Bulbar muscle weakness – dysarthria and dysphagia
• Neck and spine – 'dropped' head and scoliosis
• Respiratory musculature weakness – breathlessness, especially lying flat
• Heart – exercise intolerance, palpitations and blackouts

Onset of muscle weakness and family history

Many muscle diseases are inherited, and the onset of muscle weakness can typically be traced back to early childhood with delayed motor milestones (sitting, walking, feeding) or difficulty keeping up with peers and playing sports. A full family history is essential. Inherited muscle diseases include:

• X-linked: Duchenne muscular dystrophy, Becker's muscular dystrophy and Emery–Dreifuss dystrophy
• autosomal dominant: facio-scapulo-humeral dystrophy, scapuloperoneal dystrophy and myotonic dystrophy
• autosomal recessive: limb-girdle dystrophy, all deficiencies of enzymes of glycolytic and lipid metabolism
• mitochondrial: sometimes maternal inheritance. Chronic progressive external ophthalmoplegia and Kearns–Sayre syndrome.

INVESTIGATION OF MUSCLE DISEASE

The diagnosis may be possible from the clinical features in some causes of muscle disease. Other helpful tests include:

• **serum creatine phosphokinase (CPK; creatine kinase, CK):** this is often significantly raised in many dystrophies and in inflammatory muscle disorders, e.g. polymyositis
• **EMG:** needle examination will reveal 'myopathic units' (small, short-duration, spiky polyphasic units). There may be evidence of myotonic discharges in myotonias, and an increase in spontaneous activity (fibrillation potentials and positive sharp waves) in primary myopathies and inflammatory muscle disease
• **muscle biopsy:** this can yield information about fibre type (type I or II), inflammation, and dystrophic and histochemical changes. Electron microscopy is sometimes required

Fig. 28.2	Hereditary and acquired myopathies	
Hereditary myopathies	Muscular dystrophies	Duchenne, Becker's facio-scapulo-humeral, limb-girdle, Emery–Dreifuss, oculopharyngeal
	Myotonic disorders	Myotonic dystrophy
	Metabolic myopathies	Glycogen storage diseases (most common is McArdle's disease) Defects of fatty acid metabolism
	Channelopathies	Periodic paralysis
	Mitochondrial myopathies	Chronic progressive external ophthalmoplegia Kearns–Sayre syndrome MELAS (myopathy, encephalopathy, lactic acidosis, and stroke-like episodes) MERFF (myoclonic epilepsy with red ragged fibres)
Acquired myopathies	Inflammatory	Polymyositis Dermatomyositis Inclusion body myositis
	Metabolic or endocrine myopathies	Cushing's syndrome Hyper- or hypothyroidism Hypokalaemia
	Drug-induced	Zidovudine (AZT), steroids, statins, amiodarone, alcohol
	Paraneoplastic	Often necrotizing
	Critical illness	Probably multifactorial

- **MRI**: this is now used to demonstrate the patterns of muscle involvement, which may be helpful in differentiating the dystrophies and selecting a muscle to biopsy
- **genetic testing**: an increasing number of the hereditary myopathies (see Fig. 28.2) can be diagnosed by a genetic test.

SPECIFIC DISEASES

Myopathies can be subdivided as in Figure 28.2. Important examples are discussed below.

Hereditary myopathies

Muscular dystrophies

Duchenne muscular dystrophy
Duchenne muscular dystrophy is an X-linked recessive disease caused by an absence of dystrophin, a protein that is vital for connecting the cytoskeleton of muscle cells to the extracellular matrix through the membrane. It occurs in 1 in 4000 liveborn males. It also affects skeletal and cardiac muscle.

Clinical features Patients with Duchenne muscular dystrophy display no abnormality at birth, but the condition is apparent by the fourth year. The child is usually wheelchair-bound by 10 years old and death is usual by the age of 20, from respiratory failure or cardiac complications including cardiomyopathy and arrhythmias.

There is initially proximal muscle weakness with pseudohypertrophy of the calves caused by the accumulation of fat and connective tissue. The weakness then spreads. When rising to an erect position, there is a characteristic manoeuvre in which the patient has to 'climb' his legs with his hands (Gower's sign) (Fig. 28.3). The gait is waddling, and patients can have difficulty rising from sitting, crouching or lying.

Diagnosis The diagnosis of Duchenne muscular dystrophy is often made clinically. The CK is grossly elevated (often 10 000 U/L). The EMG is myopathic and muscle biopsy shows fatty infiltration and absence of staining for dystrophin. An accurate and rapid DNA diagnosis is now available, allowing reliable identification of carrier status and prenatal diagnosis if required.

Management There is no cure for Duchenne muscular dystrophy, so the management is supportive. Steroids may provide short-term improvement. Genetic counselling is important. Carrier females may have a raised CK and mildly myopathic EMG, but without any clinical symptoms or signs.

Becker's muscular dystrophy
Becker's muscular dystrophy is also an X-linked recessive condition, with similar characteristics to Duchenne muscular dystrophy, but it has a much milder course. Dystrophin is altered rather than absent. It occurs in approximately 1 in 20 000 live male births.

Clinical features The symptoms of Becker's muscular dystrophy begin in the first decade, although often are not noticed until later. Children continue to walk into their teens and early adult life. Cramps associated with exercise are common. The effects of the cardiomyopathy can be worse than the skeletal weakness and patients are predisposed to developing arrhythmias. These patients often succumb to the cardiac effects before the skeletal muscle problems.

Fig. 28.3 Gower's sign. This involves having to climb up the legs with the hands to overcome pelvic muscle weakness. It is found in any condition with pelvic muscle weakness.

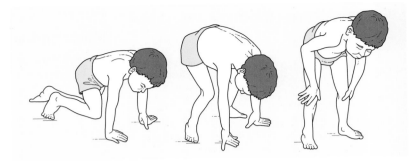

Other muscular dystrophies

Other muscular dystrophies include facio-scapulo-humeral dystrophy (autosomal dominant), limb-girdle dystrophy (autosomal recessive or dominant), Emery–Dreifuss (X-linked, autosomal dominant or recessive) and oculopharyngeal dystrophy (autosomal dominant). The clinical presentations vary from mild and slowly progressive to rapidly fatal.

Myotonic disorders

Myotonic dystrophy (dystrophia myotonica)

Myotonic dystrophy type 1 is the most common adult muscle disease, with a prevalence of 1 in 7000 in the UK. It is an autosomal dominant inherited condition, caused by an expanded trinucleotide repeat (CTG) within the myotonin protein kinase gene on chromosome 19. This trinucleotide repeat disorder exhibits 'anticipation', whereby successive generations are more severely affected. Myotonic dystrophy is unusual in that it is the female transmission of the mutation that results in more severely affected offspring rather than paternal transmission, which is seen in other forms of anticipation. The features may be very mild in some cases if the length of the expanded repeat is only just above normal.

It is a multisystem disease resulting in (Fig. 28.4):

- progressive proximal and distal muscle weakness especially in the upper limbs
- myotonia (worse in the cold) – this can be elicited either through voluntary contraction or through percussion myotonia; tapping the thenar eminence with a tendon hammer causes the thumb to be drawn across the palm, followed by slow relaxation

Fig. 28.4 Clinical features of myotonic dystrophy.

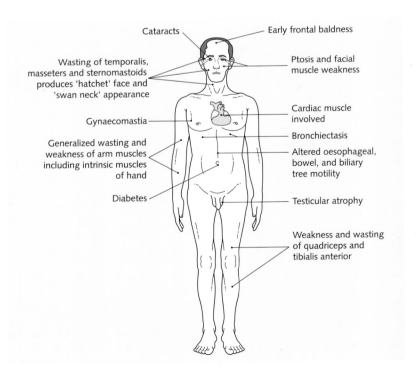

Cataracts

Early frontal baldness

Wasting of temporalis, masseters and sternomastoids produces 'hatchet' face and 'swan neck' appearance

Ptosis and facial muscle weakness

Gynaecomastia

Cardiac muscle involved

Bronchiectasis

Generalized wasting and weakness of arm muscles including intrinsic muscles of hand

Altered oesophageal, bowel, and biliary tree motility

Diabetes

Testicular atrophy

Weakness and wasting of quadriceps and tibialis anterior

- myopathic facies – weakness and thinning of the face and sternomastoids
- ptosis
- cataracts
- frontal balding
- dysarthria and dysphagia – caused by bulbar muscle weakness
- mild intellectual impairment and sleep disturbance
- cardiomyopathy and conduction defects
- impaired gastrointestinal motility due to smooth muscle involvement
- gynaecomastia and testicular atrophy
- glucose intolerance/diabetes mellitus.

The features develop between the ages of 20 and 50 years, and progress gradually. Diagnosis is based on genetic testing and management includes treatment of the associated disorders.

> **COMMUNICATION**
>
> Patients with myotonic dystrophy are often polysymptomatic and hypersomnolent. It is important to ask about and investigate for nocturnal hypoventilation and test for diabetes as these are two common causes of fatigue and sleepiness. Patients are also prone to cardiac conduction deficits and therefore require regular ECGs (at least yearly or when symptomatic).

Metabolic myopathies

Any disturbance of the biochemical pathways that support ATP levels in muscle will cause exercise intolerance, with pain during exercise and extreme fatigue. Continued exercise will lead to destruction of muscle (rhabdomyolysis) and the release of myoglobin, which may cause the patient's urine to turn red-orange and renal failure can ensue. There are a large number of specific enzyme deficiencies which are classified as either glycogen storage diseases or defects of fatty acid metabolism (see Fig. 28.2).

Periodic paralyses

The periodic paralyses are rare and belong to a group of disorders known as channelopathies. They are characterized by episodes of sudden weakness with alterations in serum potassium levels.

Hypokalaemic periodic paralysis
Hypokalaemic periodic paralysis is an autosomal dominant condition that is most commonly caused by abnormalities in L-type calcium channels due to mutations in the CACNA1S gene. Patients present between

10 and 20 years of age and may remit after 35 years of age. Attacks of generalized weakness develop after a heavy carbohydrate meal or after a period of rest following strenuous exertion (e.g. the following morning). During an attack, the serum potassium falls to below 3.0 mmol/L. Attacks may last from 4 to 24 hours. The weakness responds to treatment with potassium replacement. Prophylactic treatment involves the use of potassium supplements or potassium-sparing diuretics. Some older patients can develop a permanent weakness that progresses slowly over years.

The condition is rarely fatal, as the respiratory and bulbar muscles tend to be spared. Cardiac and eyelid involvement are also rare. Similar weakness with hypokalaemia may occur in thyrotoxicosis.

Hyperkalaemic periodic paralysis
Hyperkalaemic periodic paralysis is an autosomal dominant condition that is caused by abnormalities of voltage-gated sodium channels SCN4A.

It becomes apparent between 5 and 15 years of age and tends to remit after 20 years of age; however, a chronic proximal myopathy may persist. The attacks of weakness, especially of proximal muscles, become apparent 30 minutes to 2 hours after exercise and during fasting. They tend to be less severe than in hypokalaemic periodic paralysis and last less than an hour.

During an attack, the serum potassium is raised above 5.0 mmol/L. Attacks may be terminated by intravenous calcium gluconate or by salbutamol.

Mitochondrial myopathies

The final oxidative pathway involves the respiratory chain in mitochondria, which have their own DNA. Abnormalities of mitochondrial DNA (maternally inherited) cause a wide range of different conditions affecting muscle, the CNS, PNS and other systems within the body. Mutations in nuclear genes encoding mitochondrial proteins are now being described and may also present with a muscle disorder.

Inflammatory myopathies

Polymyositis and dermatomyositis

Polymyositis and dermatomyositis are conditions in which there is inflammation within the muscle. There may be associated connective tissue disease (25%) or underlying carcinoma (10%), especially if skin changes are present (dermatomyositis).

Clinical features
Polymyositis and dematomyositis usually present in the fourth to fifth decade, with women more commonly affected than men. Proximal muscle weakness is the cardinal symptom (difficulty rising from a chair or

climbing stairs). Pain and tenderness of the muscles occurs in less than half the patients.

The associated skin changes (dermatomyositis) include:

- macular erythema on the face, especially in the periorbital area, where it is heliotrope (blue-violet) in colour
- erythematous plaques over the dorsal aspects of the fingers (Gottron's papules)
- nail-fold haemorrhages
- photosensitivity.

As the disease progresses, there may be widespread wasting and weakness, with bulbar dysfunction and respiratory muscle weakness. Patients with polymyositis can also develop interstitial fibrosing lung disease.

Investigations

Investigations for polymyositis and dermatomyositis include the following:

- Erythrocyte sedimentation rate (ESR): raised
- CK: usually highly raised
- EMG: myopathic picture, but may include fibrillations
- Muscle biopsy: muscle fibre necrosis with an inflammatory infiltrate, which is distinct for polymyositis and dermatomyositis
- Autoantibodies (anti-Jo, antinuclear antibodies, rheumatoid factor, ENAs): present in up to 25% of patients
- Investigation for underlying carcinoma (chest X-ray as a minimum).

Treatment

Corticosteroids and other immunosuppressive drugs (e.g. azathioprine, cyclophosphamide) reduce the symptoms in about 75% of cases of polymyositis and dermatomyositis that are not associated with malignancy. Removal of an associated tumour may cause complete remission. Intravenous immunoglobulin may be useful in patients with severe dermatomyositis.

There is full recovery in about 10% of patients. The remainder of patients have varying degrees of disability and the disease may become inactive or 'burnt out' after a few years. When associated with connective tissue disease, the prognosis is linked to the course of this disease.

HINTS AND TIPS

Patients with an inflammatory myopathy often have neck weakness and this is one cause of presentation with a 'dropped head', i.e. forward flexion of the neck. Other causes are motor neuron disease and myasthenia gravis.

Inclusion body myositis

This disorder is the most common cause of muscle disease in people aged over 50 years, occurs more frequently in men, and often presents with weakness and wasting of the flexor muscles of the forearm and hand, causing difficulty grasping objects. The proximal muscles can also become involved, particularly the quadriceps (difficulty climbing stairs), and the oesophagus may be affected as the disease progresses. Extraocular and cardiac muscle involvement are rare, though respiratory muscles may be affected in approximately 10% of patients. There is an association with diabetes, but not with an underlying malignancy.

The investigation of choice is the muscle biopsy as characteristic inclusions are seen in muscle fibres, along with features of an inflammatory myopathy. There is no definitive treatment for the condition, and the disease is progressive, with death from respiratory compromise or an aspiration pneumonia.

Acquired electrolyte and endocrine myopathies

A wide range of diseases (especially endocrinological), acquired biochemical abnormalities and drugs can result in myopathy (Fig. 28.2). The weakness tends to be proximal. Most cases are reversible with treatment of the primary condition or removal of the drug.

Thyrotoxicosis

Patients often have greater shoulder than pelvic girdle involvement. Reflexes are brisk. Fasciculations and atrophy may be present.

Cushing's syndrome

A proximal myopathy can be seen in patients who are taking long-term steroids or who have an underlying steroid-secreting neoplasm.

Hypokalaemia

Hypokalaemia can be associated with a painless proximal myopathy. This is often caused by potassium-losing drugs, including liquorice.

Vitamin D deficiency

Proximal muscle pain and wasting can occur in the context of vitamin D deficiency. The weakness often improves over several weeks with vitamin replacement.

Drug-induced myopathies

Statins are increasingly recognized to be associated with a variety of muscle disorders, ranging from asymptomatic raised creatine kinase through to muscle pain and overt myopathy. The causative statin should be stopped in all but the mildest cases and a different statin commenced and monitored. Steroids are a common cause of drug-induced myopathy. Chloroquine, amiodarone and doxorubicin can all cause a dose-related vacuolar myopathy associated with proximal weakness. The causative drug should be stopped.

Zidovudine (AZT) is used in the treatment of HIV infection and can cause a dose-related proximal myopathy associated with mitochondrial dysfunction. Recovery usually occurs after the drug is stopped.

Paraneoplastic myopathy

A necrotizing myopathy can occur with malignancies, especially colorectal, lung and breast, independent of either polymyositis or dermatomyositis.

Critical Illness myopathy

Patients who are ventilated can sometimes develop a severe myopathy. It can present as an inability to wean off the ventilator and may be associated with prolonged use of paralysing agents. It is a symmetric proximal myopathy, but the neck flexors may be involved and respiratory failure occurs in 80% of cases. Patients often show a slow improvement. Muscle biopsy shows myosin loss in muscle fibres and the cause of this remains uncertain.

- Define stroke and TIA
- Understand the vascular supply to the brain and spinal cord
- Describe the main stroke syndromes
- Understand the management of stroke and TIA – what risk factors are treatable?
- Understand the presentation and management of subarachnoid haemorrhage

CEREBROVASCULAR DISEASE

Cerebrovascular disease is a significant cause of mortality and morbidity in the developed world. Strokes of all types rank third as a cause of death and are surpassed only by heart disease and cancer. Stroke is a syndrome of clinical features, but an accurate diagnosis requires the localization of the anatomical territory involved, the underlying pathology (infarction or haemorrhage), the mechanism (e.g. embolism), the underlying aetiology (e.g. atherosclerosis) and contributing risk factors (e.g. smoking).

Definitions

Stroke

Stroke is a focal, neurological deficit caused by a compromise of the cerebral circulation. The onset is sudden and the symptoms last longer than 24 hours, if the patient survives.

Transient ischaemic attack

A transient ischaemic attack (TIA) is a focal, sudden-onset, neurological deficit lasting less than 24 hours, with complete clinical recovery, caused by focal hypoperfusion within the brain. The distinction of a TIA from a stroke is largely arbitrary, as the mechanisms underlying both may be identical, and the main difference is that of duration. However, the differential diagnosis of transient events encompasses other causes of transient neurological symptoms (Fig. 29.1).

Up to 15% of patients with TIA may suffer a stroke within the first 2 weeks. It is now possible to clinically stratify patients presenting with TIAs into high- or low-risk categories. High-risk patients merit immediate assessment and investigation within 24 hours.

Types of stroke

The main subdivisions of stroke (Fig. 29.2) are cerebral infarction (ischaemic stroke) and intracranial haemorrhage (haemorrhagic stroke). About 80% of strokes are caused by infarction, which may affect all or a part of a vascular territory, occupy the border zone between arterial supplies, or occupy only a small area of brain supplied by a penetrating vessel (lacunar stroke). Ischaemic and infarcted brain can occasionally become haemorrhagic. 'Haemorrhagic transformation' is important to recognize because it is a cause of later deterioration in a patient with an ischaemic stroke. In 12% of cases stroke is caused by primary haemorrhage (intracerebral haemorrhage or ICH) within the brain which may affect deep structures or more superficial lobes of the brain. In 8% of stroke cases, bleeding occurs primarily within the subarachnoid space (subarachnoid haemorrhage or SAH). Sometimes a SAH can be complicated by cerebral infarction due to vasospasm. Cerebral venous thrombosis is a rare cause of stroke but can present with either cerebral infarction or haemorrhage or both in venous territories of the brain.

Incidence of stroke

The incidence of stroke is approximately 150–200 cases per 100 000 persons per annum in the UK, and approximately 20% of patients will die within 30 days. The incidence of TIA is 30 cases per 100 000 persons per annum, although many probably go unreported. The rates increase markedly with advancing age and 20–25% of individuals over the age of 45 years will have a stroke.

Fig. 29.1 Differential diagnoses of transient ischaemic attacks (TIAs)/stroke mimics

Differentials	Notes
Hypoglycaemia	Can present with focal neurology including hemiparesis
Mass lesions, e.g. abscess, tumour	Can present acutely
Benign positional vertigo	Vertigo affected by head position
Epilepsy	Post-ictal paralysis, history of seizure
Migraine	Aura consists of positive symptoms, evolves over minutes, lasts <1 hour, associated with headache. TIAs consist of negative symptoms and reach maximum deficit within 1 minute
Multiple sclerosis	Can present acutely with focal neurology
Transient global amnesia	

Fig. 29.2 Types of stroke and relative frequency

Type	Frequency	Subtype
Cerebral infarction	~80%	Territorial Border zone Lacunar
Intracerebral haemorrhage	~12%	Lobar Deep Posterior fossa
Subarachnoid haemorrhage	~8%	
Cerebral venous thrombosis	Rare	

Aetiology of stroke

The causes of stroke are as follows (the first five are responsible for the majority of cases):

- **Atherosclerosis:** this causes thrombotic stroke in large extracranial arteries, most commonly the bifurcation of the carotid arteries or intracranial arteries arising from the circle of Willis, especially the origin of the middle cerebral artery.
- **Cardiac or carotid embolism:** embolic stroke usually arises from pieces of ruptured atherosclerotic plaques or cardiac thrombus. The bifurcation of the common carotid and the akinetic segments of myocardium, e.g. after a heart attack or in atrial fibrillation, are the most common sources of emboli. Valvular heart disease is another important cause.
- **Arterial dissection:** in the younger population, dissection of either the carotid or vertebral arteries is a relatively common cause of stroke. This may occur spontaneously or there may be a history of injury to the neck such as sudden twisting movements or flexion–extension injuries such as 'whiplash'. Emboli from mural thrombosis associated with the dissection is a common mechanism of stroke in this setting.
- **Intracerebral haemorrhage:** this is most often secondary to chronic untreated hypertension, but can be caused by other factors, e.g. trauma, anticoagulant therapy, neoplasia, and coagulation disorders, such as haemophilia or abnormalities of platelet number or function.
- **Lipohyalinosis of small arteries:** this degenerative process especially affects small perforating arteries that supply structures deep to the cortex, e.g. basal ganglia, internal capsule and pons. It usually occurs in patients with chronic untreated hypertension. Occlusion of these penetrating arteries causes subcortical infarcts, less than 1.5 cm in diameter, which are called 'lacunes'. Occasionally, their rupture can lead to a small, but clinically devastating, haemorrhage.
- **Non-atherosclerotic diseases of the vessel wall and haematological conditions:** these are rarer than the above causes but should always be considered, especially in young patients who present with stroke. Causes include rheumatoid vasculitis, systemic lupus erythematosus, polyarteritis nodosa and temporal arteritis (in the elderly). Infections involving the base of the brain, such as TB meningitis, can occlude large blood vessels. Any prothrombotic haematological condition can cause a thrombotic stroke.

Risk factors

- **Hypertension:** this is a major factor in the development of ischaemic and haemorrhagic stroke.
- **Diabetes mellitus:** this increases the risk of cerebral infarction twofold and should be treated aggressively because it is a recognized risk factor for atherosclerosis.
- **Cardiac disease:** in addition to cardiac causes of embolic strokes, (e.g. atrial fibrillation, cardiomyopathy, arrhythmias and valve disease) the presence of coronary artery disease is a marker for atherosclerosis elsewhere and is therefore a marker for stroke.
- **Hyperlipidaemia:** this is less significant for stroke than for coronary artery disease.
- **Smoking:** cessation of smoking lowers the risk of ischaemic stroke.

- **Family history:** close relatives are at slightly greater risk than non-genetically related family members of a stroke patient.
- **Obesity and diet:** these are probably less significant for stroke than for coronary artery disease.
- **Oral contraceptive:** this may increase risk of thromboembolic stroke, cerebral venous sinus thrombosis and subarachnoid haemorrhage in individuals with other risk factors.

Vascular anatomy

A knowledge of the arterial blood supply to the brain and of the common sites for atheromatous plaque formation is important for an appreciation of the various presentations and significance of cerebrovascular disease.

The circle of Willis (Fig. 29.3) is supplied anteriorly by the two carotid arteries and posteriorly by the basilar artery, which is formed by the union of the two vertebral arteries (Fig. 29.4). It is therefore common to classify strokes into those affecting the anterior (carotid) and posterior (vertebrobasilar) circulations.

The most common sites for atheromatous plaques are:

- the origin of the internal carotid arteries
- within the carotid syphon
- the origin of the vertebral arteries.

The anterior, middle and posterior cerebral arteries arise from the circle of Willis. These supply specific portions of the cerebral hemispheres (Figs 29.5, 29.6 and 29.7); thus, reduction in perfusion in each territory will cause different and specific deficits.

Clinical syndromes

Transient ischaemic attacks

Examples of the types of deficits that can occur in TIAs are listed in Figure 29.8. The symptoms typically represent loss of function (negative symptoms), are maximal at onset and last 5 to 30 minutes. Any cause of an ischaemic stroke can cause a TIA, although rarely microhaemorrhages can cause TIA-like symptoms. The most common cause is embolic.

Middle cerebral artery occlusion

The middle cerebral artery is the largest branch of the internal carotid artery and supplies the largest area of the cerebral cortex (see Fig. 29.5). It is the most commonly involved artery in stroke. As well as supplying

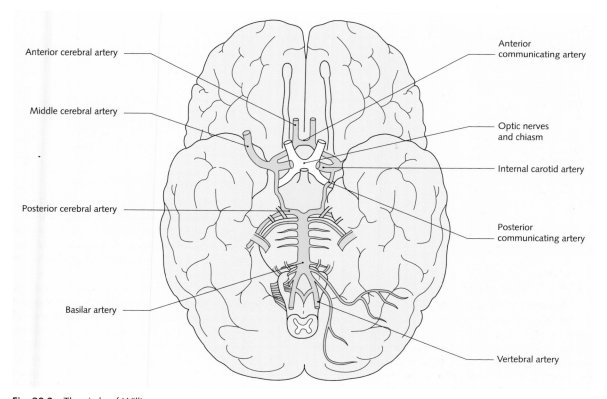

Anterior cerebral artery

Middle cerebral artery

Posterior cerebral artery

Basilar artery

Anterior communicating artery

Optic nerves and chiasm

Internal carotid artery

Posterior communicating artery

Vertebral artery

Fig. 29.3 The circle of Willis.

Fig. 29.4 The vertebrobasilar and carotid arteries. The vertebral and basilar arteries give off three cerebellar arteries, which supply the brainstem and cerebellum.

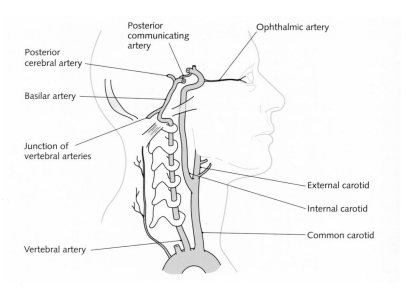

Fig. 29.5 The distribution of the three major cerebral arteries (lateral and tomographic views).

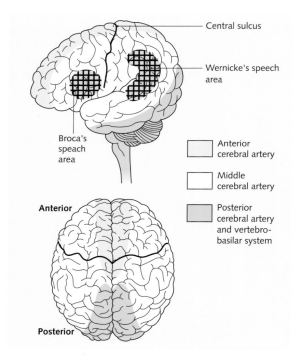

occlusion of the left middle cerebral artery. Non-dominant lesions often cause visuospatial problems, e.g. inattention. Lesions of either side can be associated with a hemianopia.

The signs of a middle cerebral artery occlusion are listed in Figure 29.9. Initially, the limbs are flaccid and areflexic. After a variable period, the reflexes recover and become exaggerated, and the plantar responses become extensor, with spastic limb tone. There is variable recovery of weakness over the course of days, weeks or months. The most common cause of occlusion is thromboembolism or, in Asians/Africans stenosis, at the origin of the middle cerebral artery. Total occlusion can lead to severe malignant oedema, which may need surgical decompression with a hemicraniectomy.

Anterior cerebral artery occlusion

The anterior cerebral artery is a branch of the internal carotid artery and runs above the optic nerve to follow the curve of the corpus callosum. The two arteries are linked by the anterior communicating artery and thus the effect of occlusion depends on the relation with respect to the anterior communicating artery (see Figs 29.3 and 29.7). Occlusion proximal to the anterior communicating artery is normally well tolerated because of adequate cross-flow and thus few symptoms result. Occlusion distal to the anterior communicating artery causes contralateral weakness and cortical sensory loss in the leg (see Chs 15 and 16). Incontinence is often present, and occasionally a contralateral grasp and other primitive reflexes. It is relatively uncommon for the anterior cerebral artery to be purely involved in stroke;

the motor and sensory cortices, the middle cerebral artery supplies the areas of the cortex pertaining to the comprehension (Wernicke's area) and expression (Broca's area) of speech (see Figs 29.5 and 29.6). These areas are found in the dominant hemisphere only, and thus, in the majority of right-handed individuals, speech production will be affected only when there is

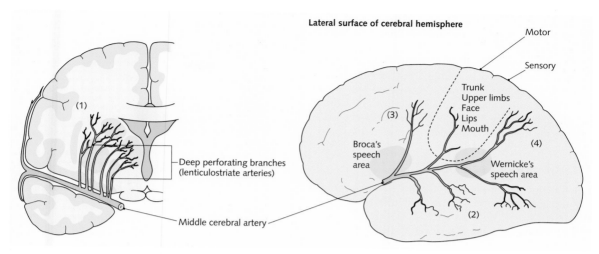

Lateral surface of cerebral hemisphere

Fig. 29.6   The middle cerebral artery is the largest branch of the internal carotid artery. It gives off (1) deep branches (perforating vessels – lenticulostriate), which supply the anterior limb of the internal capsule and part of the basal nuclei. It then passes out to the lateral surface of the cerebral hemisphere at the insula of the lateral sulcus. Here it gives off cortical branches: (2) temporal, (3) frontal and (4) parietal.

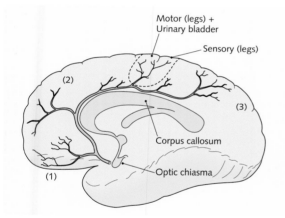

Fig. 29.7   Medial surface of the right cerebral hemisphere. The anterior cerebral artery is a branch of the internal carotid and runs above the optic nerve to follow the curve of the corpus callosum. Soon after its origin, the vessel is joined by the anterior communicating artery. Deep branches pass to the anterior part of the internal capsule and basal nuclei. Cortical branches supply the medial surface of the hemisphere: (1) orbital, (2) frontal and (3) parietal.

Fig. 29.8 Clinical features of transient ischaemic attacks (TIAs)	
Anterior circulation (carotid arteries)	**Posterior circulation (vertebrobasilar arteries)**
Amaurosis fugax Dysphasia Contralateral hemiparesis Contralateral homonymous visual field loss Any combination of the above	Diplopia, vertigo Dysarthria/dysphagia Unilateral/bilateral or alternating paresis or sensory loss Binocular visual loss Ataxia Loss of consciousness (rare) Any combination of the above

Fig. 29.9   Signs of middle cerebral artery occlusion
Contralateral hemiplegia (including the lower part of the face and relative sparing of the leg) Contralateral cortical hemisensory loss Dominant hemisphere (usually left): aphasia Non-dominant hemisphere: neglect of contralateral limb and dressing apraxia Contralateral homonymous hemianopia Conjugate eye deviation (towards the side of the lesion)

it is often due to occlusion more proximally in the internal carotid, or unusual aetiologies such as vasospasm.

Posterior cerebral artery occlusion

The posterior cerebral arteries are the terminal branches of the basilar artery. In addition to cortical branches to the medial inferior temporal lobes and occipital and visual cortices, there are perforating branches that supply the midbrain and thalamus. Occlusion is typically embolic and most patients are in atrial fibrillation.

The effect of occlusion depends on the site:

- Proximal occlusion: which includes midbrain syndrome (Weber's syndrome), third nerve palsy and contralateral hemiplegia.

- Thalamic or temporal lobe involvement may cause confusion, memory impairment and hemisensory disturbance.
- Cortical vessel occlusion: homonymous hemianopia with macular sparing (the macular area is additionally supplied by the middle cerebral artery).
- Bilateral occlusion: Anton's syndrome (cortical blindness) is rare. The patient is blind but lacks insight into the degree of visual loss and often denies it.

Carotid artery occlusion

Often an internal carotid artery occlusion does not present as a stroke due to the presence of a collateral blood supply from the circle of Willis. A stroke will only occur if the collateral supply is inadequate or thrombosis spreads or embolizes to involve the middle cerebral artery or its branches. Thus, clinically, carotid artery occlusion may present similarly to a middle cerebral artery stroke.

Lacunar stroke

Lacunar infarction is caused by occlusion of small penetrating vessels to the subcortical deep white matter, internal capsule, basal ganglia or pons. Although these vessels supply a very small area, a number of extremely important structures pass through this space. A very small lesion can cause a marked neurological deficit. Lacunar infarcts are most commonly caused by lipohyalinosis and microatheroma affecting the small perforating vessels, as opposed to embolic disease. Most patients have hypertension, diabetes or hypercholesterolaemia. Clinically, patients present with unilateral weakness or sensory loss affecting at least two of the face, arm or leg. There are no cortical signs (e.g. confusion, dysphasia, neglect, apraxia, hemianopia, conjugate eye deviation) and no cognitive difficulties. A CT brain may not detect lacunar infarcts, and MRI is more sensitive. Multiple lacunar infarcts in multiple domains can cause vascular dementia (see Ch. 18).

Vertebral and basilar artery occlusion – brainstem stroke

Vertebral and basilar artery occlusion are typically due to atheromatous disease. Multiple patterns of deficit can arise depending on the exact location of the lesion with respect to the long tracts (i.e. corticospinal, medial and lateral leminisci, brainstem connections to the cerebellum, and cranial nerve nuclei). Possible clinical features are summarized in Figure 29.10.

Specific brainstem syndromes
Lateral medullary syndrome (posterior inferior cerebellar artery syndrome; Wallenberg's syndrome) Lateral medullary syndrome (Fig. 29.11) is the most widely

Fig. 29.10 Features of brainstem infarction

Clinical features	Structures involved
Upper motor neuron hemiparesis or tetraparesis	Corticospinal tracts (pyramidal tracts)
Hemisensory or bilateral sensory impairment	Medial lemniscus or spinothalamic tracts
Diplopia	3rd, 4th (midbrain), and/or 6th (pons) cranial nerves or nuclei or their connections, e.g. median longitudinal fasciculus
Facial sensory loss	5th cranial nerve nucleus (midbrain, pons, medulla)
Lower motor neuron facial weakness (upper and lower face)	7th nerve nucleus (pons)
Nystagmus, vertigo	Vestibular nuclei (pons and medulla) and connections
Dysphagia, dysarthria	9th and 10th cranial nerve nuclei (medulla)
Dysarthria, ataxia, vomiting, hiccoughs	Cerebellum and cerebellar brainstem connection
Horner's syndrome (meiosis, ptosis, enophthalmos and disturbed sweating)	Sympathetic fibres in lateral brainstem
Altered consciousness	Reticular formation

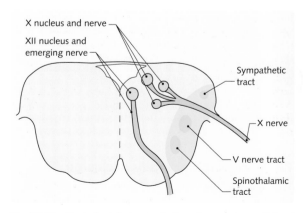

Fig. 29.11 Posterior inferior cerebellar artery syndrome (lateral medullary syndrome).

recognized brainstem syndrome. Clinical features comprise sudden-onset vertigo, vomiting, nystagmus, ipsilateral ataxia (cerebellar connections), ipsilateral facial numbness (fifth cranial nerve descending tract), ipsilateral Horner's syndrome (sympathetic tract), contralateral loss of pain and temperature sensation in the limbs (ascending spinothalamic tract) and dysarthria and dysphagia (tenth nerve). See also Ch.16.

'Locked-in syndrome' This is caused by a bilateral infarction in the ventral pons, with or without medullary involvement. The patient is conscious (intact brainstem reticular formation), but is mute and paralysed. Patients can often move their eyes because of sparing of the third and fourth cranial nuclei in the midbrain.

Weber's syndrome Weber's syndrome is caused by a lesion in one-half of the midbrain, resulting in an ipsilateral third nerve palsy (III nucleus) and contralateral hemiplegia (descending pyramidal tract above the decussation).

Border zone ischaemia

Hypoperfusion of the brain (e.g. hypovolaemia due to blood loss or hypoxia due to cardiac arrest) can cause border zone or 'watershed' infarction in terminal areas of arterial supply. The parieto-occipital cortex between the middle and posterior cerebral artery territories is especially vulnerable, as is the area between the anterior and middle cerebral arteries, hippocampi and basal ganglia.

Primary intracerebral haemorrhage

The most common non-traumatic causes include chronic hypertension, ruptured intracranial aneurysms and vascular malformations. Cerebral amyloid angiopathy is an important cause of superficial, lobar haematomas in older patients. When in conjunction with chronic hypertension, primary intracerebral haemorrhage often occurs in the internal capsule and/or basal ganglia, but it can occur in any part of the cortex, as well as in the pons and cerebellum. The clinical signs depend on the location, but are often associated with mass effect and, therefore, reduced conscious level. It is otherwise very difficult to clinically differentiate a haemorrhage from an infarct.

HINTS AND TIPS

Neurosurgical evacuation of haematomas or shunting of hydrocephalus can be life-saving, particularly in posterior fossa cerebellar haemorrhages, which can cause fatal brainstem compression and hydrocephalus.

Investigation of stroke and transient ischaemic attack

Initial investigations

The following routine investigations should be performed:

- Full blood count (FBC): polycythaemia; infection
- Renal function and electrolytes: patients with electrolyte disturbances may rarely present as stroke mimics with focal or global dysfunction
- Clotting screen: all patients with haemorrhagic stroke and those on anticoagulants
- Erythrocyte sedimentation rate (ESR); C-reactive protein (CRP): inflammatory disease
- Thyroid function tests: all patients with atrial fibrillation
- Blood sugar: hypoglycaemia and diabetes mellitus
- Fasting lipids
- Blood culture: if endocarditis or a superadded infection is suspected
- Autoantibodies and coagulation studies in young patients: connective tissue or vasculitic disease or prothrombotic disorder
- Electrocardiography (ECG): arrhythmia, myocardial ischaemia/infarction and left ventricular hypertrophy secondary to hypertension
- Chest X-ray: neoplasia and enlarged heart.

Special investigations

Imaging

All patients should have a computed tomography (CT) or a magnetic resonance imaging (MRI) of the brain. CT is more commonly available acutely and can differentiate between an ischaemic and a haemorrhagic stroke. It can also reveal stroke mimics such as subdural haematomas or tumours. CT may appear normal, depending on the time from onset of the stroke to imaging and the size and severity of the infarct. Only ~75% of infarcts are ever visible on CT. CT is a critical tool in determining a patient's suitability for thrombolysis.

MRI should be considered if the clinical signs localize to the posterior fossa (i.e. brainstem and cerebellum) because these regions are poorly visualized by CT due to artefacts caused by the surrounding bone. MRI should also be considered in patients who may have had a small stroke, which may not be visible on CT, or where the diagnosis is uncertain. Sophisticated sequences such as diffusion weighted imaging (DWI) can differentiate acute from chronic infarcts, while T2* sequences can detect microhaemorrhages. Vascular reconstructive imaging using CT angiography (CTA) and MR angiography (MRA) is helpful in visualizing the intra- and extracranial carotids and the posterior circulation to look for atheromatous disease, dissections and aneurysms.

The UK National Stroke Strategy calls for the urgent imaging of stroke patients who satisfy the criteria for thrombolysis, with a maximum 'door to needle time' of 60 minutes. In high-risk TIAs, investigations should be completed within 24 hours. NICE guidance lists other scenarios in stroke patients in whom urgent imaging is critical. These include a depressed level of consciousness (GCS < 13), severe headache at onset, progressive or fluctuating symptoms, papilloedema/neck stiffness/fever, history of head trauma and patients taking anticoagulants or who have a known bleeding tendency.

Carotid Doppler

The carotid Doppler is an extremely effective, non-invasive means of demonstrating internal carotid artery stenosis when carotid thromboembolism is suspected. A carotid endarterectomy is considered if there is greater than 50–70% stenosis in the vessel, and a history of a non-disabling ischaemic stroke or TIA within the last 6 months. The longer the period free of symptoms, the smaller the overall benefit from surgery and NICE recommends that suitable patients undergo surgery within a maximum of 2 weeks of onset of stroke or TIA symptoms. If the patient is left with a very dense hemiplegia and other cortical problems (e.g. dysphasia), there is little value in performing carotid Doppler as there is little functional brain left to protect.

Cerebral angiography

The advent of carotid Doppler and MRA has meant that conventional cerebral angiography is used infrequently in stroke patients, primarily to locate intracerebral aneurysms, and for the diagnosis of cerebral vasculitides, which are both still poorly detected with MRA. In patients with a recent completed stroke, angiography should not be considered until 1–2 weeks have elapsed.

Echocardiography and Holter monitoring

Echocardiography is useful in patients with suspected cardiogenic embolism and may define wall-motion abnormalities or the presence of atrial or ventricular thrombus. Holter monitoring or more prolonged monitoring using a REVEAL device may confirm paroxysmal atrial fibrillation in patients with suspected cardiogenic embolic stroke, but normal ECG.

Management of stroke

The management of stroke can be divided into the management of acute stroke in hyperacute stroke units and thrombolysis in appropriate cases. Beyond this, admission to an organized stroke unit is critical, for the prevention of secondary complications, risk factor management, secondary prevention of stroke and rehabilitation.

Thrombolysis

Thrombolysis is the first treatment that has been shown to be effective in acute stroke. Trials have shown that intravenous recombinant tissue plasminogen activator (rt-PA) given within 4.5 hours of onset of ischaemic stroke confers a 1 in 8 chance of a significant recovery, and a 1 in 18 chance of symptomatic intracranial haemorrhage. Knowing the time of onset of stroke is, therefore, crucial and there is almost a linear decline in functional recovery as the stroke to needle time extends, even within the window of 4.5 hours. In patients who wake up with stroke, time of onset is unknown, and they are therefore unsuitable for thrombolysis.

Other management aims

- Prescribe an antiplatelet medication after a haemorrhage has been excluded. NICE now recommends the use of clopidogrel or, in those intolerant to it, the combination of aspirin and dipyridamole. Antiplatelet treatment helps prevent early stroke recurrence, and reduces death and disability at follow-up. For people who have a contraindication or intolerance to both clopidogrel and aspirin, dipyridamole alone is recommended as a treatment option.
- Prevent development of complications, e.g. aspiration pneumonia, pressure sores, dislocated shoulders, thromboembolism and depression.
- Rehabilitate the patient, e.g. physiotherapy, occupational therapy and speech therapy.
- Control hypertension only if it is severely elevated, i.e. systolic >220 mmHg and diastolic >120 mmHg. An acute drop in blood pressure can reduce perfusion to an already ischaemic brain.
- Risk factor management – encourage the patient to stop smoking, correct lipid abnormalities with statins and good glycaemic control in diabetic patients.
- Remove or treat embolic source, e.g. anticoagulation, antibiotics for endocarditis or endarterectomy. Note: anticoagulation is indicated for cardiac embolus, but only once a cerebral haemorrhage has been excluded and not for at least 7 days after an acute event, to prevent a haemorrhagic infarct.

Management of transient ischaemic attacks

The management of TIAs is based on the secondary prevention of stroke and risk factor management. NICE recommend that all patients who have had a TIA should be treated with modified-release dipyridamole plus aspirin. In those with a contraindication or intolerance to aspirin, dipyridamole alone is recommended as a treatment option. The management of other risk factors such as hypertension are equally important. Anticoagulants are indicated in patients with a known cardiac source of embolus and atrial fibrillation, once a scan has excluded haemorrhage. Those patients with significant carotid stenosis should be treated with a carotid endarterectomy within 48 hours.

Prognosis

The mortality of stroke is approximately 12 and 19% at 7 and 30 days after stroke, respectively. In the first few days death is usually the result of cerebral oedema from infarction or mass effect from haemorrhage causing brainstem compression, coma and death. Subsequently, mortality results from complications (e.g. chest infection, pulmonary embolus) and from other atherosclerotic disease (e.g. myocardial infarction). There are no reliable clinical prognostic indicators.

Among the survivors, gradual improvement usually occurs most rapidly in the first 4 to 6 weeks, though it may continue for as long as rehabilitation input continues. Approximately 50% of survivors remain dependent at 1 year, and about one-third of patients may return to independent mobility, but even these patients often have subtle-to-overt cognitive deficits (e.g. poor memory or concentration).

INTRACRANIAL HAEMORRHAGE

Intracranial haemorrhage can be subdivided by site:
- Primary intracerebral haemorrhage (considered in the section on cerebrovascular disease)
- Subarachnoid haemorrhage
- Subdural and extradural haemorrhage.

Subarachnoid haemorrhage

Subarachnoid haemorrhage is caused by spontaneous (rather than traumatic) arterial bleeding into the subarachnoid space. The incidence of subarachnoid haemorrhage is 10–15 cases per 100 000 persons per year and the average age of onset is about 50 years.

Causes
- Intracranial aneurysms: 85%
- Non-aneurysmal perimesencephalic haemorrhage (haemorrhage into basal cisterns): 10%
- Arteriovenous malformation: 5%.

Risk factors
- Family history/genetic factors
- Smoking
- Hypertension.

Clinical features
- Patients complain of a severe headache of instantaneous onset (like a sudden 'blow to the head'). The patient often describes it as the worst headache they have ever had. Some patients may report acute headaches just prior to presentation and these 'warning' headaches may represent aneurysmal enlargement or minor rupture.
- Transient or prolonged loss of consciousness or seizure may follow immediately.
- Nausea and vomiting often occur due to raised intracranial pressure.
- Drowsiness or coma may continue for hours to days.
- Signs of meningism occur after 3–12 hours: neck stiffness on passive flexion; positive Kernig's sign (lifting the leg and extending the knee with the patient lying supine, stretches the nerve roots and causes meningeal pain).
- Focal signs due to intraparenchymal extension of blood or vasospasm causing ischaemia and infarction may be present, e.g. limb weakness, dysphasia.
- Papilloedema may be present and may be accompanied by subhyaloid and vitreous haemorrhage visible on fundoscopy.

Investigation

CT scanning is the investigation of choice and shows subarachnoid or intraventricular blood in up to 95% of patients who present within 24 hours. Beyond that, the sensitivity of CT decreases to 80% at 3 days, 50% at 1 week and 30% at 2 weeks. A lumbar puncture should be carried out if the clinical suspicion of a subarachnoid haemorrhage is high, but CT is normal and only if the patient is alert and orientated without focal signs, i.e. no evidence of raised intracranial pressure. In a patient with a mass lesion, lumbar puncture can precipitate transtentorial herniation or 'coning' and should not be performed. The diagnosis of subarachnoid haemorrhage can be made when the cerebrospinal fluid (CSF) is uniformly bloodstained or xanthochromic (straw-coloured supernatant), due to breakdown products of haemoglobin accumulating over a period of 6 hours or more. Xanthochromia determined by spectrophotometry will be positive in all patients between 12 hours and 2 weeks. An extra 5% of cases of subarachnoid haemorrhage can be diagnosed after lumbar puncture.

Angiography is carried out at the earliest convenience in most patients, but is delayed in patients with a poor clinical condition. Angiograms are required to localize aneurysms and arteriovenous malformations prior to intervention and to confirm the cause of the diagnosis. Formal cerebral angiography provides better resolution than CT angiography.

Immediate management

- General supportive care: regular neurological observations, bedrest and fluid replacement, analgesia for headache, and avoidance of hypotension and hypertension
- Nimodipine (a calcium-channel blocker): reduces risk of delayed ischaemia secondary to vasospasm.

Subsequent management

Berry aneurysms are the most common finding at angiography. These can be dealt with neurosurgically by clipping of the aneurysm neck or by endovascular coiling. Arteriovenous malformations can be treated conservatively, or with direct surgery, radiosurgery, endovascular embolization or a combination of these.

Prognosis

Subarachnoid haemorrhage has a poor prognosis, with an overall mortality rate of almost 50%, and 30% of survivors have major neurological deficits. The risk of rebleeding from aneurysms is high in the first 2 weeks, and then declines. In arteriovenous malformations the risk is lower but persists, while perimesencephalic bleeds carry the lowest risk of rebleeding.

Subdural and extradural haemorrhage

Both subdural and extradural haemorrhage can be fatal unless treated promptly.

Subdural haematoma

Subdural haematoma occurs as a result of rupture of cortical veins bridging the dura and brain. It is almost invariably caused by trauma to the head in a patient with a shrunken brain (e.g. elderly and alcoholics).

In an acute subdural haemorrhage, there can be rapid accumulation of blood with a space-occupying effect, leading to rapid transtentorial 'coning'.

With a chronic subdural haematoma, the initial injury may be minor and there may be a latent interval, from days to months, between injury and symptoms. Chronic subdural haematoma is common in the elderly and in alcoholics. Symptoms can be indolent and fluctuate and include headache, drowsiness (a key feature) and confusion. However, focal deficits (usually hemiparesis), seizures, stupor and coma can occur.

Extradural haemorrhage

Extradural haemorrhage is caused by a traumatic tear in the middle meningeal artery, usually associated with a temporal or parietal skull fracture.

Blood accumulates rapidly in the extradural spaces, over minutes to hours. After a lucid period, the patient may then develop focal signs, coma and transtentorial coning, leading to death.

Management

Diagnosis is by CT scan (Fig. 29.12).

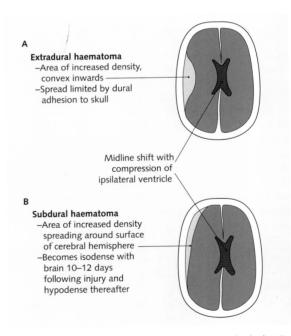

A

Extradural haematoma
–Area of increased density, convex inwards
–Spread limited by dural adhesion to skull

Midline shift with compression of ipsilateral ventricle

B

Subdural haematoma
–Area of increased density spreading around surface of cerebral hemisphere
–Becomes isodense with brain 10–12 days following injury and hypodense thereafter

Fig. 29.12 (A) Extradural haematoma: biconvex, high-density lesion abutting the inner margin of the skull. Midline ventricular shift and sulcal effacement can occur in both subdural and extradural haematomas if they are sufficiently large. (B) Subdural haematoma: crescent-shaped, high-density lesion lying adjacent to the inner margin of the skull. As the haematoma ages, it can become isodense with the brain substance.

Urgent surgical drainage is undertaken for acute subdural or extradural haematoma. Chronic subdural haematoma is often evacuated through burr holes as an elective procedure.

CEREBROVASCULAR INVOLVEMENT IN VASCULITIS

Vasculitis causing stroke may be secondary to infections (e.g. meningitis) or connective tissue disorders (e.g. systemic lupus erythematosus, polyarteritis nodosa), or rarely may be caused by a primary angiitis of the CNS, without systemic or extracranial features. All of these conditions rarely present solely as a stroke, and there may be other neurological or systemic features. However, they should always be considered in young patients, or patients with unusual features.

Investigations

Investigations should include ESR, CRP, autoantibodies, imaging (MRI), cerebral angiography, CSF analysis and, if appropriate, biopsy of the skin, muscle, kidney or other affected organ. If there is a strong suspicion of vasculitis confined to the CNS and angiography shows no diagnostic features, a biopsy of the brain and meninges may be necessary to make the diagnosis.

Treatment

Treatment is with steroids and other immunosuppressive drugs such as cyclophosphamide.

CEREBRAL VENOUS THROMBOSIS

Blood from the brain is drained by cerebral veins, which empty into dural sinuses, which subsequently drain into the internal jugular veins.

Venous sinus thrombosis is associated with:

- pregnancy, puerperium, oral contraception
- haematological diseases, e.g. polycythaemia, thrombophilia
- dehydration, e.g. prolonged vomiting
- infection: the middle ear, paranasal sinuses and face all drain into the dural sinuses
- inflammatory disorders, e.g. Behçet's disease, sarcoidosis, systemic lupus erythematosus
- meningitis.

The superior sagittal sinus is most commonly involved, followed by the lateral sinus and cavernous sinus, although all are uncommon.

Clinical features

The clinical features of thrombosis in the major sinuses and cerebral veins are variable. The most common presentations are headache, motor and sensory deficit, seizures, altered consciousness and papilloedema. The thrombosis within the sinus may lead to venous infarction, which is often haemorrhagic, in the territory draining into the affected sinus.

Cavernous sinus thrombosis

Cavernous sinus thrombosis warrants a special mention because it has a distinctive clinical picture. The cavernous sinus drains venous blood from the eye and many important structures run by or through it, including the carotid artery and the third, fourth, fifth (ophthalmic division) and sixth cranial nerves. In classic, acute cases of cavernous sinus thrombosis, there is proptosis, chemosis and painful ophthalmoplegia.

Diagnosis

Diagnosis can be made with CT angiogram or MRI supplemented with MR venography images.

Treatment

NICE recommend that anticoagulation is used and it is safe even in those with haemorrhagic infarction. Symptomatic treatments include anticonvulsants, antibiotics (if associated with infection) and methods to reduce intracranial pressure.

DISSECTION

Arterial dissection should always be considered as a cause of stroke in young patients. Dissection is due to a tear in the intima of the vessel wall, which causes development of a subintimal or intraluminal haematoma. The haematoma can embolize to produce a stroke and most cases involve the extracranial carotid or vertebral arteries. Although there may be an underlying connective tissue disorder, the majority of these patients develop dissections either spontaneously or secondary to trivial neck trauma or manipulation. Clinically, patients present with a history of minor neck trauma and pain, preceding development of a stroke. The association of a Horner's syndrome with stroke should alert one to the possibility of carotid dissection. MRI and MRA are diagnostic, and dissection is typically treated with antiplatelet medication. There is no evidence for the use of anticoagulants.

VASCULAR DISEASE OF THE SPINAL CORD

The blood supply to the spinal cord is complex. The main vessels are the paired posterior spinal arteries, which run down the posterior surface of the cord, and the single anterior spinal artery, which runs down the median fissure anteriorly (Fig. 29.13).

During development, five to eight radicular arteries become predominant and provide most of the flow to the spinal cord through the anterior spinal artery. The largest is the artery of Adamkiewicz, which enters at the T9–T11 level and supplies the major portion of blood to the lower thoracic cord and lumbar enlargement.

The midthoracic region is most vulnerable because the supply to the anterior spinal artery often consists of only one significant radicular artery and because there is a poor anastomotic network at this level.

The posterior spinal arteries have a rich collateral supply and, therefore, the posterior part of the cord is relatively protected from the effects of vascular disease, including the dorsal columns.

Figure 29.14 shows the vascular supply of the cord in cross-section and indicates the supply of the major pathways.

Anterior spinal artery syndrome

If the anterior spinal artery becomes occluded, the supply to the anterior two-thirds of the cord is disrupted, causing anterior spinal artery syndrome, resulting in disruption of the corticospinal and spinothalamic tracts bilaterally (see Fig. 29.14).

Causes

- Small vessel disease, e.g. diabetes, polyarteritis, systemic lupus erythematosus

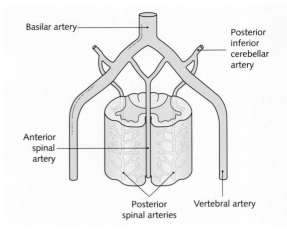

Fig. 29.13   Vascular supply of the spinal cord.

- Arterial compression or occlusion, e.g. disc fragments, extradural mass, dissecting aortic aneurysm, aortic surgery
- Embolism, e.g. aortic angiography, decompression sickness
- Hypotension: the arterial watershed at the midthoracic region is especially susceptible to hypoperfusion, e.g. pericardiac arrest.

Clinical features

The clinical features of anterior spinal artery syndrome are dependent on the level of the lesion and include:

- segmental pain at onset: usually in the back and around the trunk
- sphincter disturbance: usually urinary retention but incontinence of bladder and bowel can occur
- flaccid paraparesis, which progresses to spasticity over days (corticospinal tracts). Tetraparesis is

Fig. 29.14   Cross-sectional view of the vascular supply of the spinal cord.

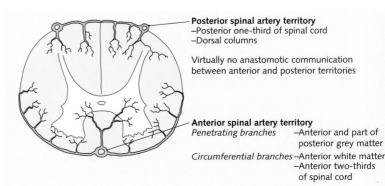

Posterior spinal artery territory
–Posterior one-third of spinal cord
–Dorsal columns

Virtually no anastomotic communication between anterior and posterior territories

Anterior spinal artery territory
Penetrating branches   –Anterior and part of posterior grey matter
Circumferential branches –Anterior white matter
–Anterior two-thirds of spinal cord

less common because the thoracic cord is most vulnerable

- areflexia below the level of the lesion, which progresses to hyperreflexia and extensor plantar responses over days
- loss of pain and temperature sensation up to the dermatome level at which the lesion occurred (spinothalamic tracts).

Note: vibration and joint-position sense are not affected as the dorsal columns are supplied by the posterior spinal artery.

Management

Treatment is symptomatic. The prognosis for recovery is variable but usually poor.

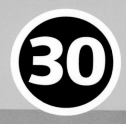
Objectives

- Understand the common types of brain tumour and their relative frequencies
- Describe the clinical features/presentation of brain tumours
- Describe how brain tumours are investigated and managed
- Describe the neurological complications of cancer

Intracranial tumours can be defined as benign or malignant lesions within the cranial cavity. They can be:

- **primary:** primary intracranial tumours account for approximately 10% of all neoplasms and represent 60% of all intracranial neoplasms. They can be derived from neuroepithelial cells (primarily gliomas), the meninges (meningiomas), nerve sheath cells (schwannomas), the anterior pituitary (adenomas) or blood vessels (haemangiomas)
- **secondary:** metastatic carcinoma (e.g. lung, breast) or lymphoma.

The relative frequencies of the most common intracranial tumours are shown in Figure 30.1. Epidemiologically there are two peaks in the incidence of brain tumours: childhood and in the eighth decade of life.

TYPES OF INTRACRANIAL TUMOUR

Gliomas

Gliomas are malignant, intrinsic brain tumours originating from astrocytes and oligodendrocytes. They usually occur within the cerebral hemispheres. They virtually never metastasize outside the CNS and spread only by direct extension. There are many different types. The most common are presented below.

Astrocytoma

Astrocytomas arise from astrocytes and are the most common primary brain tumour. They can be separated histologically into four grades dependent on the degree of malignancy (grade I, slow-growing over years; grade IV, death within months).

Oligodendroglioma

Oligodendrogliomas arise from oligodendrocytes and form slow-growing, sharply defined tumours that

may become calcified. Variants include an anaplastic form and a mixed astrocytoma/oligodendroglioma (oligoastrocytoma).

Glioblastoma multiforme

A glioblastoma multiforme is a highly malignant tumour with no cell differentiation, preventing identification of its tissue of origin. Life expectancy is usually less than a year.

Ependymoma

Derived from ependymal cells and choroid plexus, ependymomas can arise anywhere throughout the ventricular system or spinal canal, but usually in the fourth ventricle or cervical spine or conus medullaris. They are divided into three grades, depending on histology. They spread through cerebrospinal pathways and infiltrate surrounding tissue. Overall, in adults, they have a better survival rate than other gliomas.

Meningiomas

Meningiomas are mostly benign tumours that arise from the arachnoid membrane and granulations and may grow to a large size, usually over many years. They peak in the sixth decade of life, and are more common in women. They tend to compress adjacent brain structures rather than infiltrate. Calcification is common and they may erode adjacent bone. They are rare below the tentorium cerebelli. The most common sites are parasagittal, olfactory groove, tuberculum sellae and sphenoidal wing.

Primary central nervous system lymphoma

This is a rare form of B-cell non-Hodgkin's lymphoma accounting for about 5% of all primary brain tumours. It is more common in male patients over 60 years age,

Fig. 30.1 Relative frequencies (RF) of the most common intracranial tumours

Tumour	RF (%)
Metastases	40
Gliomas	33
Meningiomas	8
Pituitary adenomas	8
Schwannomas	3
Haemangioblastomas	3
Others (includes primitive neuroectodermal tumours, primary CNS lymphoma, germ cell tumours, craniopharyngiomas, chordomas and chondrosarcomas)	5

and especially in immunosuppressed patients such as those with HIV. It arises in the brain, spinal cord and leptomeninges, and 20% of patients can have intraocular involvement at diagnosis. Lesions are typically multifocal and enhance on imaging. Treatment options include chemotherapy and radiotherapy, but surgery has no role.

HINTS AND TIPS

Steroid treatment of CNS lymphomas usually causes a marked reduction in mass effect, contrast enhancement and can cause temporary regression of the tumour. This can confuse the radiological diagnosis and biopsy targeting. Where possible, steroid treatment should be avoided prior to biopsy.

Pituitary tumours

Pituitary tumours may cause endocrine dysfunction that is not always apparent to the patient. They may also present with visual symptoms due to chiasmal compression and can result in bitemporal hemianopia (see Ch. 8). The visual failure may progress and become irreversible if the tumour is left untreated.

The most common types of pituitary tumour include:

- prolactinomas: usually microadenomas
- non-functioning adenomas
- growth-hormone-secreting adenomas (causing acromegaly and usually macroadenomas)
- ACTH-secreting adenomas or hyperplasia: Cushing's disease.

COMMUNICATION

Pituitary apoplexy occurs when there is acute infarction or haemorrhage into the pituitary in the presence of tumour, causing a sudden headache, diplopia, visual loss and reduced conscious level. It is more common in pregnancy, trauma and diabetic ketoacidosis. Management includes steroids and decompressive surgery.

Nerve sheath tumours – neurofibromas and schwannomas

Schwannomas arise from Schwann cells; neurofibromas arise from non-myelinating Schwann cells and other cells in the peripheral nerves such as fibroblasts. The principal intracranial site of schwannomas is in the cerebellopontine angle, where they arise from the vestibular portion of the eighth cranial nerve sheath (Fig. 30.2). They are a common finding in neurofibromatosis type 2, when they can be bilateral, although they are usually sporadic and unilateral. Clinical features of a vestibular schwannoma include ipsilateral sensorineural deafness and fifth nerve involvement (sometimes only loss of the corneal reflex, with no sensory symptoms), then later facial weakness (seventh nerve) and ipsilateral cerebellar signs. Ultimately, contralateral pyramidal signs and hydrocephalus may develop. In general, these tumours are more common arising from spinal nerve roots.

Haemangioblastomas

Haemangioblastomas are derived from blood vessels and occur within the cerebellar parenchyma or spinal cord. They are found in von Hippel–Lindau disease in association with similar tumours in the retina and cystic lesions in the pancreas and kidney.

Metastases

Metastases are the most common intracranial tumour, especially in the elderly. The most common primaries are from the lung, breast and melanomas. More than half are solitary lesions at presentation, but there are usually many micrometastases that cannot be seen with magnetic resonance imaging (MRI) or computed tomography (CT) scanning.

CLINICAL FEATURES OF INTRACRANIAL TUMOURS

Mass lesions or space-occupying lesions within the cranium may present with one or more of the following features:

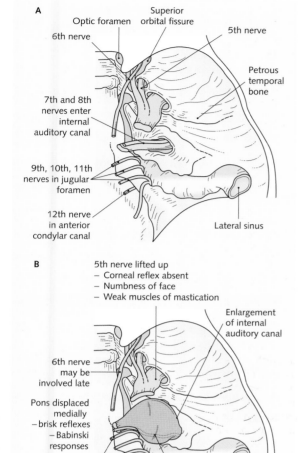

A

Superior
Optic foramen orbital fissure

6th nerve   5th nerve

                                          Petrous
                                          temporal
                                          bone
7th and 8th
nerves enter
internal
auditory canal

9th, 10th, 11th
nerves in jugular
foramen

12th nerve
in anterior   Lateral sinus
condylar canal

B   5th nerve lifted up
               – Corneal reflex absent
               – Numbness of face
               – Weak muscles of mastication

                                    Enlargement
                                    of internal
                                    auditory canal

6th nerve
may be
involved late

Pons displaced
medially
– brisk reflexes
– Babinski
responses

9th nerve
may be
involved late

                        Right lobe of cerebellum
                        compressed – ipsilateral
                        ataxia of limbs – unsteady
                        gait, falling to right side

Fig. 30.2 Acoustic neuroma. Vestibular schwannoma. (A)
A view from above of an opened skull with the brain removed,
showing the middle cranial fossa and its relation to the cranial
nerves and lateral sinus. (B) The spatial effect of a neuroma
on the surrounding cranial nerves.

- Effects of raised intracranial pressure: headache,
  vomiting and papilloedema
- Focal neurological signs occurring singly or in various combinations, caused by the direct effects of
  the tumour (compression, infiltration or oedema)
- Diffuse cerebral symptoms: seizures and cognitive
  impairment.

Primary and secondary intracranial tumours are the
most common cause of these symptoms, but any space-
occupying lesion can present similarly, e.g. cerebral abscess,
tuberculoma, subdural or intracerebral haematoma.

Raised intracranial pressure

Raised intracranial pressure can be due to mass effect
(direct tumour infiltration and vasogenic oedema),
haemorrhage into the tumour or obstruction of cerebrospinal fluid pathways. It produces the classic triad
of headache, vomiting and papilloedema. However,
these features, especially papilloedema, are relatively
infrequent early presentations, as the symptoms usually imply obstruction to the cerebrospinal fluid pathways. The full picture is more common early in
posterior fossa tumours, when the flow of cerebrospinal fluid is disrupted and lesions are usually within a
very confined space. Early morning headache, which
improves with an upright posture, is a common first
symptom of intracranial tumours, although focal neurological signs and symptoms often occur without
headache.

The raised pressure can also cause symptoms and
signs distant to the tumour, including:

- herniation
- false localizing signs.

Herniation

There may be compression of the medulla by herniation of the cerebellar tonsils through the foramen magnum ('coning'), which leads to impairment of
consciousness, respiratory depression, bradycardia,
decerebrate posturing and death (Fig. 30.3). This is
called 'tonsillar herniation'. Similarly, the uncus of
the temporal lobe may herniate through the tentorial
opening (see Fig. 30.3). This is called 'uncal herniation'
and the resulting compression of the third nerve is the
cause of the dilating pupil on the side of the tumour,
then later bilaterally. There may also be ipsilateral
hemiparesis (see below).

Fig. 30.3 Herniation of (A) the temporal lobe (supratentorial tumours) and (B) the cerebellar tonsils (infratentorial tumours; coning).

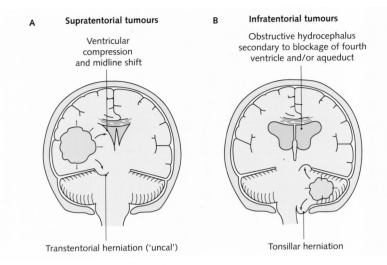

A **Supratentorial tumours**
Ventricular compression and midline shift

B **Infratentorial tumours**
Obstructive hydrocephalus secondary to blockage of fourth ventricle and/or aqueduct

Transtentorial herniation ('uncal')

Tonsillar herniation

False localizing signs

These are 'false' in that they are distant to the site of the mass and caused by the raised pressure. They include:

- sixth nerve palsy: this is caused by compression of the nerve during its long intracranial course. It is often unilateral initially, then bilateral
- third nerve palsy: caudal herniation of the uncus of the temporal lobe causes pupillary dilatation and then later ophthalmoplegia
- hemiparesis on the same side as the tumour: this is caused by compression of the brainstem on the free edge of the tentorium in uncal herniation.

False localizing signs are very important because they indicate an increase in pressure with brain shift and require urgent investigation and treatment, which may include surgery.

Focal neurological signs

Focal neurological signs may be caused by direct effects of the tumour (compression, infiltration or oedema) or be false localizing signs (as discussed above). The direct effects will depend on the site of the tumour.

Seizures

Partial seizures, whether simple or complex, are characteristic of many focal hemispheric lesions. They may then secondarily generalize to a tonic–clonic seizure. The seizures caused by tumours are often difficult to control with drugs, but are often helped by steroids in the acute setting.

INVESTIGATIONS

HINTS AND TIPS

Lumbar puncture is contraindicated in any case of suspected or definite intracranial mass because it can lead to herniation ('coning') and prove fatal.

Imaging of the head is essential if an intracranial tumour is suspected. However, as many intracranial tumours are metastatic, more systemic investigations may also be necessary (e.g. chest X-ray, CT scan of chest, abdomen, pelvis and mammography).

Computed tomography

CT scans should be carried out with contrast, as enhancement of a lesion (which may not be visible precontrast) adds to the discriminating ability.

However, CT scans show only the presence and site of a mass, and whether there is oedema, shift or hydrocephalus; they do not provide much information about the type of tumour. Different intracranial masses, i.e. tumours (benign and malignant), cerebral abscesses and tuberculomas, all have characteristic, but not entirely diagnostic, appearances (Fig. 30.4).

Magnetic resonance imaging

MRI usually provides more anatomical information about soft tissue and tumour delineation than CT scanning, and is always the investigation of choice for suspected posterior fossa mass lesions and pituitary

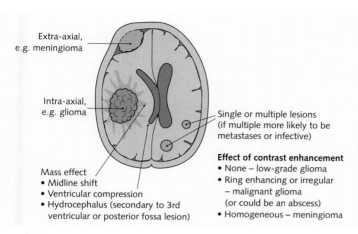

Fig. 30.4 CT scan features of various intracranial tumours.

Extra-axial,
e.g. meningioma

Intra-axial,
e.g. glioma

Single or multiple lesions
(if multiple more likely to be
metastases or infective)

Effect of contrast enhancement
• None – low-grade glioma
• Ring enhancing or irregular
  – malignant glioma
  (or could be an abscess)
• Homogeneous – meningioma

Mass effect
• Midline shift
• Ventricular compression
• Hydrocephalus (secondary to 3rd
  ventricular or posterior fossa lesion)

tumours. Small metastases and meningeal lesions may also be missed by CT scans. CT provides more information about calcification and bony abnormalities.

Specialized neuroradiology

Modern imaging techniques such as magnetic resonance spectroscopy (MRS), MRI perfusion techniques, diffusion weighted imaging (DWI) and positron emission tomography (PET) are able to provide complementary biological information about blood flow and cellular ultrastructure that can guide the choice of treatments and assessment of response. They can be particularly helpful in tumour grading and the distinction between tumour recurrence and radiation necrosis.

Stereotactic brain biopsy

A frame is positioned on the head with identifiable external reference (fiducial) markers. CT or MRI can then be used to place a biopsy needle into the precise coordinates of the lesion. The subsequent histological findings help determine further management.

TREATMENT

A multidisciplinary approach is critical to the management of patients with brain tumours.

Cerebral oedema and raised intracranial pressure

The oedema round the tumour can be reduced with the use of oral corticosteroids (usually dexamethasone). In a neurosurgical emergency setting, raised intracranial pressure can be rapidly reduced with the use of intravenous corticosteroids or intravenous mannitol. Raised intracranial pressure due to hydrocephalus may be treated with insertion of a ventriculoperitoneal shunt or third ventriculostomy.

Seizures

Seizures are treated with anticonvulsants, but are often difficult to control and the patient may be left with mild ongoing partial seizures and/or secondary generalized seizures.

Surgery

Benign tumours (e.g. meningiomas) can often be removed entirely. The location of benign tumours is critical and sometimes not all of the tumour can be removed, especially if it is in a difficult anatomical position (e.g. sphenoid wing). Malignant tumours cannot be totally removed and, therefore, they are usually only debulked for palliation, if they are in an amenable position.

Radiotherapy and chemotherapy

Radiotherapy is usually recommended for gliomas and radiosensitive metastases to provide palliation. Chemotherapy can be curative or palliative, and is combined with surgery and/or radiotherapy.

PROGNOSIS

The prognosis for brain tumours depends on tumour type and grade, tumour location and size, and patient age and performance status at diagnosis. There is an overall 1-year survival of less than 50% for high-grade malignant tumours. Benign tumours, especially meningiomas, neurofibromas and pituitary tumours, can often be removed entirely and therefore cured.

NEUROLOGICAL COMPLICATIONS OF CANCER

The neurological complications of cancer are the second most common cause of admission to hospital for oncology patients. Neurological complications arise for a number of reasons:

- Direct or indirect (metastatic) invasion of the brain or spinal cord
- Leptomeningeal metastases – these are most commonly associated with breast, small-cell lung cancer, lymphoma and melanoma. They can present with multifocal symptoms and meningism, without obvious masses on brain imaging. Cytological examination of CSF is the most valuable diagnostic test, but should be carried out at least three times with at least 10 mL of fluid each time for adequate sensitivity

- Delirium – this can be caused by many different factors, including direct effects of the tumour, toxic/metabolic encephalopathy or drug effects
- Vascular disorders – patients with cancer are at increased risk of both ischaemic and haemorrhagic strokes
- Infections – patients with cancer may be immunosuppressed and may be susceptible to infection of the CNS by atypical organisms
- Paraneoplastic disorders – paraneoplastic disorders are rare neurological complications of cancer, but are important to recognize as they can cause significant neurological disability and often present before the cancer itself becomes symptomatic. They can affect any part of the nervous system, and result from indirect immune-mediated effects of systemic cancer, rather than direct or metastatic invasion of the cancer. These immune responses may be associated with specific antineuronal antibodies in CSF and serum (Fig. 30.5)

Fig. 30.5 Paraneoplastic neurological syndromes and antibodies

Antibody	Syndrome	Most common associated cancer
Well characterised paraneoplastic antibodies		
Anti-Hu (ANNA-1)	Encephalomyelitis (inc. cortical, limbic, brainstem encephalitis), cerebellar degeneration, myelitis, sensory neuronopathy, and/or autonomic dysfunction	SCLC
Anti-Yo (PCA-1)	Cerebellar degeneration	Gynecological, breast
Anti-Ri (ANNA-2)	Cerebellar degeneration, brainstem encephalitis, opsoclonus-myoclonus	Breast, gynecological, SCLC
Anti-Tr	Cerebellar degeneration	Hodgkin's lymphoma
Anti-CV2/CRMP5	Encephalomyelitis, cerebellar degeneration, chorea, peripheral neuropathy	SCLC, thymoma
Anti-Ma proteins	Limbic, hypothalamic, brainstem encephalitis, cerebellar degeneration	Germ-cell tumors of testis, lung cancer
Anti-amphiphysin	Stiff-person syndrome, encephalomyelitis	Breast, lung cancer
Antibodies that can occur with or without cancer		
Anti-AChR	Myasthenia gravis	Thymoma
Anti-VGCC	Lambert–Eaton myasthenic syndrome, cerebellar dysfunction	SCLC
Anti-NMDAR	Multistage syndrome with memory and behavioral disturbances, psychosis, seizures, dyskinesias, and autonomic dysfunction	Teratoma
Anti-AMPAR	Limbic encephalitis, psychiatric disturbances	Misc solid tumours
Anti-GABA	Seizures, limbic encephalitis	SCLC
Anti-VGKC	Limbic encephalitis, seizures, Morvan's syndrome	Thymoma, SCLC, misc solid tumours
Anti-GlyR	Encephalomyelitis with muscle spasms, rigidity, myoclonus	Often no associated cancer

ANNA=antineuronal-nuclear antibody, PCA=purkinje cell antibody, VGCC=voltage gated calcium channel antibody, VGKC=voltage gated potassium channel antibody, nAChR=neuronal acetyl-choline receptor, SCLC=small cell lung cancer

- Neurotoxicity of chemotherapy and radiotherapy – chemotherapeutic agents can affect all levels of the nervous system. Many cause a peripheral neuropathy, which is usually sensory and axonal in nature. Radiotherapy to the brain can also give rise to neurological toxicity and predispose patients to secondary tumours, sometimes many years after treatment.

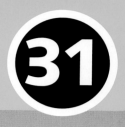
- Describe the presentation, differential diagnosis and management of meningitis
- Describe the clinical presentation and management of encephalitis
- Consider the predisposing causes for cerebral abscess
- Understand how HIV may affect the nervous system
- Be aware of the manifestations of TB within the nervous system

This chapter will consider only the most common and important infections of the nervous system. General conditions will be considered first, followed by diseases caused by individual organisms.

GENERAL CONDITIONS

Meningitis

The term 'meningitis' typically refers to inflammation of the meninges caused by an infective agent; however, it can also be applied to inflammation caused by malignant cells, inflammatory disease (e.g. sarcoidosis), drugs, contrast media and blood following subarachnoid haemorrhage. All of these causes can have a similar presentation to infective causes of meningitis. Infective agents can reach the meninges from direct spread (e.g. from sinuses, the nasopharynx or the inner ear), through fractures of the skull or, more commonly, from the bloodstream (haematogenous).

Causative agents

Infective meningitis can be caused by a variety of organisms, including bacteria, viruses, fungi and parasites.

Bacteria

The organisms causing bacterial meningitis vary with age and the predisposing factors of the host (Fig. 31.1). The three most common meningeal pathogens accounting for more than 80% of cases are:

- *Haemophilus influenzae*
- *Neisseria meningitidis*
- *Streptococcus pneumoniae*.

Clinical features

The classic clinical triad of 'meningism' is:

- headache

- photophobia
- neck stiffness.

Patients with bacterial meningitis classically present with fever, headache, neck stiffness and signs of cerebral dysfunction (confusion, delirium, decreasing consciousness). Symptoms have typically developed over the course of a few days or hours. Neck stiffness or meningisim may be subtle or marked, and may be accompanied by Kernig's or Brudzinski's signs. Kernig's sign is positive when there is painful extension of the knee with the hip flexed at 90° and Brudzinski's sign is positive when there is involuntary lifting of the legs with the patient supine and the neck flexed passively.

The absence of any of these findings does not exclude a diagnosis of bacterial meningitis. The clinical picture may change quickly, with rapid clinical decline seen over the course of a few hours. In a severe infection there may be cerebral oedema and raised intracranial pressure, leading to confusion, fluctuating conscious levels, seizures and cranial nerve palsies. In the elderly or immunocompromised patient, signs may be subtle, and patients may present with fever and confusion, but no specific evidence of meningeal irritation. In all subgroups of patients presenting with confusion or altered mental state it is essential to exclude bacterial meningitis before ascribing to another cause, i.e. urinary sepsis.

Fig. 31.1 Causes of bacterial meningitis depending on specific age groups and risk factors

Age group	Organism
Neonate < 1 month	Group B streptococcus, *Escherichia coli, Listeria monocytogenes, Klebsiella* species
1–23 months	Group B streptococcus, *Escherichia coli, Streptococcus pneumoniae, Neisseria meningitidis, Haemophilus influenzae*
2–50 years of age	*Streptococcus pneumoniae, Neisseria meningitidis*
Over 50 years of age	*Streptococcus pneumoniae, Neisseria meningitidis, Listeria monocytogenes,* aerobic Gram-negative bacilli
Immunocompromised	*Streptococcus pneumoniae, Neisseria meningitidis, Listeria monocytogenes,* aerobic Gram-negative bacilli (including *Pseudomonas aeruginosa*)
Risk factor	
Pregnancy	*Listeria monocytogenes*
Diabetes	*Streptococcus pneumoniae, Staphylococcus aureus,* Gram-negative bacilli
Alcoholism	*Streptococcus pneumoniae, Listeria monocytogenes*
Head trauma; postneurosurgery	*Staphylococcus aureus,* coagulase-negative staphylococci, aerobic Gram-negative bacillli (including *Pseudomonas aeruginosa*)

Viral meningitis

Viruses are the major cause of aseptic meningitis syndromes (predominant CSF lymphocytosis and negative routine stains and culture). At presentation it is often difficult to differentiate from bacterial meningitis as patients typically present with similar symptoms of headache, fever, neck stiffness and photophobia. Where there is any doubt, treatment for bacterial meningitis should be instituted and changed accordingly once results are known. Viral meningitis can be acute or subacute and is usually self-limiting, lasting between 4 and 10 days. Headaches may persist for some weeks, but serious sequelae are rare. If the virus proceeds to affect the brain substance, the patient can become very unwell with meningoencephalitis/encephalitis (see below).

Enteroviruses are the leading cause of viral meningitis, accounting for 85–95% of all cases in which a pathogen is identified. This encompasses a large group of viruses including echoviruses and coxsackieviruses. Other common viral pathogens causing meningitis include mumps virus and the herpesviruses including HSV-1 and -2, and VZV. HSV meningitis is most commonly associated with primary genital infection with herpes simplex type 2. Mollaret's meningitis or recurrent benign lymphocytic meningitis is almost always associated with HSV-2. In any sexually active individual presenting with aspetic meningitis it is important to consider HIV, which can be seen as part of the primary infection or in already infected individuals. In the immunocompromised, CMV, EBV, HHV-6 and 7 are important pathogens. It is important to take a good travel history as travel abroad will change the viral differential.

Tuberculous meningitis

Tuberculosis meningitis (TBM) typically causes a chronic meningitis, developing over a few weeks to months. Symptoms are initially non-specific, with gradual onset of headache and malaise. Meningeal symptoms follow, progressing to seizures, cranial nerve palsies and cerebral dysfunction. Fifty per cent of patients will have an abnormal CXR, so look for evidence of TB elsewhere. Cerebral imaging with CT or MRI may reveal associated hydrocephalus, basal meningeal enhancement, infarcts or tuberculomas.

Fungal meningitis

Cryptococcal meningitis is the most common fungal meningitis in Europe and is associated with immunocompromised individuals, particularly those with advanced HIV. The presentation is similar to TBM.

Diagnosis

Lumbar puncture (LP) is the gold standard diagnostic tool. This should be carried out immediately to prevent delay in treatment. If there are signs of raised intracranial pressure, a computed tomography (CT) scan should be carried out first so that the risk of coning can be assessed. Figure 31.2 lists the patients that should undergo CT prior to lumbar puncture.

Fig 31.2 Who should undergo CT prior to LP?
Immunocompromised
History of central neurological disease
New-onset seizures
Papilloedema
Abnormal level of consciousness
Focal neurological deficit

Fig. 31.3 CSF findings in meningitis

	Normal	Bacterial	Viral	Tuberculous
Appearance	Clear	Turbid/pus	Clear/turbid	Turbid/viscous
Neutrophils	Nil	200–10 000/mm^3	Nil/few	0–200/mm^3
Lymphocytes	<5 mm^3	<50/mm^3	10–100/ mm^3	100–300/mm^3
Protein	0.2–0.4 g/L	0.5–2.0 g/L	0.4–0.8 g/L	0.5–3.0 g/L
Glucose	>1/2 blood glucose	<1/3 blood glucose	<1/2 blood glucose	<1/3 blood glucose

The diagnosis of bacterial meningitis depends on the cerebrospinal fluid (CSF) examination performed after LP. Normal CSF opening pressures are between 10 and 18 mmHg. Pressures are typically elevated in bacterial meningitis and may be grossly elevated in cases of tuberculous or cryptococcal meningitis. Figure 31.3 gives the typical CSF findings in meningitis.

The appearance of the CSF also gives important clues. A cloudy CSF is due to presence of significant concentrations of white blood cells, red blood cells, bacteria, and/or protein and is always abnormal.

Staining of cerebrospinal fluid

- A Gram stain should be performed immediately to diagnose bacterial meningitis. The higher the concentration of bacteria in the CSF, the more likely the Gram stain will yield a positive result. Typical Grams seen in bacterial meningitis include Gram-positive diplococci (*Streptococcus pneumoniae*), Gram-negative diplococci (*Neisseria meningitidis*), Gram-negative coccobacilli (*Haemophilus influenzae*) and Gram-positive rods (*Listeria monocytogenes*)
- Request a Ziehl–Neelsen stain when TBM is suspected. Acid-fast bacilli are visualized in only 20% of cases of TBM
- Request an Indian-ink stain when cryptococcal meningitis is suspected.

Cerebrospinal fluid culture

- CSF cultures are positive in 70–85% of patients who have not received prior antimicrobial therapy, but cultures may take up to 48 hours for organism identification.
- When TBM or fungal meningitis is suspected, dedicated TB and fungal cultures should be setup.
- In the case of TBM, a positive culture is achieved in less than 50% of cases and can take up to 6 weeks to grow. It is especially important that sufficient quantities are put up for TB culture (approx. 10 mL) and repeated LPs are almost always required.

Other required tests

- Paired CSF and blood glucose
- CSF protein

- Blood cultures, throat swab, EDTA blood sent for PCR for *N. meningitidis* and *S. pneumoniae* (essential when bacterial meningitis is suspected).

Polymerase chain reaction

- Polymerase chain reaction (PCR) can be carried out on CSF, EDTA blood and throat swabs in cases where bacterial meningitis is suspected. When PCR is used results can be available in hours.
- CSF PCR is the gold standard test for viral meningitis. A typical viral panel would include testing for enterovirus, HSV and VZV. Any further tests would require discussion with microbiology/virology.

Serology

Due to the advent of PCR, this is used much less frequently. However, serology performed on blood is a useful way of diagnosing cases of HIV, mumps and enterovirus meningitis.

Imaging

Chest X rays, CTs or MRIs may be necessary to define the extent of spread or other involved areas.

Complications

Consciousness is not severely impaired in uncomplicated meningitis, although a high fever may cause delirium. Marked changes in conscious level, focal neurological signs, seizures and papilloedema indicate that complications may be developing or that an alternative diagnosis should be considered (e.g. cerebral abscess or encephalitis). Such cases often require urgent imaging and discussion with a neurosurgical unit and admission to critical care. Complications include:

- hydrocephalus due to obstruction of CSF outflow, leading to raised intracranial pressure: this is especially common in TB meningitis
- cerebral oedema
- venous sinus thrombosis
- subdural empyema
- cerebral abscess
- arteritis and endarteritis: TB can often inflame the origin of the cerebral vasculature as it rises from the

base of the brain. In severe cases, this can lead to occlusion of the artery causing a large vessel stroke. Meningitis can also inflame the smaller arteries within the meninges, causing further damage from ischaemia.

Treatment

Bacterial meningitis is a medical emergency. Each hour of delay increases the likelihood of a fatal outcome or permanent neurological deficit.

If there is any suspicion that a patient may have bacterial meningitis, treatment should be started immediately after LP. If there is going to be more than a 30-minute delay prior to performing the LP, treatment should be commenced and the LP performed at the earliest opportunity.

The empirical treatment of community-acquired meningitis is with a third-generation cephalosporin (either cefotaxime or ceftriaxone). Cover with ampicillin ± gentamicin can be added in cases where *Listeria* is suspected.

In more complicated circumstances, for example if the patient is immunocompromised, post neurosurgery, has recently travelled abroad or has been recently hospitalized, cases should be discussed urgently with the oncall microbiologist as treatment regimes will differ depending on the presumed pathogen. Once the results of the LP are known, treatment can then be tailored appropriately.

The role of adjunctive dexamethasone in adults with bacterial meningitis

Steroids may be useful in decreasing the inflammatory response during bacterial meningitis, which is a major factor contributing to morbidity and mortality. Current evidence suggests that adjunctive dexamethasone should be initiated in all adult patients with suspected or proven pneumococcal meningitis (*S. pneumoniae*). The addition of dexamethasone results in a decreased rate of associated neurological sequelae. Dexamethasone should only be continued if the CSF Gram stain reveals Gram-positive diplococci, or if blood or CSF cultures are positive for *S. pneumoniae*. There is no evidence to recommend adjunctive dexamethasone in adults with meningitis caused by other bacterial pathogens.

Tuberculous meningitis

Tuberculous meningitis is treated for 12 months usually with a combination of isoniazid, rifampicin, pyrazinamide and ethambutol with pyridoxine (to protect against the peripheral nerve side-effects of isoniazid) for 2 months and with isoniazid and rifampicin for a further 10 months. Adjunctive dexamethasone has been shown to reduce mortality by 30%. Treatment is highly specialized and always requires the involvement of an infection expert.

Viral meningitis

The treatment of viral meningitis is largely supportive. The use of aciclovir in cases of HSV meningitis is controversial.

Infection control, notification and chemoprophylaxis of contacts

Bacterial meningitis, suspected or confirmed, is a notifiable disease. Patients with suspected bacterial meningitis should be nursed in respiratory isolation, with staff and visitors using masks, gloves and gowns until 48 hours after initiation of antibiotics. Chemoprophylaxis should be offered to household, school or work contacts and medical staff involved in the initial resuscitation of patients with *Haemophilus influenzae* (rifampicin) or *Neisseria meningitidis* (ciprofloxacin). Liaison with Infection Control, Occupational Health and the Health Protection Agency is essential.

Encephalitis

Definition

- Encephalitis is characterized by inflammation of the brain parenchyma in association with clinical evidence of neurological dysfunction. Traditionally, a pathological diagnosis, CSF and parenchymal changes on imaging are now used as surrogate markers.
- 'Meningoencephalitis' is a term used to describe the encephalitic component with associated meningeal inflammation.
- 'Encephalopathy', in contrast, is defined by a disruption of brain function in the absence of a direct inflammatory process in the brain parenchyma. Causes include metabolic disturbances, hypoxia, drugs, organ dysfunction or systemic infections.

Aetiology

The causes of encephalitis comprise:

- direct infection of the CNS
- post-infectious/post-immunization causes
- non-infectious causes (such as paraneoplastic antibody-associated encephalitis).

The reported incidence in Western settings ranges from 0.7 to 12.6 cases per 100 000 adults. In the UK less than half of patients presenting with encephalitis had an infectious cause. In immunocompetent individuals the top five causes of encephalitis were HSV, ADEM (see Ch.32), antibody-associated encephalitis, *M. tuberculosis* and VZV. In the immunocompromised, VZV followed by HSV were the main causes.

In both groups just under 40% of individuals with confirmed encephalitis had an unknown aetiology.

Fig. 31.4 Infective causes of encephalitis	
Viruses	
Herpes viruses	HSV-1 and 2 VZV, EBV, CMV (mainly immunocompromised) HHV-6 and 7 (immunocompromised and children)
Enteroviruses	Enterovirus 70 and 71 Poliovirus Coxsackieviruses Echoviruses Parechovirus
Paramyxoviruses	Measles virus Mumps virus
Others	Influenza viruses Adenoviruses Rubella virus
Associated with travel	West Nile virus Japanese encephalitis Tick-borne encephalitis virus Dengue viruses Rabies
Bacteria	
	Mycobacterium tuberculosis *Mycoplasma pneumoniae* *Chlamydophila*

Infectious causes of encephalitis

The most common infective causes of encephalitis are viruses, and bacteria to a lesser extent (see Fig. 31.4). Viruses enter the CNS either via the bloodstream (most viruses) or via peripheral nerves (HSV, VZV, polio, rabies).

Clinical features

Encephalitis can be difficult to differentiate from acute meningitis, as patients with each syndrome will often present with fever, headache and altered conscious levels. Focal neurological signs and seizures are common. Disturbance of consciousness ranges from stupor, to confusion and coma.

Diagnosis

- CSF examination is essential. A lymphocytosis usually predominates (10–2000 cell/mm³), but the CSF may be acellular or contain neutrophils. The CSF protein is usually mildly or moderately elevated, with a normal CSF to serum glucose ratio. In cases of haemorrhagic encephalitis, red blood cells may be detected in the CSF.
- All patients with suspected encephalitis should have a CSF PCR test for HSV (1 and 2), VZV and enteroviruses as this will identify 90% of cases due to known viral pathogens. In HSV encephalitis, HSV PCR may be negative in the first few days of illness, but a second CSF taken 3–7 days later will often be positive, even if aciclovir has been started.
- Further testing should be directed towards specific pathogens as guided by clinical features. An HIV test (blood serum) should be performed on all patients with encephalitis or suspected encephalitis, regardless of risk factors.
- Serological testing of both the CSF and blood may occasionally reveal some causes of encephalitis. These should be requested in liaison with microbiology, virology or infectious diseases.
- MRI is the imaging of choice in encephalitis, being more sensitive and specific than CT. Bilateral temporal lobe changes are virtually pathognomonic for HSV encephalitis, but are a late development.
- EEG is a sensitive indicator of cerebral dysfunction and may uncover concomitant non-convulsive seizures. In HSV encephalitis, there may be a temporal lobe focus demonstrating stereotypical sharp and slow wave complexes occurring at intervals of 2–3 seconds.
- A septic screen with blood and CSF cultures is also essential in excluding other pathogens such as bacterial and fungi.
- Brain biopsy should be considered in cases where the diagnosis remains unknown and the clinical situation continues to deteriorate despite aciclovir.

HINTS AND TIPS

Consider the diagnosis of antibody-mediated encephalitis in all patients with suspected encephalitis. Delays in diagnoses result in poor outcomes.

Treatment

- Intravenous aciclovir should be initiated if the initial CSF and/or imaging suggests viral encephalitis, or within 6 hours of admission if these results are not yet available, or if the patient is very unwell or deteriorating. This can be continued or stopped according to later CSF PCR results.
- In patients with proven HSV encephalitis, IV therapy should be continued for 14–21 days, and a repeat LP performed at this time to confirm the CSF is negative for HSV by PCR. If the PCR is still positive, aciclovir should be continued.
- Institute other antivirals/antibiotics as per presumed/confirmed aetiologies. Treatment is otherwise supportive, including seizure control and intubation with sedation if necessary.
- Treatment of ADEM and antibody-mediated encephalitis will require immunomodulatory such as steroids, intravenous immunoglobulins, or plasma exchange.

Prognosis

Prognosis, in terms of neurological sequelae and death, is dependent on the aetiological cause. The overall mortality rate is 7–10% in industrialized countries. Even if not fatal, individuals often have severe physical, cognitive, emotional, behavioural and social difficulties.

HSV causes the most severe viral encephalitis in the UK, with high mortality and morbidity rates. Early treatment with aciclovir improves outcome in adults with HSV encephalitis, reducing mortality from 70 to 20–30%.

Cerebral abscess

Definition

A cerebral abscess is a focal encapsulated area of infection within the cerebrum or cerebellum. The abscess passes through several stages, from localized suppurative cerebritis to complete encapsulation. There may be solitary or multiple abscesses.

Aetiology

Infection can reach the brain by local spread, via the bloodstream, or by being directly inoculated, i.e. through trauma or neurosurgery. Disease states that predispose to cerebral abscess formation include:

- otitis media/mastoiditis
- sinusitis
- bacterial endocarditis
- dental sepsis
- chronic lung infections
- congenital heart disease, especially those with 'right to left' shunts.
- trauma or neurosurgery
- infections in immunocompromised patients.

Causative organisms

Bacteria are the usual causative organisms; however, in immunocompromised patients, other organisms (e.g. fungi and parasites) are more common. Anaerobic and microaerophylic organisms are the main pathogens:

- *Streptococcus* species, especially *S. viridans* and *S. milleri*
- *Bacteroides* species
- *Fusobacterium*
- Enterobacteriaceae, e.g. *Escherichia coli* and *Proteus* species
- *Staphylococcus aureus*

The following organisms are important in immunocompromised patients:

- *Toxoplasma*
- *Aspergillus*
- *Candida*
- *Listeria*
- *Cryptococcus*.

Clinical features

The history in patients with cerebral abscess is usually short (less than 1 month) and progressive. Brain abscesses present as space-occupying lesions with features of raised intracranial pressure:

- Headache
- Vomiting
- Deterioration in conscious level
- Papilloedema.

There may also be focal features associated with the space occupation:

- Seizures (occur in 30% of cases)
- Focal neurological signs, depending on location of abscess.

There may also be symptoms of systemic infection (e.g. pyrexia, malaise) or of focal infection (e.g. cough, earache), but these may not be present, particularly in immunocompromised patients.

Diagnosis

CT scanning or, if available, MRI, is the investigation of choice. Lumbar puncture is contraindicated in the presence of a mass lesion because of the risk of herniation. Other investigations include X-rays/CT of the chest, sinuses and middle ear, which may reveal the primary source of the infection. A full septic screen, including blood cultures, is essential. The classic appearance seen on a CT scan with contrast comprises:

- 'ring enhancement' of the lesion, which is usually spherical
- central area of low density
- surrounding area of oedema.

In addition, there may be ventricular compression and midline shift due to a mass effect.

Treatment

- Discuss all cases with the regional neurosurgical centre: a diagnostic aspirate ± surgical drainage will likely be required.
- Commence empirical antibiotics based on the most likely pathogen; all cases should be discussed with microbiology. A third-generation cephalosporin with metronidazole would be appropriate for community-acquired infections, pending rationalization, once antimicrobial sensitivities are known.
- Treat any source of infection, e.g. drainage of chronic sinus infection, mastoiditis, dental abscess.
- Exclude risk factors for immunosuppression and perform an HIV test if appropriate.

- Adjunctive corticosteroid therapy in those with significant oedema and mass shift.
- Antiepileptics where appropriate.

Prognosis

Mortality rates have vastly improved since the advent of CT scanning, surgical drainage and antimicrobial therapy. However, even with appropriate therapy, the mortality rate can range from 0 to 24%. Poor prognostic indicators include:

- reduced preoperative level of consciousness
- brain herniation
- rupture of the abscess into the ventricles or subarachnoid space
- immunocompromised patient
- poor general medical condition, e.g. severe pulmonary disease.

Of survivors, 25–50% have neurological sequelae, 30–50% have persistent seizures, 15–30% have a persistent hemiparesis and 10–20% have disorders of speech and language.

SPECIFIC ORGANISMS AND THEIR ASSOCIATED DISEASES

Tuberculosis

TB is caused by a bacterium called *Mycobacterium tuberculosis*. It is spread via the respiratory route, and coughed or sneezed out by someone with infectious tuberculosis. TB in organs other than the lungs is rarely infectious to others. Neurological TB results from haematogenous spread of TB from other sites, principally the lungs.

Diagnosis

- TB is diagnosed in a number of ways. A definite diagnosis of neurological TB requires culturing the TB bacterium from CSF or other samples.
- Tuberculin testing and/or interferon-gamma immunological testing are used for diagnosing latent TB, and should not be used to diagnose active cases of TB. They may be helpful in proving past exposure to TB in suspected cases.
- Imaging is an essential part of the diagnosis. A chest X-ray may show signs of associated pulmonary involvement. Spinal/brain CT or MRI are favoured when there are sings of neurological involvement.

Neurological complications of tuberculosis

- Tuberculous meningitis complicated by hydrocephalus, cranial nerve palsies and cerebral infarcts (see above)
- Tuberculoma (brain and spine)

- Spinal TB (Pott's disease of the spine)
- Spinal arachnoiditis causing myelopathy and radiculopathy.

Tuberculoma

Tuberculomas are inflammatory masses in the brain, which can be present at diagnosis or develop during treatment. They may produce focal neurological symptoms and signs.

Spinal tuberculosis (Pott's disease)

Spinal TB accounts for half of all the sites of bone and joint TB seen in England and Wales. It can cause significant morbidity secondary to spinal cord compression from extradural abscesses and/or vertebral collapse. Symptoms include back pain, fever, night sweats, weight loss and signs of spinal cord compression in advanced cases. Aspiration of paraspinal abscesses and/or biopsy from spinal sites may be required to obtain material for diagnosis, culture and sensitivity.

Spinal arachnoiditis

Spinal arachnoiditis may result from downwards spread of intracranial infection or from direct spread from epidural infection. The presentation is of a spreading myelitis with root involvement: that is, weakness (pyramidal and radicular), root pain, sensory loss and sphincter disturbance.

Treatment

Treatment for spinal TB comprises conventional antituberculous therapy for a minimum of 6 months. If there is direct parenchymal or spinal cord involvement (i.e. spinal cord tuberculoma), management should be as for meningeal TB. Spinal decompression may be required in cases of severe spinal cord compression.

Syphilis

Syphilis is caused by the motile spirochaete *Treponema pallidum*. Transmission occurs from direct contact with an infectious lesion (usually through sexual contact), during pregnancy from mother to child, or via infected blood products. Syphilis is divided into acquired or congenital cases. Acquired syphilis is classified into early and late stages. Prior to the antibiotic era, approximately one-third of individuals would develop late symptomatic syphilis.

Early:

- Primary
- Secondary
- Early latent < 2 years of infection.

Late:

- Late latent > 2 years of infection
- Tertiary (including gummatous, cardiovascular and neurological).

Conditions associated with neurosyphilis

The main syphilitic syndromes that affect the nervous system are described below.

Asymptomatic neurosyphilis (early/late)

Up to 30% of patients with primary and secondary syphilis may have abnormalities of their CSF, but no neurological symptoms or signs. The clinical significance of this is unknown.

Meningovascular (2–7 years)

Patients may present in a number of ways:

- Focal arteritis causing infarction/meningeal inflammation. Signs depend on the site of involvement
- Acute basal meningitis with hydrocephalus, cranial nerve palsies and papilloedema
- Focal meningitis: when a gumma presents as an expanding intracranial mass, favouring the meninges rather than parenchyma and presenting with seizures, raised intracranial pressure and focal signs
- Meningovascular meningitis causing an obliterative endarteritis and periarteritis and presenting as a 'stroke', most often in a young person.

Tabes dorsalis (15–20 years)

Tabes dorsalis is a late presentation of syphilis, causing a meningoradiculitis with degeneration of the dorsal columns and pupillary involvement. The classic features include:

- Lightning pains: irregular, severe, sharp stabbing pains, usually in the lower limb, chest, or abdomen, caused by dorsal root involvement
- Visceral crises: abdominal pain, diarrhoea and tenesmus
- Argyll Robertson pupils: small, irregularly shaped pupils that do not react to light but do accommodate
- Ptosis: with compensatory over-activity of the frontalis muscle
- Optic atrophy
- Impaired vibration and joint-position sense and reduced deep pain
- Patchy loss of pin-prick and temperature sensation
- Trophic skin lesions and Charcot joints (painless joint damage)
- Sensory ataxia: positive Romberg's test and stamping gait
- Hypotonia and reduced reflexes
- Extensor plantar responses in spite of absent ankle jerks: caused by the combination of radiculopathy and upper motor neuron involvement.

General paralysis of the insane (10–20 years)

General paralysis of the insane develops 10–20 years after primary infection and, as its historical name indicates, involves psychiatric abnormality and weakness. There are two phases:

- Preparalytic: with progressive dementia
- Paralytic: with involvement of the corticospinal tracts and extrapyramidal system.

Clinical features include:

- dementia: usually similar to that associated with Alzheimer's disease, but occasionally involves manic behaviour or delusions of grandeur
- seizures and incontinence
- pupil abnormalities: pupils are large, unequal and unreactive in 75% of cases; the remainder have Argyll Robertson pupils
- tremor of tongue ('trombone' tongue)
- dysarthria
- hypertonia with brisk reflexes and extensor plantar responses.

Diagnosis

In late syphilis a thorough clinical examination should be undertaken, especially of the cardiovascular and neurological systems.

Serological testing

Serological diagnosis for syphilis consists of treponemal and non-treponemal tests. Specific (treponemal) tests include:

- treponemal enzyme immunoassay (EIA) to detect immunoglobulin (IgG or IgM)
- T. pallidum haemagglutination assay (TPHA)
- T. pallidum particle agglutination assay (TPPA)
- fluorescent treponema antibody absorbed test (FTA-abs).

Non-treponemal tests include:

- Cardiolipin tests (VDRL/RPR).

A treponemal test, most commonly the EIA or TPPA, is used for screening. A quantitative VDRL/RPR should be performed when treponemal tests are positive, as this helps diagnose the stage of disease and indicates the need for treatment. A VDRL/RPR titre of >16 and/or a positive IgM test indicates active disease and the need for treatment. The VDRL/RPR and EIA-IgM are often negative in late syphilis.

Evaluation of neurological syphilis

CSF examination is recommended only when neurological or ophthalmic signs or symptoms are present and syphilis serological tests are positive:

- The white cell count (>5 cells/mm^3) is usually raised in symptomatic neurosyphilis
- A negative treponemal test on CSF excludes neurosyphilis. A positive test is highly sensitive for neurosyphilis, but lacks specificity
- A positive CSF VDRL/RPR is diagnostic of neurosyphilis.

Neurological imaging should be performed on all patients who have symptoms/signs consistent with neurosyphilis.

Treatment

Procaine penicillin IM od plus probenecid is given for 17 days. Established neurological disease can be arrested, but may not be reversed. Alternative agents include doxycycline, amoxicillin and ceftriaxone. Treatment of all cases should be discussed with infectious diseases or genitourinary medicine.

Jarisch–Herxheimer reactions (severe allergic reactions) may occur following treatment and high-dose steroid cover is often given with the penicillin. All patients diagnosed with syphilis should have partner notification discussed at the time of treatment by a trained healthcare professional.

Human immunodeficiency virus

HIV can cause neurological involvement either directly or via induced immunosuppression, resulting in opportunistic infections or AIDS-related malignancies. Both the central and peripheral nervous system can be affected.

Central nervous system involvement

The most important feature in determining the differential diagnosis when evaluating a neurological complaint in an HIV-infected individual is the degree of immunosuppression in the host (see Fig. 31.5). Central lesions can further be classified according to whether there is associated mass effect.

Fig. 31.5	Approach to patient with HIV and neurological features
CD4 cell count	**Differentials**
>500/μL	Benign and malignant brain tumours
200 to 500/μL	HIV-associated cognitive and motor disorders
<200/μL	Opportunistic infections and AIDS-associated tumours: • *Toxoplasma* encephalitis • Primary CNS lymphoma • Progressive multifocal leucoencephalopathy (PML) • HIV encephalopathy • CMV encephalitis • Cryptococcal meningitis

Central nervous system lesions with mass effect

The two leading diagnoses associated with mass effect in developed countries are *Toxoplasma* encephalitis and primary CNS lymphoma:

- CNS toxoplasmosis is the most commonly encountered neurological opportunistic infection. Patients present with fever, headache, altered mental state and focal neurological complaints or seizures. The CD4 cell count is often <100 cell/μL. Lesions are often multiple, with ring enhancement present in approximately 90%. Surrounding oedema with mass effect is often seen. It can uncommonly present with diffuse encephalitis not associated with focal abscess formation.
- Primary CNS lymphoma is similar in presentation to, and can often be very difficult to initially distinguish from, CNS toxoplasmosis.

Other rarer infections which can cause lesions with mass effect include bacterial brain abscesses, cryptococcomas, neurocysticercosis, tuberculosis or fungal infections.

CNS lesions without mass effect

- Progressive multifocal leucoencephalopathy (PML) is caused by JC virus, a papovavirus that reactivates in the setting of advanced immunosuppression. PML causes a relentlessly progressive central demyelination with a poor prognosis. Differentials include HIV encephalopathy, cytomegalovirus encephalitis and primary CNS lymphoma.
- HIV encephalopathy typically presents with memory and psychomotor speed impairment, depressive symptoms and movement disorders. Although it rarely presents with mass lesions it can be similar in presentation to PML.

Dementia in HIV-infected patients

Neurological impairment has recently been classified into three conditions;

- Asymptomatic neurocognitive impairment (ANI): individuals who score one standard deviation below the mean on at least two areas of a standardized neuropsychological test
- HIV-associated mild neurocognitive disorder (MND): individuals who in addition to meeting the criteria for ANI demonstrate some mild impairment in daily functioning. The prevalence is estimated at 20–30% of patients with HIV who have no specific neurological symptoms and may be missed without formal neuropsychological testing
- HIV-associated dementia (HAD): individuals who show marked impairment on neuropsychological testing and in daily functioning. The incidence of HAD has declined since the introduction of highly

active antiretroviral therapy (HAART), from 20–30% to 10–15% of those with advanced HIV infection.

Traditionally, little attention has been played to the contribution of age-related neurodegenerative diseases to cognitive impairment in HIV. In developed countries patients are now living longer.

It is estimated that 50% of AIDS cases will be >65 years of age by 2015.

Peripheral nervous system involvement

Peripheral neuropathy

HIV may be associated with the following peripheral neuropathies:

- Distal symmetrical polyneuropathy: the most common type of neuropathy. It is usually a late feature, with pain and paraesthesia of the feet. Treatment is symptomatic.
- Chronic inflammatory demyelinating polyradiculoneuropathy (CIDP): an early feature. It comprises a subacute, predominantly motor polyneuropathy, affecting proximal muscles more than distal, without painful dysaesthesia. Plasmapheresis may help, unlike in forms of CIDP in non-HIV-positive patients.
- Guillain–Barré syndrome (GBS): the acute counterpart of CIDP. This is an early feature that can occur at seroconversion. It has the same clinical features as seronegative GBS, but with a high CSF lymphocyte count. Plasmapheresis may help.
- Multifocal neuropathy: nerve infarction leads to sudden-onset sensory and motor deficits. Herpes zoster and CMV radiculitis must be excluded.
- Mononeuritis/mononeuritis multiplex: asymmetrical mix of motor and sensory defects occurring over several weeks. Exclude CMV infection if CD4 cell count < 50 cell/μL.
- Antiretroviral toxic neuropathy: associated with didanosine and stavudine, which are now rarely used.

Myopathy

Myopathies caused by HIV include:

- polymyositis: indistinguishable from seronegative polymyositis. Immunosuppressive treatment results in improvement
- type 2 fibre muscle atrophy: frequent finding on biopsy in patients with proximal weakness and normal creatine kinase (CK) levels
- drug-induced myopathy, especially from zidovudine.

Poliomyelitis

Polio virus is one of the enteroviruses; it is a picornavirus (pico, small; rna, RNA) transmitted via the oral-faecal route. It has an incubation period of 7 to 14 days, and 90–95% of infections are asymptomatic. In a small minority of patients, polio virus causes a selective destruction of anterior horn cells/motor neurons, characterized by severe back, neck and muscle pain. Paralysis occurs in only about 0.1% of all poliovirus infections.

Europe has been declared offically polio-free since 2001. In 2010 there were 1300 cases worldwide, with the major foci of disease in South Asia, West and Central Africa and the Horn of Africa.

Clinical features

There is considerable variation in symptoms:

- Asymptomatic (95%): with resultant immunity
- Abortive poliomyelitis (4–5%): a self-limiting illness with gastrointestinal and mild upper respiratory symptoms and pyrexia
- Non-paralytic poliomyelitis (0.5%): features of abortive poliomyelitis with meningism. Recovery is complete
- Paralytic poliomyelitis (0.1%): initially there are features of abortive poliomyelitis, which subside and then recur with meningism and myalgia. There is subsequent asymmetrical paralysis with no sensory involvement. Respiratory failure is due to paralysis of the respiratory muscles. The lower limb or limbs are most commonly affected, especially in children. Bulbar symptoms can occur with cranial nerve involvement. When paralytic poliomyelitis occurs before puberty, the patient is often left with a wasted, shortened limb.

Diagnosis of paralytic poliomyelitis

Poliomyelitis is suspected based on the clinical presentation and CSF findings. Paralytic poliomyelitis is distinguished clinically from GBS by the lack of sensory signs and the asymmetry.

CSF findings are similar to those in other viral meningitides (raised protein, increased number of lymphocytes and normal glucose), but there are usually increased numbers of polymorphs initially.

The virus may be grown from throat swabs and stool. It is rarely isolated from CSF. The diagnosis can also be confirmed by PCR amplification of poliovirus RNA from CSF or serologically.

Treatment of paralytic poliomyelitis

Treatment is supportive. Patients with paralytic poliomyelitis should be isolated and contacts immunized. Respiratory failure may develop, requiring mechanical ventilation. Patients with bulbar involvement require close monitoring of cardiovascular status because of the association with blood pressure fluctuations, circulatory collapse and autonomic dysfunction.

Prognosis

Lack of ventilatory support for respiratory paralysis is the usual cause of death, but otherwise mortality rates are very low. Improvement in muscle power can commence a week after paralysis and continue for up to 1 year. Bulbar palsies usually recover well. Some muscles may remain permanently paralysed and fasciculations may persist. In affected limbs in children, bone growth is retarded, resulting in a wasted, shortened limb.

Vaccination

Routine immunization from 2 months of age occurs in the UK. In areas of the world where polio is endemic, primary immunisation is performed with the Sabin oral poliovirus vaccine (live attenuated). Live virus will be excreted in the stool after immunization and therefore great care must be taken to avoid transmission of infection to immunocompromised and non-vaccinated individuals. The Sabin vaccine causes polio in one out of 2.5 million cases, and thus has been replaced by the Salk vaccine (inactive) in non-endemic countries such as the UK.

Post-polio syndrome

A deterioration in function with atrophy in the affected as well as unaffected limbs can occur many years after the primary infection (usually between 20 and 40 years). The cause is uncertain, but theories include progressive degeneration of reinnervated motor units, persistence of poliovirus in neural tissue, and induction of autoimmunity with subsequent destruction of neural structures.

Lyme disease

The causative agent in Lyme disease is the spirochaete (spiral bacteria) *Borrelia burgdorferi*, which is transmitted by the bite of infected ticks of the *Ixodes ricinus* complex. It is acquired in temperate regions of the Northern Hemisphere, usually forested, woodland or heathland areas. The organism is prevalent throughout Europe and North America (e.g. Lyme, Connecticut, where the disease was first recognized).

Clinical features

There is evidence for variation in the types of clinical presentation caused by different genospecies of the ticks. The most common manifestation of Lyme disease is a slowly expanding rash called erythema migrans, which spreads out from a tick bite, after 5 to 14 days (range 3–30 days). It is not usually painful or itchy,

and may enlarge over several weeks if not treated with antibiotics, but will eventually disappear without treatment. Other symptoms may include tiredness, headaches and muscle or joint aches and pains.

If the infection is untreated, organisms may spread in the bloodstream and lymphatics to other parts of the body, including the nervous system. In the UK the most common complications are neurological, which occur in 10–15% of untreated individuals. These include:

- cranial nerve palsies, particularly a facial palsy
- lymphocytic 'viral-type' meningitis
- meningoencephalitis
- radiculopathy causing pain, altered sensation or weakness of a limb.

A small number of untreated patients may progress to late neuroborreliosis, with brain and spinal cord damage. Treatment given at an early stage will minimize progression to this unusual, but serious, complication. It is estimated that late Lyme encephalomyelitis occurs in no more than 1 in 1000 untreated cases.

Diagnosis

It is important that a patient's risk of exposure to ticks is properly assessed before requesting diagnostic tests. Assess a patient's risk of exposure to ticks rather than simply ask about tick bites, as many tick bites go unnoticed. Tests should not be used for 'screening' if there is little evidence that infection, either clinically or epidemiologically, has occurred, as the predictive value of a positive result is very low in this situation. False-positive results can occur with many other infections and inflammatory conditions (glandular fever, rheumatoid arthritis and syphilis), which leads to misdiagnosis and inappropriate treatments.

Usually, tests look for the presence of antibodies to *Borrelia burgdorferi*, rather than the organism itself. Antibodies may not be present in the first few weeks after infection, but it is rare for tests to be negative in late-stage disease. Antibody tests on CSF are useful in suspected neuroborreliosis. If initial screening tests are positive, more detailed and specific tests, usually immunoblots (Western blots), should be performed by reference laboratories to establish whether these results are true positives or false positives.

Treatment

In the majority of individuals, symptoms usually resolve or improve within months, even without treatment. However, prompt treatment helps resolve symptoms more rapidly and patients with painful radiculopathy usually have markedly reduced symptoms and analgesia requirements shortly after starting antibiotics.

The most widely recommended treatment regimes are for:

- oral antibiotics, doxycycline 200 mg od, amoxicillin 500 mg tds or cefuroxime 500 mg bd for 2 weeks for erythema migrans and isolated facial palsy
- oral doxycycline 200 mg od or IV ceftriaxone 2 g od is recommended in acute neuroborreliosis for 14 days
- intravenous treatment with ceftriaxone 2 g IV od for 28 days is recommended for late neurological presentations.

Prognosis

Clinical features of late neuroborreliosis may be slow to resolve. Re-treatment may be indicated in occasional cases, but there is no evidence that prolonged or multiple courses of antibiotics are valuable.

A small minority of patients may continue to have prolonged subjective symptoms after appropriate treatment, similar to chronic fatigue syndrome or fibromyalgia. In such cases prolonged or multiple courses of antibiotics are not indicated. Referral to specialist clinics should be considered. Relief may be gained from intensive physiotherapy or cognitive behavioural therapy.

Prion diseases

Prion diseases are neurodegenerative diseases that have long incubation periods and progress relentlessly once clinical symptoms appear. Five human prion diseases are currently recognized:

- Kuru
- Creutzfeldt–Jakob disease (CJD)
- Variant Creutzfeldt–Jakob disease (vCJD)
- Gerstmann–Sträussler–Scheinker syndrome (GSS)
- Fatal familial insomnia (FFI).

These human prion diseases share common neuropathological features, including neuronal loss, proliferation of glial cells, absence of an inflammatory response and the presence of small vacuoles within neuropil, which produces a spongiform appearance. Bovine spongiform encephalopathy (BSE), one of a number of prion infections affecting animals, has focused public attention on these diseases with its possible link to variant CJD.

Prions are small infectious pathogens containing protein, but which lack a nucleic acid. They are characteristically resistant to a number of normal decontaminating procedures, and disinfection and sterilization of prion-contaminated medical instruments requires specific procedures.

Prion diseases are associated with the accumulation of an abnormal form of host protein, designated the prion protein (PrP). These changes are due to both variation in amino acid sequence as well as glycosylation of the prion protein. Transport of the abnormal prion protein to the nervous system, once it appears in the host, occurs via axons and appears to be neurotoxic, leading to apoptosis and cell death.

Creutzfeldt–Jakob disease

CJD is the most common of the human prion diseases. Sporadic, familial, iatrogenic and variant forms of CJD are all recognized.

Sporadic Creutzfeldt–Jakob disease

Sporadic CJD occurs with a frequency of 1 case per 1 000 000 population per year worldwide, and accounts for 85–95% of all cases of CJD. Onset of disease is usually between 57 and 62 years of age. Rapidly progressive mental deterioration and myoclonus are the two cardinal features of sCJD.

Variant Creutzfeldt–Jakob disease

New – vCJD – was first described in 1996. As of 2012, there have been a total of 224 cases of probable vCJD reported worldwide. Available evidence suggests that vCJD represents bovine-to-human transmission of BSE, with most patients acquiring the disease through ingestion of infected meat products. Variant CJD presents with a progressive cognitive decline, with prominent neuropsychiatric features often accompanied by sensory symptoms. It presents at a younger age and has a more protracted course than sCJD (14 versus 4 to 5 months).

Since 1989, when the specified bovine offal (SBO) ban was first introduced, the use of all tissues most likely to contain the infective agent of BSE in products for human consumption, such as the brain, spinal cord, thymus, tonsils, spleen, intestines and, more recently, bones, are prohibited.

Iatrogenic Creutzfeldt–Jakob disease

Iatrogenic CJD has occurred following the use of cadaveric human pituitary hormones, dural graft transplants, corneal transplants, liver transplants and the use of contaminated neurosurgical instruments or stereotactic depth electrodes. Exact incubation periods for iatrogenic CJD are unknown but are estimated to be between 9 and 10 years.

Diagnosis

Brain biopsy remains the gold standard diagnostic test for CJD, but is often unnecessary. A compatible clinical presentation with MRI, EEG and CSF analysis are in most cases sufficient to exclude other causes and establish CJD as the probable diagnosis:

- The main histopathological features of prion disease are spongiform change, neuronal loss without inflammation and accumulation of abnormal prion protein, which is detected by immunohistochemical techniques on brain tissue.
- MRI can often demonstrate a high T2 and FLAIR signal in the caudate and putamen in sCJD. In vCJD there may be high signal in the pulvinar and dorsomedial thalamus. In both forms of the disease, diffusion weighted imaging may be more sensitive, and also show cortical changes.

- A characteristic EEG pattern of periodic synchronous bi- or triphasic sharp wave complexes is observed in 67–95% of patients with sCJD, less so in vCJD.
- Detecting 14-3-3 protein in CSF is a specific test finding for sCJD, but has low sensitivity.

Treatment

There is no effective treatment for CJD, which is uniformly fatal. Death usually occurs within 1 year of symptom onset.

HINTS AND TIPS

A rapidly progressive dementia (over weeks or months), especially with myoclonus, should always be considered to be prion disease unless an alternative diagnosis can be made. This has implications for how all samples from the patient, including blood and CSF, are handled by medical and laboratory staff.

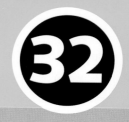
- Understand the epidemiology and possible pathogenic mechanism of multiple sclerosis (MS)
- Describe the neurological systems typically affected by MS
- Understand the investigations needed to make a firm diagnosis of MS
- What are the differential diagnoses of white matter disease?
- Understand the pharmaceutical and non-pharmaceutical management of patients with MS

Multiple sclerosis (MS) is the most common autoimmune, inflammatory, demyelinating disease of the central nervous system.

EPIDEMIOLOGY

MS occurs worldwide, but is particularly common in North America, Australia and northern Europe. It affects about 80 000 people in the UK, and has a prevalence of approximately 1 in 800.

The disease usually occurs in young Caucasian adults, the peak age of onset for the relapsing–remitting form of the disease being between 20 and 30 years; this may convert to secondary-progressive MS at a mean age of 40 to 44 years. More females than males are affected in all forms of the disease.

PATHOGENESIS

MS is a heterogeneous disorder with variable clinical and pathological features reflecting different pathways to disease. The major mechanisms that cause disease are inflammation, demyelination and axonal degeneration in the later stages of the disease. A large number of hypotheses exist regarding the pathogenesis of MS and the exact cause remains uncertain. Immunological mechanisms undoubtedly play a role, although the causation is probably multifactorial. Risk factors include genetic factors, viral infections and other environmental factors.

PATHOLOGY

Areas of demyelination are found in the white matter of the brain and spinal cord. These areas are called plaques. The lesions lie in close relationship to post-capillary venules (perivenular). There is a particular predilection for certain sites within the CNS:

- Periventricular region of the cerebral hemispheres
- Corpus callosum
- Brainstem (including medial longitudinal fasciculus), cerebellum and cerebellar peduncles
- Cervical cord
- Optic nerves.

There is myelin destruction with relative preservation of axons. An inflammatory infiltrate containing mononuclear cells and lymphocytes is found. Interstitial oedema occurs in acute lesions. Remyelination is rare and the mechanism of functional recovery is uncertain. It is postulated that chronic demyelination may eventually account for the loss of axons and subsequently the cell bodies. This may explain the clinical irreversibility of some of the relapses.

CLINICAL FEATURES

MS can present in a multitude of ways and no single presentation is diagnostic. It is most commonly characterized by relapse, which is defined as the acute or subacute onset of clinical dysfunction that usually reaches its peak from days to several weeks, followed by a remission during which the symptoms and signs resolve to a variable extent. Three main patterns of disease progression are recognized:

- Relapsing and remitting: clearly defined relapses with full recovery or with some residual deficit upon recovery. Relapses are more common in early disease, and there is no disease progression during the periods between relapses. This makes up 85–90% of cases initially.
- Secondary progressive: when the disease starts with a relapsing–remitting picture, but eventually recovery from each successive relapse becomes less complete,

Fig. 32.1 Good prognostic factors in multiple sclerosis

- Caucasian ethnic origin
- Relapsing–remitting form of disease
- Monosymptomatic onset of disease (including no bowel or bladder symptoms at onset)
- Complete recovery from first attack
- Low relapse rate in the first 2 years after disease onset
- Long interval between the first two attacks
- Minimal lesion load on MRI at presentation

and there is progression of disease between relapses causing the development of long-term disability. Approximately 40% of patients presenting with relapsing–remitting disease eventually develop secondary progressive disease 10 years after disease onset. It is the progression of disease, rather than incomplete recovery from relapses, which causes disability.

- Primary progressive: disability worsens gradually from onset without true relapses or remissions, with a cumulative disability from the onset. Approximately 10–30% of patients may present with this form of disease.

There is a marked variability in the disease progression. Overall, studies have shown that the median time from disease onset to walking with a cane is 28 years. About 20% of patients with relapsing–remitting MS develop little or no disability after 10 years. Patients with primary progressive disease who tend to have a later age of onset, and more even sex distribution, have a worse prognosis for ultimate disability compared with relapsing–remitting patients. Once the progressive phase has begun, primary and secondary progressive patients decline at the same rate, and need a walking aid after a median of 6 years. Overall, the life expectancy of MS patients is reduced by 6–7 years compared with the general population, and severe disability is a major risk factor for premature death. Prognostic factors for MS are shown in Figure 32.1. Pregnancy does not worsen the prognosis for those women with MS, and in fact there may be a reduction in relapse rates during pregnancy, which is probably compensated for by a higher relapse rate in the immediate period after delivery.

The most common presentations of MS are discussed below and shown in Figure 32.2.

Optic and retrobulbar neuritis

Optic neuritis presents as subacute visual loss, usually unilateral, associated with a central scotoma and pain on ocular movement. Recovery is usual over a few weeks. The ophthalmological findings depend on whether the lesion is in the optic nerve head (papillitis) or in the optic nerve behind the eye (retrobulbar neuritis). In the former, a pink swollen disc is seen, whereas in the latter, the disc looks normal.

There are usually no residual symptoms following optic neuritis, although a relative afferent pupillary defect, small central scotomata and defects in colour vision may be demonstrated. Following an attack, optic atrophy (pale disc) often develops several weeks later.

Optic neuritis may be an isolated event, or it may be a forerunner for further episodes of CNS demyelination, i.e. MS. Up to 70% of cases fall into the latter category.

In some patients, optic nerve demyelination may be asymptomatic and only discovered clinically by the presence of optic atrophy or by the use of visual evoked potentials (see Ch. 3).

Fig. 32.2 Common presenting symptoms in multiple sclerosis

Location	Frequency	Nature of symptoms
Spinal cord	50%	Motor – weakness, clumsiness, tonic spasms Sensory – numbness, tingling, burning, band-like sensation, Lhermitte's phenomenon, altered temperature sensation Sphincter – urinary urgency/hesitancy/retention/incontinence, constipation, faecal incontinence, erectile dysfunction
Optic nerve (unilateral in 90%)	25%	Visual loss, blurred vision, reduced colour vision, pain on eye movement
Brainstem/ cerebellum	20%	Dysarthria, dysphagia, diplopia, vertigo, facial numbness/weakness, trigeminal neuralgia, deafness, ataxia (trunk and limbs), nystagmus, pyramidal weakness due to corticospinal tract involvement, patchy sensory loss, tonic spasms
Cerebral hemispheres	5%	Hemiparesis, hemisensory loss, visual field deficit, dysphasia, seizures, cognitive impairment

Papillitis can look similar to papilloedema through an ophthalmoscope. Papillitis causes early and profound loss in vision, with a central scotoma, impaired colour vision and pain on eye movement. In papilloedema, visual deterioration occurs only at a late stage, when there is enlargement of the blind spot and sometimes constriction of the fields.

Brainstem/cerebellar presentation

Demyelination may initially affect the brainstem, including the cerebellar connections and medial longitudinal fasciculus (see Ch. 9) in the brainstem. Classical presentations include those described in Figure 32.2.

Spinal cord lesion (myelopathy)

A spinal cord lesion is the most common presentation and results in a spastic paraparesis (thoracic cord) or tetraparesis (cervical cord), often with tonic spasms of the limbs. There is associated difficulty walking and sensory loss. Bladder symptoms are extremely common.

Lhermitte's symptom, in which there is a brief, electric-shock-like sensation down the limbs on flexion of the neck, may be present. It is indicative of lesions within the spinal cord, which can occur with processes other than demyelination, e.g. vitamin B_{12} deficiency before treatment.

The symptoms and signs of MS tend to get worse with heat, e.g. in the bath or during hot weather (Uthoff's phenomenon).

Other symptoms

Patients with significant subcortical MRI lesion load can also present with subtle cognitive deficits. Seizures, fatigue and depression are also more common in patients with MS.

DIFFERENTIAL DIAGNOSIS

The differential diagnoses that should be considered when presented with a relapsing–remitting CNS condition include systemic lupus erythematosus (SLE), sarcoidosis, Behçet's disease, neurosyphilis and Lyme disease. The differential diagnoses that should be considered in patients with a progressive presentation include structural lesions, vitamin B_{12} deficiency, paraneoplastic syndromes and hereditary disorders, such as the leucodystrophies, spinocerebellar ataxias and hereditary spastic paraparesis.

There are also multiple causes of optic neuritis, brainstem syndromes and myelopathy, and these must be excluded on initial presentation.

Neuromyelitis optica (NMO) is a relapsing, autoimmune condition in which patients present with a demyelinating optic neuritis and myelitis either simultaneously, or with an interval between them. Patients are typically positive for antibodies to aquaporin 4, and have a worse prognosis than those patients with MS. Treatment requires prolonged courses of steroids and immunomodulation.

INVESTIGATIONS

There is no diagnostic test for MS, but the clinical suspicion is supported by the following three tests.

Magnetic resonance imaging

Computed tomography (CT) scans do not accurately pick up areas of demyelination, whereas magnetic resonance imaging (MRI) is far more sensitive at showing the white matter disease. Hyperintense lesions are seen on T2-weighted images, typically in periventricular areas, the corpus callosum and juxtacortical white matter in the brain. Widespread MRI abnormalities are often seen at presentation, in spite of the symptoms being isolated to one or two sites. Similar hyperintense lesions may be seen in cerebrovascular disease, neurosarcoidosis, vasculitis and lymphoma. Contrast enhancement of some lesions (suggesting active disease) and not of others on the same MRI suggests that the lesions are separated in time as well as space, which is an important criterion for making the diagnosis of MS.

Cerebrospinal fluid examination

A mild lymphocyte pleocytosis may be present, especially during relapses. The protein may be slightly elevated. However, the presence of 'oligoclonal bands' (several intense bands of staining for IgG on Western blotting) in the CSF but not in the serum is highly suggestive of MS. Oligoclonal bands in the CSF and often the serum (i.e. matched bands) may also be found in many chronic infective or inflammatory conditions involving the CNS.

Evoked potentials

Visual evoked potentials

If there has been demyelination at any time along the optic nerve (i.e. optic neuritis), whether symptomatic or asymptomatic, the conduction of visual images (usually a changing checkerboard) to the occipital cortex will be delayed. The normal response takes about 100 milliseconds.

Somatosensory evoked potentials

Measurement of somatosensory evoked potentials (SSEPs) may detect a delay in central sensory pathways.

Brainstem auditory evoked potentials

Measurement of brainstem auditory evoked potentials (BAEPs) during auditory testing may detect brainstem lesions.

DIAGNOSIS

The diagnosis of MS is based on the McDonald criteria. This basically states that typical lesions should be disseminated in time and space: that is, have occurred in the CNS in different places and at different times. Often this may be clear from the history and examination, but if not, laboratory investigations may provide the necessary evidence. In patients presenting with a single clinical attack (clinically isolated syndrome or CIS), dissemination in space may be shown by the MRI finding of a specified number of non-enhancing typical MS lesions in the brain or spinal cord (or oligoclonal bands in the CSF). If that same MRI or a follow-up MRI shows new or enhancing lesions, or the patient develops a second clinical attack, the criteria dissemination in time is fulfilled and MS can be diagnosed.

MANAGEMENT

Treatments for acute relapses

Corticosteroid therapy

Steroid therapy, usually given intravenously as methylprednisolone, is the mainstay treatment used for severe acute relapses. This may shorten the duration of the relapse, but does not affect eventual clinical outcome.

Disease-modifying treatment

Beta-interferon and glatiramer acetate

Interferon-β1a and 1b and glatiramer acetate are drugs that suppress or modulate the immune system. The UK NICE and the ABN (Association of British Neurologists) guidelines suggest that they are used in ambulant patients with relapsing–remitting MS, where at least two relapses have occurred in the preceding 2 years, and in whom there is no progression between relapses. Patients with secondary progressive MS may also be treated if their disability is primarily due to their relapses which must occur at least annually. All three drugs are given as regular injections, and side-effects can include flu-like symptoms, injection site reactions and the development of neutralizing antibodies. The effect of these drugs is to reduce relapse rates by about one-third over two years, and they may reduce the development of disability through prevention of those relapses, though the effect is modest. They do not modify progressively increasing disability that is unrelated to relapses. Furthermore, it is unknown whether these drugs reduce the accumulation of disability over the long term, and whether they prevent or slow entry into the secondary progressive stage of the disease.

Other immunomodulatory agents

In patients with aggressive or rapidly evolving relapsing–remitting MS, or in patients in whom beta-interferon/glatiramer acetate has failed, ABN and NICE guidance suggest consideration can be given to the use of other, more powerful immunomodulatory agents. Natalizumab is a monoclonal antibody that has been found to reduce the risk of sustained progression of disability by ~40% over 2 years, and that of relapses by ~70% over 12 months. However, this drug is associated with an increased risk of opportunistic infections, including progressive multifocal leucoencephalopathy (PML), which can be fatal. Currently, the overall risk for this infection is a 1.5 per 1000 patients, but the specific risk depends also on the duration of natalizumab treatment, prior immunosuppressant treatment, and previous infection with JC virus.

Mitoxantrone is another immunosuppressant which has been licensed for progressive MS as well as relapsing–remitting MS. It too has significant toxicity, including cardiotoxicity and leukaemia. For this reason it is generally only used in patients with rapidly advancing disease who have failed other therapies, or as an alternative to natalizumab.

Fingolimod is the latest disease-modifying treatment to be licensed for MS. It is an oral medication taken daily that prevents lymphocytes from crossing the blood–brain barrier and causing damage to nerve cells in the brain and spinal cord. NICE guidelines recommend its use in highly active relapsing–remitting MS: that is, patients who have an unchanged or increased relapse rate, or ongoing severe relapses compared to the previous year, despite treatment with beta interferon. It reduces relapse rates by 52% compared to beta-interferon, and disability progression by about 30% compared to placebo. The most common side-effects associated with the drug include flu-like symptoms and elevated liver function tests. More rarely, cardiac arrhythmias, diminished respiratory function, tumour development and macular oedema can occur. An ophthalmological evaluation is therefore recommended 3 to 4 months after treatment initiation, along with regular blood tests and clinical follow-up. Patients should also take their first dose under medical supervision with blood pressure and heart rate monitoring.

> **HINTS AND TIPS**
>
> Patients presenting with clinically isolated syndromes can be a therapeutic problem. In many countries disease-modifying treatment is offered to those patients with an initial demyelinating episode, and an abnormal MRI scan suggesting a high probability (~60%) of conversion to MS. Although there is some evidence that disease-modifying treatment may delay conversion to clinically definite MS, it is unknown whether such treatments prevent or delay long-term disability. If the initial MRI is normal, the likelihood of developing MS is ~20%, and a repeat MRI should be obtained between 3 and 6 months.

Symptomatic treatment

An overview of the types of symptomatic treatment that are relevant in MS is shown in Fig. 32.3.

OTHER CENTRAL DEMYELINATING DISEASES

A number of other rarer diseases can cause demyelination within the CNS, but their presentation is very different from MS. These include:

- **Acute disseminated encephalomyelitis (ADEM):** this monophasic syndrome presents following a viral illness or vaccination. It is fatal in as many as 30% of cases. The areas of white matter change can occur simultaneously in several parts of the CNS, and are often confluent and more symmetrical than in MS. Rarely, the lesions are haemorrhagic. Patients may also have other features that are unusual for MS, including fever, encephalopathy, seizures and a lack of oligoclonal bands in the CSF. Despite these features, this condition can be difficult to distinguish from an initial presentation of MS
- **Progressive multifocal leucoencephalopathy (PML):** caused by JC papovavirus infection, especially in immunocompromised patients, e.g. 4% of patients with HIV
- **Leucodystrophies:** metachromatic leucodystrophy (disorder of arylsulphatase A enzyme), adrenoleucodystrophy (accumulation of very long chain fatty acids [VLCFAs])

Fig. 32.3 Symptomatic treatment in multiple sclerosis

Symptom	Treatment
Cognitive dysfunction	Disease-modifying treatment Cognitive rehabilitation techniques
Depression	Psychotherapy and/or pharmacotherapy
Pain	Mechanical pain – NSAIDs, transcutaneous electrical stimulation (TENS), physiotherapy Neurogenic pain – anticonvulsants (e.g. gabapentin, pregabalin, carbamazepine, amitriptyline), antidepressants (e.g. amitriptyline), TENS
Ataxis and tremor	Physiotherapy and occupational therapy Medications – clonazepam, propranolol, isoniazid
Fatigue	Treatment of any underlying depression or nocturia Physiotherapy – graded exercise programmes Medications – amantadine or modafinil
Bladder dysfunction	Detrusor hyper-reflexia causing urinary frequency and urgency – anticholinergics, e.g. oxybutynin, intravesical botulinum toxin Detrusor-sphincter dyssynergia causing retention – intermittent self-catheterization Nocturia – antidiuretic hormone analogue DDAVP (desmopressin)
Spasticity	Physiotherapy Medications – baclofen, tizanidine, dantrolene (care must be taken not to reduce tone too far as may exacerbate weakness)
Paroxysmal symptoms	e.g. muscle spasms, burning dysaesthetic pains, trigeminal neuralgia, and other brief brainstem symptoms – best treated with sodium channel blockers such as carbamazepine

- **SSPE (subacute sclerosing panencephalitis):** this is a rare and deadly delayed complication of measles virus infection
- **Vitamin B$_{12}$ deficiency:** can cause central demyelination
- **Central pontine myelinolysis (CPM):** this is associated with too rapid a correction of sodium in patients who are hyponatraemic and often have a history of alcohol abuse. Demyelination occurs within the pons and the clinical presentation can vary from no symptoms to ataxia to a profound tetraplegia and pseudobulbar palsy.

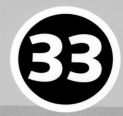
● **Objectives**

- Understand the common neurological complications that may arise from rheumatological, endocrine, haematological, renal, gastrointestinal and cardiac disease
- Be aware of the neurological complications that may arise from sarcoidosis and Behçet's disease

ENDOCRINE DISORDERS

Diabetes mellitus

Diabetes mellitus is by far the most common endocrinological and metabolic cause of neurological symptoms and signs involving the whole nervous system.

Hypoglycaemia and hyperglycaemia

Hypoglycaemia can be caused by oral hypoglycaemics, insulin or insulin-secreting tumours. It can cause confusion, dysarthria, altered behaviour, agitation, seizures and, rarely, focal neurological signs. If not treated promptly it will lead to coma. Similarly, hyperglycaemia due to diabetic ketoacidosis, or hyperosmolar non-ketotic hyperglycaemia, can also cause coma. Any patient in a coma should immediately have his or her glucose measured.

Cerebrovascular disease

Patients with diabetes have a higher risk of developing cerebrovascular disease than the general population. This includes large vessel (e.g. middle cerebral artery occlusion) and small vessel diseases (e.g. pseudobulbar palsy syndrome, gait apraxia and multi-infarct dementia).

Visual loss

Visual loss in diabetes may be due to retinal disease and haemorrhage, cataracts or vascular disease (e.g. central retinal artery occlusion).

Peripheral nerve lesions

Peripheral neuropathy is a very common finding in diabetes. The most common types of neuropathy are:

- distal symmetrical polyneuropathy (sensory greater than motor)
- painful proximal asymmetrical motor neuropathy ('diabetic amyotrophy'): this syndrome is probably due to a lumbosacral plexopathy

- compression mononeuropathies, e.g. carpal tunnel syndrome
- multifocal neuropathy ('mononeuritis multiplex'): diabetes is the commonest cause of this syndrome, which may affect peripheral nerves in the limbs or individual cranial nerves, especially the third, sixth and seventh (see Ch. 22)
- autonomic neuropathy.

Hyperthyroidism

Hyperthyroidism can be caused by immune disease (Graves' disease), thyroiditis, multinodular goitre or pituitary tumours. Clinical features of Graves' disease often include exophthalmos with ophthalmoplegia. This is due to inflammatory infiltration and oedema of the periorbital fat and connective tissues.

A high-frequency, postural, upper limb tremor is characteristic of hyperthyroidism, and a proximal myopathy may also be present. Hyperthyroidism can cause upper motor neuron signs, especially in the legs, including spasticity, clonus, weakness, brisk reflexes and extensor plantars. Lower motor neuron features can also be present, including muscle atrophy accompanying severe weight loss. It can therefore sometimes be difficult to differentiate hyperthyroidism from motor neuron disease. Neuropsychiatric symptoms may also be present, including seizures, anxiety, confusion and emotional lability.

In addition, atrial fibrillation is common and may result in embolic cerebral infarction.

Hypothyroidism

Carpal tunnel syndrome is common in hypothyroidism. Myopathy, neuropathy, cerebellar ataxia and encephalopathy can all occur. It is the most common treatable cause of dementia, arising in 2–4% of elderly patients.

Pituitary gland

Pituitary tumours are common but many are small, asymptomatic microadenomas. Macroadenomas can cause neurological symptoms by mass effect and give rise to headache, hydrocephalus and raised intracranial pressure, and visual disturbances, such as a bitemporal hemianopia due to compression of the optic chiasm. Lateral extension can cause compression of cavernous sinus structures, including cranial nerves III, IV, V(i) and VI. Pituitary adenomas are hormone secreting in two-thirds of cases and, of these, 65% secrete prolactin, 15% secrete growth hormone and the remainder secrete adrenocorticotrophic hormone, gonadotrophins or thyroid-stimulating hormone. The specific conditions a patient may present with depend on the hormones secreted by the tumour and include acromegaly and Cushings's disease. Investigations of patients with suspected pituitary tumours should include measurement of visual acuity and fields, endocrine assessments and magnetic resonance imaging (MRI).

Hypopituitarism can result from a number of conditions, including tumours, infections (e.g. tuberculosis), head injury and inflammatory conditions such as sarcoidosis. Pituitary apoplexy describes a syndrome of acute headache, nausea, vomiting, hypotensive collapse and sudden bilateral visual loss. It is typically due to haemorrhage into a pituitary macroadenoma.

The posterior pituitary secretes antidiuretic hormone (ADH), which is important for plasma osmoregulation. Diabetes insipidus results from dysfunction of the posterior pituitary and reduced ADH secretion, causing thirst, polyuria and polydipsia. Common causes include trauma, tumours, sarcoidosis and infections.

Electrolyte imbalances

Electrolyte imbalances (sodium, potassium, magnesium, calcium) can cause disturbances of both the central and peripheral nervous systems. The clinical severity of the presentation tends to be greatest when the abnormality has developed rapidly. Treatment should not only correct the electrolyte disturbance but also identify the underlying cause. Central pontine myelinosis can arise in the context of a severe electrolyte disorder, especially with the rapid correction of sodium abnormalities (see Ch. 32).

HAEMATOLOGICAL DISORDERS

Anaemias

Anaemia can cause non-specific neurological symptoms, including fatigue, dizziness, syncope, headache, irritability and impaired concentration. Rarely it may cause focal neurological deficits if there is significant intra-/extracranial vascular stenosis. Iron deficiency anaemia is also associated with idiopathic intracranial hypertension and restless leg syndrome. Vitamin B_{12} deficiency can also cause a number of neurological features, including a peripheral neuropathy, myelopathy, encephalopathy, optic neuropathy, dementia and ophthalmoplegia. Sickle cell disease, as well as causing anaemia, can also predispose to cerebrovascular disease.

Proliferative conditions

Leukaemia can cause neurological disease either directly by invasion of the nervous system via the blood circulation, lymphatics or meninges, or indirectly via infection or haemorrhage. Meningeal leukaemia can present as a subacute meningitis with associated cranial neuropathies. Plasma cell dyscrasias are caused by the proliferation of a single clone of immunoglobulin-secreting plasma cells. They include myeloma, Waldenström's macroglobulinaemia, monoclonal gammopathy of unknown significance, plasmacytoma and plasma cell leukaemia. They are associated with peripheral neuropathies and, therefore, all patients with an unexplained neuropathy should be screened for a paraprotein. Both Hodgkin's and non-Hodgkin's lymphomas commonly spread to the CNS. Primary CNS lymphoma is rarer, but more common in immunosuppressed patients. Polycythaemia is an increased red cell mass and may be primary or secondary. It is a risk factor for focal, acute vascular syndromes. Similarly, thrombocythaemia is an increased platelet count, and associated with an increased risk of thrombosis and haemorrhage within the CNS.

Clotting disorders

Thrombotic thrombocytopenic purpura, antiphospholipid antibody syndrome and the thrombophilias can all predispose patients to cerebrovascular events. Patients may present with fluctuating conscious levels, seizures, encephalopathy or focal neurological deficits.

GASTROINTESTINAL DISORDERS

A small percentage of patients with inflammatory bowel disease will develop neurological complications, most typically a demyelinating peripheral neuropathy. Vascular complications can also occur due to hypercoagulability, and include cerebral venous thrombosis and ischaemic strokes. In coeliac disease up to 10% of patients may have neurological complications, the most common of which are ataxias and neuropathies. Whipple's disease, although rare, can also be associated with a number of neurological complications, including dementia, myoclonus and supranuclear ophthalmoplegia.

The most important neurological complication of liver disease is hepatic encephalopathy. This typically presents as delirium, which progresses to stupor and coma. Seizures, rigidity, pyramidal signs and primitive reflexes may also be present.

RENAL DISORDERS

Renal disease can be associated with neurological disorders in several ways. Firstly, many vasculitides, connective tissue disorders and genetic diseases affect both the kidneys and nervous system. Secondly, renal failure itself can have neurological consequences. These include uraemic encephalopathy, electrolyte disorders and uraemic neuropathy. The latter tends to be a peripheral sensorimotor, axonal neuropathy. Finally, the treatment of renal disease can have neurological complications; dialysis can be associated acutely with confusion, and chronic dialysis can rarely cause dementia. Following renal transplant and immunosuppression, a range of infections may occur: particularly, fungal and lymphoma of the central nervous system develops in 5% of transplant cases. Ciclosporin, a common immunosuppressant, can cause tremor, seizures, encephalopathy, neuropathy and myopathy.

VASCULITIDES AND CONNECTIVE TISSUE DISORDERS

In primary vasculitides and connective tissue disorders, there is inflammation of the connective tissue and blood vessels (vasculitis). Neurological complications are caused by the active vasculitis, treatment side-effects (e.g. proximal myopathy secondary to steroids) and the mechanical effects of disease or treatment (e.g. entrapment neuropathies in rheumatoid arthritis). The active vasculitis causes ischaemic damage in the brain, spinal cord, peripheral nerve and muscle. The ischaemia is caused by thrombosis and distal embolism, or direct thrombotic occlusion of arteries, capillaries or veins. Vasculitis can also cause an aseptic meningitis with a CSF lymphocytosis and mild protein elevation. Secondary causes of vasculitis include infections (e.g. HIV, fungi, TB), drugs (e.g. cocaine, amphetamines) and malignancy (e.g. lymphoma). Neurological involvement in systemic vasculitides is common, but may not be the presenting feature. In giant cell arteritis, and isolated cerebral angiitis, the first and only presentation is neurological. All connective tissue diseases and primary

vasculitides can be associated with polymyositis. For specific neurological features associated with connective tissue disorders and vasculitis see Figure 33.1.

CARDIAC DISORDERS

The neurological complications of cardiac disease are shown in Figure 33.2. Cerebral hypoperfusion secondary to heart failure, and cardiac embolization, are important underlying mechanisms. Cardiac embolism to the anterior circulation is more common than to the posterior circulation. Clinical and radiological features consistent with cardiac embolism include abrupt and maximal neurological deficit at onset (rather than in a stepwise manner), haemorrhagic transformation due to rapid reperfusion and multiple vascular territory infarcts on imaging.

OTHER MULTISYSTEM DISEASES

Sarcoidosis

Sarcoidosis is a multisystem granulomatous disorder of unknown aetiology that affects the nervous system in 5% of patients. Its pathological hallmark is non-caseating epithelioid cell granulomas. It is more common in younger patients and those of Afro-Caribbean extraction. Over 90% of patients have respiratory involvement, most commonly bilateral hilar lymphadenopathy. Other systems that can be affected include the skin (25%), eyes (25%), liver (40–70%), and heart (5–10%). The neurological consequences of sarcoidosis are numerous and are shown in Figure 33.3. Diagnosis can be difficult without a tissue biopsy, though the presence of an elevated serum and CSF angiotensin converting enzyme (ACE), bilateral hilar lymphadenopathy and a restrictive lung deficit can aid diagnosis. MRI of the brain may show parenchymatous mass lesions and meningeal or focal nodular enhancement. Treatment is with steroids and immunosuppressive agents.

Behçet's disease

This is an immune-mediated vasculitis and multisystem disease causing recurrent orogenital ulceration, skin lesions, ocular lesions (including uveitis) and a positive pathergy test. Men and those from the Eastern Mediterranean and Japan tend to be most commonly affected. Neurological involvement can take several forms: an aseptic meningitis, parenchymal involvement most commonly affecting the brainstem, and cortical venous sinus thrombosis. Pathologically, there is infiltration of the perivasculature and meninges with immune cells.

Fig 33.1 Main neurological features of systemic connective tissue disorders and vasculitis

Systemic connective tissue disease/vasculitis	Neurological complication
Polyarteritis nodosa	Peripheral neuropathy – mononeuritis multiplex CNS involvement rarer – headache, encephalopathy, psychosis, seizures, aseptic meningitis, stroke, cranial nerve palsies, ischaemic myelopathy
Churg–Strauss	Peripheral neuropathy – mononeuritis multiplex
Wegener's granulomatosis	CNS involvement – cranial nerve palsies (e.g. hearing loss, ischaemic optic neuropathy, facial and trigeminal nerve involvement) Peripheral neuropathy – mononeuritis multiplex
Sjögren's syndrome	Peripheral neuropathy – asymmetric, segmental or multifocal sensory neuronopathy (mostly affecting joint-position sense and vibration) – mononeuritis multiplex less common Autonomic neuropathy CNS involvement – cranial nerve palsies (e.g. hearing loss, trigeminal nerve involvement), myelopathy, cognitive impairment, seizures, stroke
Rheumatoid arthritis	Peripheral neuropathy – entrapment neuropathy, mononeuritis multiplex, polyneuropathy CNS involvement – atlanto-axial subluxation causing spinal cord compression, cranial nerve palsies
Scleroderma	Rare – peripheral or cranial neuropathies, headache, seizures, stroke
Systemic lupus erythematosus	CNS involvement – neuropsychiatric features (e.g. seizures, psychosis, mood changes, cognitive impairment), cranial nerve lesions, focal neurological signs, myelopathy Peripheral neuropathy
Isolated cerebral angiitis	Can present in three ways: encephalopathy; multiple sclerosis-like illness with stroke-like episodes; and intracranial mass with focal signs ± raised intracranial pressure
Giant cell arteritis	Headache Monocular blindness Strokes

Fig. 33.2 Neurological complications of cardiovascular disease

Cardiovascular disease	Neurological complication
Aortic disease (e.g. aortitis, atherosclerosis, aneurysms, dissection, coarctation)	Brain – stroke, transient ischaemic attack, hypoperfusion Spinal cord – ischaemia
Cardiac surgery	Perioperative stroke (5%) Late encephalopathy (Both complications secondary to microemboli, hypoperfusion and postoperative atrial fibrillation)
Rhythm disturbance (e.g. AF, sick sinus syndrome, tachyarrhythmias)	Cardioembolic stroke Syncope, dizziness
Primary cardiomyopathies	Associated with arrhythmias and increased tendency to ventricular thrombus formation and embolism
Valve disease (e.g. infective endocarditis)	Embolism to brain Mycotic aneurysm and haemorrhagic stroke
Atrial myxoma	Cerebral emboli

Fig. 33.3 Neurological consequences of sarcoidosis

- Cranial nerve palsies (e.g. deafness, bilateral VIIth nerve palsy, optic neuropathy)
- Aseptic basal meningitis which can cause hydrocephalus
- Intracranial mass lesions (granulomas) causing focal signs or raised intracranial pressure
- Pituitary or hypothalamic dysfunction (e.g. diabetes insipidus)
- Sarcoid encephalopathy – seizures, neuropsychiatric features and cognitive impairment
- Myelopathy with intramedullary granuloma
- Peripheral neuropathy – mononeuritis multiplex or less commonly a symmetrical polyneuropathy
- Proximal myopathy

The diagnosis can be confused with multiple sclerosis, but headaches are much more common in Behcet's disease, while optic neuritis is rare. Treatment is with steroids and immunosuppressive agents. Venous thrombosis may be treated with anticoagulation.

The effects of vitamin deficiencies and toxins on the nervous system

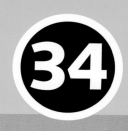

34

Objectives

- Understand the common syndromes associated with vitamin deficiencies
- Consider the wide range of medication-induced neurological disorders
- Describe the main neurological syndromes associated with other toxins

VITAMIN DEFICIENCIES

Nutritional deficiencies are particularly common in developing countries, but do occur in developed countries due to poor eating habits, alcoholism and malabsorption syndromes. The most common conditions are described below.

Vitamin B₁ (thiamine) deficiency

Deficiency of vitamin B_1 causes beriberi or Wernicke–Korsakoff syndrome.

Beriberi

Beriberi is caused by a staple diet of polished rice and results in either a polyneuropathy (dry beriberi) or marked generalized oedema with ascites and pleural effusions (wet beriberi).

Wernicke–Korsakoff syndrome

Wernicke–Korsakoff syndrome is more common in the Western world than beriberi and is caused primarily by chronic alcoholism with poor dietary intake of thiamine. An uncommon presentation is that of intractable vomiting such as that associated with pregnancy.

The syndrome is composed of an acute phase (Wernicke's encephalopathy) and a chronic phase (Korsakoff's psychosis).

The typical triad of Wernicke's encephalopathy comprises:

- ocular signs: with nystagmus and ophthalmoplegia
- ataxia: with a broad-based gait, and cerebellar signs in the limbs, especially the legs
- confusion: with disorientation, apathy, agitation, amnesia, stupor and coma.

In over 80% of cases there may also be signs of a peripheral neuropathy. In chronic cases, a slower amnestic syndrome develops, with selective impairment of short-term memory, which is made up for by confabulation (Korsakoff's psychosis). The pathology of Wernicke–Korsakoff syndrome involves symmetrical damage to the mamillary bodies, thalamus, periaqueductal grey matter and cerebellum.

Treatment for Wernicke's encephalopathy is intravenous thiamine followed by instigation of a normal diet and continued oral thiamine. Korsakoff's psychosis is also treated with oral thiamine and a normal diet, but patients are often left with a severe cognitive deficit.

Vitamin B₆ (pyridoxine) deficiency

Vitamin B_6 deficiency causes a mainly sensory neuropathy and may be precipitated during isoniazid therapy for tuberculosis. Pyridoxine supplements should, therefore, be given when isoniazid is prescribed.

Vitamin B₁₂ deficiency

Deficiency of vitamin B_{12} (cobalamin) can, rarely, result from nutritional deficiency (e.g. vegans), but is more often caused by malabsorption. The usual causes are pernicious anaemia, gastrectomy and diseases of the terminal ileum (e.g. Crohn's disease, coeliac disease, Whipple's disease, blind-loop syndrome). Up to 25% of patients with neurological damage caused by vitamin B_{12} deficiency do not have haematological abnormalities (i.e. macrocytic megaloblastic anaemia).

Vitamin B_{12} deficiency should be considered in any patient with a peripheral sensory neuropathy, myelopathy, optic neuropathy or dementia. The earliest symptom a patient may complain of is pins and needles in the feet, before signs of a myelopathy and impaired vibration and joint-position sense due to dorsal column loss develop. The combination of a myelopathy and a peripheral sensory neuropathy is called subacute combined degeneration of the cord.

Treatment with intramuscular vitamin B_{12} must be started promptly. If treatment is initiated early, there can be complete recovery; if delayed, the progression may be halted, but there is little reversal. The condition can theoretically be made worse by giving folic acid without vitamin B_{12}.

Vitamin B₃ (nicotinic acid) deficiency

Nicotinic acid deficiency causes pellagra and is found in areas where the staple diet is maize. It is also found in chronic alcoholics who present with acute delirium. The classical clinical features comprise dermatitis, diarrhoea and dementia. More widespread neurological features include pyramidal and extrapyramidal signs, and a peripheral neuropathy.

Vitamin D deficiency

This is associated with a proximal myopathy with wasting and weakness. It is most commonly seen in the elderly with poor diet and lack of sun exposure. It is also seen in immigrant populations, malabsorption syndromes, those treated with anticonvulsants and in chronic renal failure.

Vitamin E deficiency

Vitamin E is a fat-soluble vitamin that can become deficient in malabsorption syndromes, especially in cystic fibrosis, coeliac disease and diseases in which there is a reduced bile salt pool. There is a rare familial fat malabsorption syndrome with abetalipoproteinaemia associated with vitamin E deficiency.

Vitamin E deficiency primarily causes an ataxic syndrome, with areflexia and loss of vibration sense and proprioception, but sparing of cutaneous sensation. It can mimic Friedreich's ataxia.

Treatment is with oral vitamin E.

TOXINS

There are numerous toxins capable of causing neurological symptoms, many of which are drugs prescribed for other medical conditions. The most common are listed in Figure 34.1.

> **HINTS AND TIPS**
>
> In thiamine deficiency, glucose is inadequately metabolized and lactate and pyruvate accumulate. It is therefore essential to give thiamine immediately to any patient with suspected thiamine deficiency, before giving any sugar-containing substance, especially 5% dextrose or dextrose saline.

Fig. 34.1 Toxins and their neurological effects

Neurological complication	Toxin
Dementia	Alcohol, mercury, lead, manganese, aluminium, solvent abuse, tin
Acute or subacute encephalopathy	Lead, mercury, manganese, thallium, solvent abuse, arsenic, tin
Drug-induced confusional state or psychosis	Antiparkinsonian drugs, steroids, isoniazid, mercury, tricyclics, alcohol withdrawal, lithium, amphetamines, cannabis, lysergic acid diethylamide (LSD), numerous other drugs
Lowered threshold of seizures	Alcohol, amphetamines, neuroleptics, tricyclics, other antidepressants, tin
Parkinsonism	Neuroleptics, flupentixol, antiemetics, reserpine, amiodarone
Chorea and/or dystonia	L-dopa, dopamine agonists, antiemetics, neuroleptics, phenytoin, trihexyphenidyl, manganese
Tremor	β_2-agonists, lithium, sodium valproate, amiodarone, amphetamines, alcohol, levothyroxine, mercury, manganese
Cerebellar syndrome	Alcohol, phenytoin, solvent abuse, mercury, carbamazepine
Ototoxicity	Aminoglycoside antibiotics, quinine, ethacrynic acid, furosemide, overdose of aspirin
Optic neuropathy	Ethambutol, chloroquine, methyl alcohol, chloramphenicol, possibly pipe tobacco
Lens opacities	Steroids, chloroquine, amiodarone
Myelopathy	Nitrous oxide abuse, lathyrism (plant toxins), tin

Fig. 34.1 Toxins and their neurological effects – cont'd

Neurological complication	Toxin
Peripheral neuropathy	Gold, lead (motor), arsenic, thallium, mercury, alcohol, acrylamide, organophosphates, industrial solvents, medications including isoniazid, nitrofurantoin, vincristine, metronidazole, disulfiram, clioquinol, dapsone, sulphonamides, emetine, phenytoin, pyridoxine, griseofulvin, cisplatin, amiodarone, tricyclics
Neuromuscular blockade	Botulinum toxin, organophosphate compounds, 'nerve gases', penicillamine, aminoglycosides (and other antibiotics) may exacerbate myasthenia
Myopathy	Alcohol, steroids, chloroquine, statins, clofibrate, amiodarone, zidovudine (AZT)

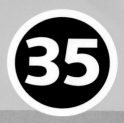
- Describe the main clinical features of neurofibromatosis type 1 and 2, tuberous sclerosis and Sturge–Weber syndrome
- Describe the main clinical features of the inherited ataxias
- Have an understanding of the inborn errors of metabolism, porphyria and Wilson's disease

The genetic basis of neurological disease has been revolutionized by two methods of identifying disease genes. The first method employs families where disease is inherited in a 'Mendelian' manner (such as autosomal dominant, autosomal recessive or X-linked). The second method, genome-wide association studies, uses hundreds and thousands of patients with the same disease to map the disease-causing mutation in human genes. As our understanding of the molecular pathophysiological role played by these variants increases, it is only a matter of time before this translates into diagnostic utility and pharmacological treatments in the clinical setting.

Inherited neurological diseases are rare, but cumulatively they make up a significant neurological burden. Many of these diseases have been described in the preceding, relevant chapters and those discussed here are a collation of the remaining diseases.

THE NEUROCUTANEOUS SYNDROMES

A number of inherited conditions involve disorders of organs derived from the ectoderm, causing tumours (benign and malignant), hamartomas (disorganized collections of blood vessels) and lesions in the skin and nervous system. Only the most common are outlined below.

Neurofibromatosis

There are a number of different types of neurofibromatosis, but types 1 (peripheral predominance) and 2 (central predominance) are the most important.

Neurofibromatosis type 1 (von Recklinghausen's disease)

Neurofibromatosis type 1 is an autosomal dominant condition caused by mutations in the neurofibromin gene (NF1) on chromosome 17. This gene encodes a protein called neurofibromin. The mutation has an incidence of 1 in 4000.

Clinically, it is characterized (Fig. 35.1) by:

- neurofibromas: lying along peripheral nerves
- café-au-lait spots: multiple pale-brown macules, especially on the trunk. They are found in the normal population, but > 5 lesions > 1.5 cm in an adult is abnormal
- cutaneous fibromas (molluscum fibrosum): subcutaneous, soft, often pedunculated, and usually multiple
- axillary freckling
- Lisch nodules: small hamartomas of the iris.

Other associated features include:

- neural tumours: there is a higher incidence of neural tumours than in the general population, e.g. meningioma, vestibular schwannomas on the eighth nerve, gliomas and spinal root neurofibroma
- skeletal abnormalities: 50% of patients have a scoliosis. There may be bone hypertrophy underlying subperiosteal neurofibromas. Local gigantism of a limb
- endocrine abnormalities: associated phaeochromocytoma, medullary carcinoma of the thyroid

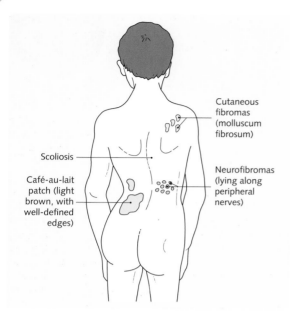

Fig. 35.1 Cutaneous manifestations of neurofibromatosis type 1.

- learning difficulty and epilepsy: in 10–15% of patients
- renal artery stenosis
- obstructive cardiomyopathy
- pulmonary fibrosis.

Neurofibromatosis type 2

Neurofibromatosis type 2 is an autosomal dominant condition caused by mutations in the NF2 gene on chromosome 22. This gene encodes a protein called merlin. The mutation has an incidence of 1 in 50 000. Clinically, it is characterized by few skin and skeletal manifestations and the presence of bilateral eighth nerve vestibular schwannomas (previously referred to as 'acoustic neuromas'). Other intracranial and intraspinal tumours may be present and include brain and spine meningiomas, ependymomas and astrocytomas.

Treatment

Intracranial tumours require excision and, if necessary, radiotherapy. Cosmetic surgery may be required for the cutaneous manifestations. Genetic counselling is important.

Tuberous sclerosis

Tuberous sclerosis is an autosomal dominant condition with an incidence of 1 in 10 000. It is characterized by skin lesions, especially adenoma sebaceum on the face (Fig. 35.2), epilepsy and varying degrees of learning disability.

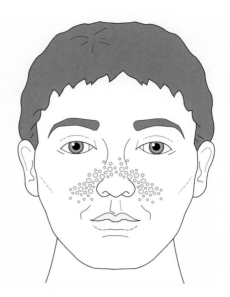

Fig. 35.2 Adenoma sebaceum: classic raised reddish nodules found over the nose and cheeks in tuberous sclerosis.

In addition to the nodular lesions on the cheeks or facial angiofibromas (previously called adenoma sebaceum), skin manifestations include depigmented patches (ash-leaf macule), 'shagreen' patches and subungual fibromas around the finger and toe nails. Slowly expanding cerebral tumours, such as hamartomatous 'tubers' and astrocytomas, can also occur and may cause seizures. Tuberous sclerosis also increases the susceptibility to systemic tumours that may affect the kidney, lung or muscle.

Treatment

The epilepsy is often quite resistant to treatment. Surgery may be required for large cerebral tumours, especially if hydrocephalus develops. Careful regular evaluation and follow-up of these patients must be made to provide a possibility of early treatment for the neoplastic complications.

Sturge–Weber syndrome

Sturge–Weber syndrome has no clear inheritance pattern. It is characterized by an extensive port-wine naevus or 'stain' on one side of the face (Fig. 35.3), usually within the first and second divisions of the trigeminal nerve, and an underlying leptomeningeal angioma. There may be atrophy of the affected hemisphere, epilepsy and congenital glaucoma.

If epilepsy is sufficiently intractable, lobectomy or even hemispherectomy may be required. The early removal of the surface lesion remains controversial.

Patients often die from the cardiac complications (heart failure and arrhythmias) rather than the neurological complications.

Ataxia telangiectasia

Ataxia telangiectasia is an autosomal recessive disorder causing progressive cerebellar ataxia, ocular and cutaneous telangiectasia and IgA immunodeficiency. Death is often by the third decade from infection or lymphoreticular malignancy.

Spinocerebellar ataxias

The predominant symptom of the spinocerebellar ataxias (also referred to as the SCAs) is one of progressive cerebellar ataxia inherited often in an autosomal dominant manner. The spinocerebellar ataxias may present as a pure ataxia (such as SCA6) or be associated with a wide range of signs, including a degenerative retinopathy (SCA7), spasticity, parkinsonism (SCA3) and a peripheral neuropathy.

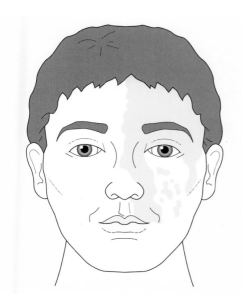

Fig. 35.3   Port-wine naevus in Sturge–Weber syndrome.

HEREDITARY ATAXIAS

There are a large number of inherited conditions accompanied by varying clinical features of cerebellar degeneration, alone or in combination with spinal degeneration, and these are referred to as the hereditary ataxias. Three of the more common conditions are outlined below, but they are all rare.

Friedreich's ataxia

Friedreich's ataxia is an autosomal recessive condition caused by an expanded trinucleotide repeat (GAA) in the intronic sequences of the frataxin gene on chromosome 9. The severity of the disease phenotype depends on the number of trinucleotide repeats. Frataxin is especially found in the spinal cord, heart and pancreas and not in the cerebellum or cerebrum.

Within the spinal cord there is progressive degeneration of the posterior columns, corticospinal tracts and dorsal and ventral spinocerebellar tracts.

Clinical features include:

- ataxia: starting in the legs, spreading to the arms
- dysarthria
- sensory neuropathy: absent ankle jerks, absent joint-position and vibration sense
- pyramidal signs: upgoing plantar responses (in spite of absent ankle jerks)
- optic atrophy
- skeletal abnormalities: pes cavus and scoliosis
- cardiomyopathy and associated arrhythmias
- diabetes.

INHERITED NEUROPATHIES

See Ch. 15.

INBORN ERRORS OF METABOLISM

Numerous rare metabolic conditions can cause abnormalities of both the central and peripheral nervous system. Two of these will be discussed briefly and some others are listed in Figures 35.4 and 35.5.

Acute intermittent porphyria

The porphyrias comprise a heterogeneous group of disorders of haem synthesis, causing an overproduction of porphyrins.

Acute intermittent porphyria, an autosomal dominant disorder occurring in adult life, is often associated with neurological complications. It can be precipitated by medications, sepsis or alcohol.

Clinical features and their frequency are as follows:

- Abdominal pain: 90%; these patients are often admitted with unexplained abdominal pain
- Peripheral neuropathy: 70%; usually an acute motor neuropathy that can present like Guillain–Barré syndrome
- Hypertension and a sinus tachycardia: 70%

Fig. 35.4 Some examples of rare metabolic encephalopathies

Disorders of phenylalanine
Phenylketonuria
Disorders of sulphur amino acid metabolism
Homocystinuria
Disorders of branched-chain amino acids
Maple syrup urine disease
Organic acidaemias
Carnitine deficiency
Methylmalonic acid deficiency
Carnitine palmityl transferase deficiency
Acyl CoA dehydrogenase deficiency
Lactic acidosis
Pyruvate dehydrogenase deficiency
Leigh's disease
Disorders of sugar metabolism
Galactosaemia
Disorders of purine metabolism
Lesch–Nyhan syndrome
Xanthine oxidase deficiency
Disorders of pyrimidine metabolism
Xeroderma pigmentosum
Porphyrias
Lipoprotein deficiencies
Abetalipoproteinaemia
Tangier disease
Disorders of copper metabolism
Wilson's disease
Menke's kinky-hair syndrome
Mitochondrial encephalopathies
MELAS/MERRF/CPEO
Peroxisomal disorders
Infantile Refsum's disease
Adrenoleukodystrophy

CPEO, chronic progressive external ophthalmoplegia; MERRF, myoclonic epilepsy and ragged red fibres; MELAS, mitochondrial encephalopathy, lactic acidosis and stroke-like episodes

Fig. 35.5 Metabolic storage diseases

Glycogen storage diseases
Pompe's disease
Cholesterol storage diseases
Cerebrotendinous xanthomatosis
Neuronal ceroid-lipofuscinosis
Late onset (Kufs' disease)
Mucopolysaccharidoses
Hurler's (type I)
Hunter's (type II)
Sphingolipidoses
Gangliosidoses
 GM1 gangliosidosis
 GM2 gangliosidosis
Niemann–Pick disease
Gaucher's disease
Krabbe's disease
Fabry's disease
Metachromatic leucodystrophy

medication that precipitates this condition should be avoided.

Wilson's disease (hepatolenticular degeneration)

Wilson's disease is a rare autosomal recessive disorder of copper metabolism. There is a deficiency of caeruloplasmin protein, which binds copper, resulting in copper deposition in various organs, especially in the liver and the basal ganglia in the brain. It is caused by mutations in the ATP7B gene, and clinical features comprise:

- movement disorders: a wide range of movements can occur, including tremor, early dysarthria, and dysphagia, dystonia, parkinsonism and chorea.
- cirrhosis of the liver
- Kayser–Fleischer ring: a fine brown deposition of copper in Descemet's membrane of the cornea, which may ultimately form a ring. This may be visible to the naked eye, but slit-lamp examination is usually necessary
- neuropsychiatric features such as depression, mania and psychosis.

Diagnosis is by measurement of a low serum caeruloplasmin and total serum copper, with elevated unbound or 'free' copper. There is high urinary copper excretion and liver biopsy may show massive copper deposition.

Treatment involves a lifelong low-copper diet and a chelating agent such as penicillamine. Liver transplantation is sometimes performed.

- Psychiatric disturbance such as mania and depression: 50%
- Seizures: 15%.

To secure the diagnosis, the urine is screened for porphobilinogen levels. However, testing the blood for reduced erythrocyte porphobilinogen deaminase and raised aminolaevulinic acid synthetase is most sensitive.

Management is largely supportive, with a high carbohydrate intake and a haematin infusion. Any

SELF-ASSESSMENT

Single best answer questions (SBAs)   257

Extended-matching questions (EMQs)   267

SBA answers   273

EMQ answers   283

Objective structured clinical examination (OSCE) stations   285

Single best answer questions (SBAs)

1. The following cranial nerves also carry parasympathetic fibres:
   a. Oculomotor.
   b. Trigeminal.
   c. Trochlear
   d. Hypoglossal.
   e. Optic

2. A 79-year-old woman, on warfarin for a previous deep vein thrombosis, falls and hits her head. She develops a mild headache and a fluctuating level of consciousness. What is the most likely diagnosis?
   a. Subarachnoid hemorrhage.
   b. Acute subdural hematoma.
   c. Stroke.
   d. Sagittal sinus thrombosis.
   e. Extradural hematoma.

3. The following clinical sign would support a diagnosis of myasthenia gravis:
   a. Brisk tendon reflexes.
   b. Muscle wasting.
   c. A 'glove and stocking' distribution of pin prick loss.
   d. Reduction in power after repeated shoulder abduction and adduction.
   e. A right-sided hemiparesis.

4. A 25-year-old woman presents a 9-month history of diffculty walking. The neurological examination identified a spastic paraparesis. Five years ago there was a 4 month history of visual loss in the right eye that was associated with some pain when her eye moved from side to side, suggestive of optic neuritis. The most likely diagnosis is:
   a. Motor neurone disease.
   b. Myasthenia gravis.
   c. Multiple sclerosis.
   d. Peripheral neuropathy.
   e. Subdural hematoma.

5. Which disease can cause both upper and lower motor neuron signs in the same patient:
   a. Guillain–Barré syndrome.
   b. Multiple sclerosis.
   c. Diabetic peripheral neuropathy.
   d. Motor neuron disease.
   e. Stroke.

6. Unilateral lower motor neuron facial weakness is a feature of:
   a. Bell's palsy
   b. Motor neuron disease.
   c. Stroke.
   d. Trigeminal neuralgia.
   e. Syringomyelia.

7. Bilateral lower motor neuron facial weakness may occur in:
   a. Stroke.
   b. Guillain–Barré syndrome.
   c. Trigeminal neuralgia.
   d. Parkinson's disease.
   e. Parasagittal meningioma.

8. A 29-year-old woman presents to her General Practitioner with frequent headaches that have caused her some concern because they interfere with her ability to work at the checkout tills in the supermarket. Which of the following would support a diagnosis of migraine:
   a. The headache is worst on waking in the morning.
   b. The onset of the headache is sudden and severe.
   c. The headache is bilateral and described as 'a tight band'.
   d. The headache is associated with recurrent loss of consciousness.
   e. A right sided throbbing headache which develops gradually.

9. A 79-year-old man presents to his GP after his wife noticed that he had slowed down and that his posture had changed in that he was bent over. The following would support a diagnosis of idiopathic Parkinson's disease:
   a. Rest tremor, bradykinesia and spasticity.
   b. Vertical supranuclear gaze palsy.
   c. Shuffling gait.
   d. Postural tremor.
   e. Urinary incontinence.

10. Which of the following medications can can be complicated by parkinsonism:
    a. Chlorpromazine.
    b. Benzhexol (Trihexyphenidyl).
    c. Bromocriptine.
    d. Sinemet^{TM}
    e. Propranolol

11. The following characteristics favour that increased tone is due to rigidity rather than spasticity and may support a diagnosis of Parkinson's disease:
    a. Tone is increased equally in flexor and extensor muscles.
    b. The plantar responses are extensor.
    c. There is a postural tremor.
    d. There is reduction of power in the limbs.
    e. There is deafness.

12. A 55-year-old lady is brought to the GP's surgery by her husband who reports that she has become increasingly forgetful and that her personality had changed. She is no longer as lively as she used to be and has lost her emotional response to important matters. This has been slowly getting worse over the past 12 months. During the consultation she is unable to sit still and is very fidgety. The diagnosis is most likely to be:
    a. Subacute sclerosing panencephalitis.
    b. Huntington's chorea.
    c. Alzheimer's disease.
    d. Normal pressure hydrocephalus.
    e. Schizophrenia.

13. A 62-year-old woman presented for the first time to the A&E department. Earlier that morning, whilst brushing her teeth she had looked in the mirror and noticed that her right eye appeared very different from the left. The right pupil was much smaller and her right eyelid had partially drooped down. The examination confirmed these were the only abnormal signs. The most likely diagnosis is:
    a. Myasthenia gravis.
    b. Holmes–Adie syndrome.
    c. A third nerve palsy.
    d. Optic neuritis.
    e. Horner's syndrome.

14. A 54-year-old man presents to the A&E department complaining of a headache which is prominent on waking in the morning and wakes him from sleep at night. He reports that he has not had headache before and feels unwell. Fundoscopy shows swollen optic discs bilaterally with loss of retinal venous pulsation. The visual examination is likely to demonstrate the following:
    a. A loss of colour vision.
    b. An enlarged blind spot.
    c. A central scotoma.
    d. A small pupil.
    e. A relative afferent pupillary defect.

15. A 20-year-lady presents to the A&E department complaining that she is unable to see anything with her left eye and that her eyeball is also painful especially when looking over to the left or right. The neurological examination identified reduced visual acuity down to 6/60 on the left, mild dysarthria and finger-nose ataxia (cerebellar signs) and a spastic paraparesis. The remainder of the cranial nerve examination is likely to demonstrate the following:
    a. An enlarged blind spot.
    b. A small pupil.
    c. A central scotoma with loss of colour vision.
    d. Papilloedema.
    e. Tunnel vision.

16. Bilateral ptosis may be a feature of:
    a. Horner's syndrome.
    b. A oculomotor nerve (third nerve) palsy due to a left posterior communicating artery aneurysm.

c. Abducent nerve (sixth nerve) palsy.
    d. Myotonic dystrophy.
    e. Graves disease.

17. The following may cause a third nerve palsy:
    a. Idiopathic intracranial hypertension.
    b. Myasthenia gravis.
    c. Multiple sclerosis.
    d. Herniation of the uncus of the temporal lobe.
    e. Pancoast tumour.

18. A 32-year-old man presented to his GP complaining of increasing weakness of his right arm and leg which had gradually developed over 7 months. He also noticed that the left hand side of his body felt odd and different from the right. The neurological examination revealed a right sided hemiparesis, with loss of vibration and joint position sense in the right arm and leg, and loss of pin prick in the left arm and leg, compatible with a Brown–Séquard syndrome. Which investigation would secure the diagnosis?
    a. Nerve conduction studies.
    b. A lumbar puncture.
    c. An MRI of the cervical spinal cord.
    d. Syphilis serology.
    e. MRI of the brain.

19. A 72-year-old man presented to the A&E department after he slipped and fell down a flight of stairs. Within an hour of the fall, he had developed severe back pain just below the scapulae. He had difficulty walking and was unable to climb the staircase because of the weakness in both legs. He had also noticed difficulty with passing urine. The following clinical sign or signs may be found in a thoracic myelopathy:
    a. Fasciculations.
    b. Normal tone.
    c. Weakness of shoulder abduction and elbow extension.
    d. Absent reflexes with flexor plantars.
    e. Sensory level on the trunk.

20. A 48 year old woman visits her GP with concerns that she has motor neuron disease because she had noticed twitching in the right thigh. Four months earlier, her sister had seen a neurologist and been diagnosed with motor neuron disease after developing weakness of the arms and legs and difficulty with swallowing. In motor neuron disease:
    a. Fasciculations are required to make the diagnosis.
    b. Abnormalities of ocular movements are a common finding.
    c. Fatigueable weakness is a feature.
    d. There should be no signs of sensory loss.
    e. Sphincter dysfunction is common.

21. Concerning the brachial plexus:
    a. In brachial neuritis, severe pain around the shoulder precedes rapid wasting.
    b. Klumpke's paralysis causes proximal arm weakness.

c. Erb's palsy is caused by a lesion to C8-T1-derived regions of the brachial plexus.
d. A brachial plexus lesion and an ipsilateral Horner's syndrome may indicate an underlying pancreatic tumour.
e. A vegan diet may precipitate brachial neuritis.

22. Causes of a mononeuropathy of the median or ulnar nerve include:
a. Hereditary motor sensory neuropathy.
b. Vincristine chemotherapy.
c. Polyarteritis nodosa.
d. Guillain–Barré syndrome.
e. Multiple sclerosis.

23. A 63-year-old woman had made an appointment to see the practice nurse in her GP's surgery. She complained of an unpleasant sensation in the toes of both feet that first started 6 months earlier and had slowly spread more proximally. She was under regular review by the practice nurse for the monitoring of Diabetes which had been diagnosed with over 10 years ago. The characteristic sign of a sensory polyneuropathy is:
a. Increased tone.
b. a glove and stocking sensory loss.
c. Proximal wasting.
d. Fasciculations.
e. Extensor plantars.

24. A lesion to the common peroneal nerve at the fibular head causes:
a. Weakness of plantar flexion.
b. If long term, wasting of the quadriceps femoris
c. Weakness of abductor pollicis brevis
d. Weakness of dorsiflexion of the foot.
e. Brisk ankle jerk.

25. Hyposmia may arise secondary to:
a. Migraine.
b. Seizures.
c. Excessive alcohol consumption.
d. A frontal meningioma.
e. Multiple sclerosis.

26. A 58-year-old gentleman was brought in by an ambulance crew to the A&E department following an out-of-hospital cardiac arrest. He had received cardio-pulmonary resuscitation at the scene by the ambulance crew and from the A&E was transferred to the intensive care unit where he had a further cardiac arrest and required both cardiac and respiratory support. The ITU Consultant confirmed brainstem death. To diagnose brainstem death the following are required:
a. Extensor response of the limbs to painful stimuli.
b. A ventilated and sedated patient.
c. Absent tendon reflexes.
d. A flat electroencephalogram (EEG).
e. Absent 'doll's eye' reflexes.

27. A 67-year-old man presented to his GP complaining of a fogging of vision in the left eye which he described as a "curtain coming down". It lasted a minute before returning back to normal. There were no other symptoms. The following is the most likely cause of his visual impairment:
a. Retinitis pigmentosa.
b. Carotid embolism.
c. Papilloedema.
d. Migrainous aura.
e. Glaucoma.

28. A 70-year-old man was brought to the A&E department by his daughter who was concerned about his mobility. Over the past 2 weeks he had been repeatedly bumping into furniture and knocking over objects on his left hand side. The examination was remarkable for bruises over the left arm and leg and a left sided homonymous hemianopia. A homonymous hemianopia may arise from a lesion of:
a. The optic chiasm.
b. The optic radiation.
c. The parietal lobe.
d. The optic nerve.
e. The temporal lobe.

29. A 68-year-old man was brought to see his GP by his wife with concerns about his change in personality in that he appeared withdrawn and was not himself. He had become irritable and aggressive towards her and his children. During a family gathering he began to undress himself in the living room. The following may be an additional feature of frontal lobe dysfunction:
a. A grasp reflex.
b. Constructional and dressing apraxia.
c. Olfactory hallucinations.
d. A receptive dysphasia.
e. Cortical blindness.

30. Dysphasia may result from a lesion of:
a. The cerebellum.
b. Broca's area.
c. The hypoglossal nerve.
d. The basal ganglia.
e. The accessory nerve.

31. The following may give rise to a pseudobulbar palsy:
a. Poliomyelitis.
b. Motor neuron disease.
c. Huntington's chorea.
d. Occlusion of the anterior cerebral artery.
e. Myasthenia gravis.

32. A 30-year-old lady described a 6 month history of poor balance and clumsy hands. Which of the following is an additional clinical feature of cerebellar dysfunction?
a. Resting tremor.
b. Spastic paraparesis.
c. Dysarthria.
d. Dysphasia.
e. Internuclear ophthalmoplegia.

33. Facial sensory loss may occur with a lesion of:
    a. The cerebellopontine angle.
    b. The facial nerve.
    c. The parotid gland.
    d. The geniculate ganglion.
    e. The occipital lobe.

34. A 16-year-old girl is brought to the A&E department after losing consciousness for minutes. She was accompanied by her father who witnessed the event. The following clinical feature may help differentiate between a seizure and a syncopal attack:
    a. The patient was lying in bed at the onset.
    b. There were brief jerks of the limbs.
    c. The tongue was bitten.
    d. There was urinary incontinence.
    e. The was prolonged malaise after the attack.

35. Conductive deafness may occur secondary to:
    a. Exposure to loud noises.
    b. Gentamicin therapy.
    c. Ménière's disease.
    d. An acoustic neuroma.
    e. Otosclerosis.

36. A 37-year-old lady made an appointment to see her GP for an annual check up. During the consultation the GP noticed an number of hyperkinetic involuntary movements of the limbs and torso. Choreic movements can be:
    a. Slow and writhing with sustained postures.
    b. Shock-like, asymetrical and irregular.
    c. Brief, twitchy and jerky.
    d. A sign of restlessness.
    e. Rhythmical and oscillatory.

37. A 21-year-old pianist noticed a fine tremor in both hands that was a little more prominent whilst playing. His GP informed him that it was a physiological tremor that is:
    a. Treated with sodium valproate.
    b. Improved by medication containing L-dopa.
    c. Usually treated by deep brain stimulation.
    d. Improved by beta-blockers.
    e. Treated with neuroleptics.

38. The upper motor neuron descends from the cortex, through the internal capsule, the cerebral peduncle of the midbrain, and through the pons to form the pyramids of the medulla. The motor decussation fibres cross over in the lower medulla, just above the foramen magnum, to descend in the contralateral corticospinal tract (the pyramidal tract), and synapse with anterior horn cells in the spinal cord. Signs of an upper motor neuron lesion are:
    a. Brisk abdominal and cremasteric reflexes.
    b. Wasted muscles.
    c. Hypertonia (spasticity).
    d. Weakness of individual muscles.
    e. Fatigable muscle strength.

39. A 58-year-old woman was transferred from the A&E department to the Stroke ward with a diagnosis of Wallenburg (or lateral medullary) syndrome. There was a 6-year history of diabetes and an ECG in the A&E department had identified a new diagnosis of atrial fibrillation. A lesion of the lateral medulla on one side may give rise to:
    a. Ipsilateral facial weakness.
    b. Horner's syndrome.
    c. Contralateral weakness of the palate.
    d. Contralateral weakness of the tongue.
    e. Ipsilateral third nerve palsy.

40. A 43-year-old lady was applying her make up one morning when she noticed the the right eye appeared different and that the pupil appeared much larger than that in the left eye. A large pupil may be seen in:
    a. A lesion in the midbrain.
    b. Elderly patients.
    c. Horner's syndrome.
    d. Terminally ill patients taking morphine for analgesia.
    e. A pontine lesion.

41. The following sign may be seen in a patient with a lesion involving the right sixth cranial nerve:
    a. A fixed dilated pupil.
    b. Ptosis.
    c. Diplopia in all positions of gaze.
    d. Reduced abduction of the right eye.
    e. An associated contralateral hemiplegia.

42. An internuclear ophthalmoplegia may be seen in:
    a. A patient who is blind.
    b. A lesion at the foramen magnum.
    c. A lesion of the medial longitudinal fasciculus.
    d. A patient with cerebellar dysfunction.
    e. A lesion in the midbrain.

43. A 23-year-old lady presented to her GP with weakness of both her arms and legs. She had diffuclty climbing a flight of stairs and hanging clothes on her washing line. Her mother had noticed that her eyelids had drooped down and at her father's birthday party the week before she was unable to blow up the party balloons due to weakness around her mouth. In a patient with a myopathy:
    a. Vibration may be impaired.
    b. The gait is characterized by 'scissoring' posture of the legs.
    c. Gower's sign may be present.
    d. Brisk reflexes are present.
    e. Clonus may be elicited on examination of the legs.

44. A 35-year-old man had been diagnosed with a vestibular schannoma (previously referred to as an acoustic neuroma) by a Neurologist after he went to his GP complaining of a pressure in his ear and poor balance. An MRI brain with gadolinium contrast identified an enhancing lesion of the 8th cranial nerve

on the right. The clinical features of a lesion of the right cerebellopontine angle may include:
a. Conductive deafness on the right side.
b. Right sided cerebellar features.
c. Right sided weakness of the lower face.
d. A pseudobulbar dysarthria.
e. Vertigo as a prominent early symptom.

45. A patient with herpes zoster infection of the geniculate ganglion may present with:
a. An upper motor neuron facial weakness.
b. Diplopia.
c. Hyperacusis.
d. Altered perception of smell.
e. Retro-orbital pain.

46. The fibres of the dorsal column pathway:
a. Carry information about temperature perception.
b. Decussate in the midbrain.
c. Are affected in the deficiency of vitamin B_1.
d. When damaged may result in a positive Gower's sign.
e. Are spared following occlusion of the anterior spinal artery.

47. A dissociated pattern of sensory loss may be seen in:
a. Brown–Séquard syndrome.
b. Anterior spinal artery occlusion.
c. A radiculopathy.
d. Occlusion of a middle cerebral artery.
e. Compression of the spinal cord by a prolapsed intervertebral disc.

48. A 53 -year-old lady with a 13 year history of insulin-treated diabetes complained that her feet felt like blocks of ice and walking on ground felt like she was walking on a pebble beach. Her GP diagnosed a diabetic polyneuropathy which:
a. Always produces symptoms.
b. Usually causes weakness rather than sensory loss.
c. Is unaffected by good blood glucose control.
d. Is less common in type II diabetes.
e. May be associated with painless foot ulcers.

49. A 42-year-old lady presented with numbness of her hands and feet that was unpleasant and interferred with her ability to sleep at night on account of the pain that she experienced in her feet. The neurological examination demonstrated a sensory peripheral neuropathy. Causes of a painful neuropathy include:
a. Diphtheria.
b. Alcohol overuse.
c. A paraproteinaemic neuropathy.
d. Charcot–Marie–Tooth disease.
e. Acute intermittent porphyria.

50. The cause of a demyelinating neuropathy is:
a. Guillain–Barré syndrome.
b. Diabetes.
c. Vincristine.
d. Cryoglobulinaemia.
e. Amyloidosis.

51. A 27-year-old lady who was 33 weeks pregnant would awake at night with an unpleasant and numb sensation of the right hand which would improve by shaking it repeatedly. Following an examination by her GP, she was diagnosed with carpal tunnel syndrome which:
a. Is associated with symptoms only in the hand.
b. Only becomes symptomatic at night.
c. Pinprick testing may be abnormal over the medial aspect of the middle finger.
d. Often causes severe wasting and weakness of the whole hand.
e. Weakness affects the first doral interossei greater than abductor pollicis brevis.

52. A 24-year-old man is reviewed by a Neurologist in the outpatient clinic and informed of a diagnosis of multiple sclerosis. He recovered from left-sided optic neuritis a year earlier and more recently had developed a progressive ataxia. An MRI of the brain and spinal cord identified a number of areas of demyelination. When discussing the prognosis the patient was informed that multiple sclerosis is more likely to have a benign course if the patient:
a. Presents with a spastic paraparesis.
b. Presents with sensory symptoms.
c. Is over 50 years old at the onset of symptoms.
d. Presents with brainstem or cerebellar features.
e. Is male.

53. The multiple sclerosis nurse specialist is counselling a 38-year-old lady who has just been given a new diagnosis of MS and discusses the different treatment options. The MS nurse informed the patient that the following medication will significantly reduce relapse rates in relapsing–remitting multiple sclerosis:
a. Beta-interferon.
b. Mycophenylate.
c. Steroids.
d. Methotrexate.
e. Cyclosporine.

54. A 17 year-old-boy is admitted to the psychiatric ward of his local hospital with acute psychosis and suicidal ideation. There was an 8 year history of intractable depression. The examination is remarkable for symmetrical parkinsonism. The following supports a diagnosis of Wilson's disease:
a. The total serum copper is raised.
b. Urinary 24-hour copper is raised.
c. Urinary 24-hour copper is low.
d. Penicillamine binds to copper and decreases the release of copper in the urine.
e. Magnesium supplementation increases copper excretion in stool and reduces copper absorption in the gut.

55. A 42-year-old woman was admitted to hospital with weakness of the arms and legs. Her muscles felt painful especially with movement and she had

over the past fortnight developed considersable fatigue. A rheumatologist diagnosed polymyositis where:
a. The creatinine kinase is usually raised.
b. Swallowing is normal.
c. Patients are hyporeflexic.
d. Distal limb muscles are affected more than than proximal muscles.
e. A heliotrope rash of the face and around the eyelids and extensor joint surfaces is common.

56. A 43-year-old lady was under review by her neurologist having presented with intermittent double vision in different directions, difficulty swallowing and weakness in her arms and legs. She had been diagnosed with myasthenia gravis which is associated with:
a. Diplopia or ptosis in over 90% of patients at some time in their illness.
b. Exercise such as repetitive shoulder abduction improves weakness.
c. Muscle cramps and myoglobinuria.
d. Type I respiratory failure.
e. Absent tendon reflexes.

57. A unilateral extensor plantar response is usually seen in:
a. Amyotrophic lateral sclerosis.
b. A cervical myelopathy secondary to cervical spondylosis.
c. Multiple sclerosis.
d. A right middle cerebral artery ischaemic stroke.
e. Subacute combined degeneration of the spinal cord.

58. A 47-year-old man was brought by his wife to casualty. He had been hallucinating that morning seeing three dogs run aross his living floor and four small children in the kitchen. Formed visual hallucinations may occur in:
a. Ocular blindness.
b. Temporal lobe pathology.
c. Occipital lobe epilepsy.
d. Migraine aura.
e. Bipolar disorder.

59. Fasciculations of muscle may be seen in:
a. Motor neuron disease.
b. Muscular dystrophy.
c. Sleep.
d. Parkinson's disease.
e. A hot bath or shower.

60. A 63 year old Indian lady was brought to the A&E department by her daughter complaining of a new and persistent headache for 2 weeks that would awake her from her sleep. She felt persistently nauseated and drowsy through the day. The casualty officer requested a CT head which showed hydrocephalus. In this case the most likely explanation for hydrocephalus is:
a. Cerebral venous sinus thrombosis.
b. Tuberculous meningitis.

c. Herpes simplex meningitis.
d. Idiopathic intracranial hypertension.
e. A sub-dural haemorrhage.

61. A primary school teacher noticed that one of his 9 year old pupils had become less attentive in class and mentioned this to the child's mother who had also noticed this and had witnessed her daughter have brief blanks spells lasting a few seconds up to three times a day. Absence seizures (formerly known as petit mal) is associated with:
a. Mental retardation.
b. Prolonged post ictal confusion.
c. Distinctive 3-per-second spike and wave dischargeon EEG.
d. Post-traumatic epilepsy.
e. Structural brain lesion on MRI.

62. Intracranial aneurysms are:
a. Multiple in 15% of cases.
b. Associated with pain and a sixth nerve palsy when involving the posterior communicating artery.
c. Associated with intracerebral haemorrhage when on the posterior cerebal artery.
d. More likely to rupture if in the anterior circulation.
e. Rarely associated with hydrocephalus if they rupture.

63. In the treatment of epilepsy, sodium valproate:
a. Is the drug of choice in pregnant women.
b. Can cause weight loss.
c. No blood tests are required to screen for liver and white blood cell abnormalities.
d. Can cause hirsuitism.
e. Is usually the drug of choice in primary generalized epilepsy.

64. A 53-year-old lady complains of difficulty walking due to poor balance that first started 6 months earlier. Her speech has become slurred and she had become clumsy, dropping and breaking cups and plates. Cerebellar disease:
a. Can be associated with Coeliac's disease.
b. Is due to Vitamin B_1 deficiency
c. Is often associated with Alzheimer's disease.
d. Is associated with an irreversible ataxia in association with phenytoin toxicity.
e. Is a recognized paraneoplastic complication of non-small cell lung cancer.

65. A 43-year-old builder complains of the suddent onset of lower back pain after lifting a sack of cement. It is a sharp shooting sensation that radiates to his right leg. Compression of the right L4 nerve root:
a. Causes pain over the anterior thigh and medial leg.
b. Causes loss of the right ankle jerk.
c. Can be confused with a common peroneal nerve lesion.
d. Is usually caused by a lateral disc protrusion at L5/S1.
e. Is associated with wasting of the hamstrings.

66. A 64-year-old lady visits her GP complaining of neck pain from the base of the back of her head radiating down to each shoulder. Rotation of her head to each side exacerbated symptoms and at night she would find it diffcult to sleep because of neck stiffness. In cervical spondylosis:
    a. There may be upper motor neuron signs in the upper limbs.
    b. Pain is far worse during the day.
    c. Headaches are a rare co-existant symptoms.
    d. Most patients have neurological signs.
    e. Neck traction may be helpful if the patient has upper motor neuron signs to relieve pressure off the spinal cord.

67. A 67-year-old lady presented to her GP with two week history of a new daily headache which she described as a dull ache. She generally felt unwell, had developed night sweats and had lost her apetite. She had also lost weight and her clothes were much looser than normal. Temporal arteritis:
    a. Is more common in men.
    b. Is often associated with optic neuritis.
    c. Can be associated with neck pain.
    d. Is ruled out with a normal erythrocyte sedimentation rate.
    e. Steroid treatment should be initiated as soon as the diagnosis is strongly suspected.

68. A 43-year-old woman is seen in the A&E department after developing double vision especially on looking to the right. She had also developed headache which was a persistent dull ache that woke her from her sleep. On examination there was bilateral papilloedema and on assessing ocular movements, the left eye failed to adduct. The sixth nerve:
    a. Carries the parasympathetic fibres to the pupil.
    b. May be affected as a 'false localizing' sign.
    c. Arises from the medulla.
    d. Travels through the superior stylomastoid foramen.
    e. Supplies the superior oblique muscle.

69. A 72-year-old right handed man was admitted to the stroke unit. A CT brain scan perfomed in the A&E department identified an infarct in the right middle cerebral artery territory. The following signs typically occur with non-dominant cortical lesions:
    a. Dysphasia.
    b. Dressing apraxia.
    c. Dyscalculia.
    d. Finger agnosia.
    e. Impaired discrimination between left and right.

70. The ulnar nerve:
    a. Is the main continuation of the posterior cord of the brachial plexus.
    b. Supplies the brachioradialis muscle.
    c. Runs in the spiral groove on the humerus where it is easily compressed.

d. If damaged usually causes numbess over the ring and little finger of the hand.
    e. Is the main motor nerve to the extensor compartments of the arm and forearm.

71. The fundoscopic examination of a 59-year-old lady who complained of headache identified blurring of the optic margins, elevation of the optic disc, loss of retinal venous pulsation and hemorrhages adjacent to the optic disc in both eyes. Bilateral papilloedema:
    a. May produce 'tunnel-vision'.
    b. Is often seen in temporal arteritis.
    c. Is also referred to as papillitis associated with optic neuritis.
    d. May be caused by a low CSF protein.
    e. Is not a cause of transient loss of vision.

72. Multiple sclerosis typically presents with:
    a. Monocular visual loss associated with pain on eye movement.
    b. Papilloedema.
    c. A homonymous hemianopia.
    d. Weakness of abductor digit mini and the first dosal interosseous muscle.
    e. Seizures.

73. 56-year-old lady is reviewed by her GP as she has expressed concerns about her headaches. She has had headaches for at least 20 years but her sister had recently been diagnosed with a brain tumor and was undergoing cranial radiotherapy under the local oncologists. Her mother died from status epilepticus which was thought to be due to a brain tumour. The headache of raised intracranial pressure is typically associated with:
    a. Worsening with coughing, sneezing or bending over.
    b. Fortification spectra.
    c. Stabbing or shooting pains.
    d. Being better on waking first thing in the morning and worse on standing.
    e. Photophobia and phonophobia.

74. The following statement is correct:
    a. The ulnar nerve supplies most of the muscles in the flexor compartment of the forearm.
    b. The ulnar nerve supplies most of the intrinsic muscles of the hand.
    c. The median nerve supplies most of the muscles in the hypothenar eminence.
    d. The radial nerve supplies the dorsal interossei.
    e. Most of the intrinsic hand muscles are supplied by nerves from the C5 and 6 spinal roots.

75. A 21-year-old lady was brought to casualty by ambulance after she had a generalised convulsion. Her mother accompanied her and also reported that her daughter often had blank spells and had developed unexplained bouts of fear and anxiety

from time-to-time associated with *deja vu*.
Temporal lobe epilepsy is associated with:
a. Repetitive conjugate eye movements.
b. Lip-smacking and chewing automatisms.
c. Jerking of the upper limbs.
d. Adopting a 'fencing posture' at the start of an episode.
e. Seeing flashes or balls of light.

76. A 27-year-old woman was brought to the A&E department by ambulance after she collapsed to the floor and lost consciousness. The event had been witnessed by a friend who told the ambulance driver that just before collapsing she suddenly developed a severe headache with neck pain. In a subarachnoid haemorrhage:
a. A lumbar puncture is contraindicated because of the risk of coning.
b. Severe hypertension should be treated immediately with antihypertensive agents.
c. A Berry aneurysm is more often found in the posterior rather anterior circulation.
d. CT head scan detect 50% of haemorrhages.
e. There is a 20% chance of rebleed within the first two weeks.

77. Alzheimer's disease:
a. Commonly presents with disorientation in time and place.
b. The patient usually has insight into memory loss.
c. Typically presents with disinhibition and apathy.
d. Geographical apraxia and language deficits are often early features.
e. Patients may accuse their spouse of being an imposter (Capgras syndrome).

78. A 32-year-old man presents to the emergency room with facial pain triggered by touching his face and mouth and because of this has been unable to shave or eat properly for 4 days. The casualy officer identifies a normal neurological examination. Trigeminal neuralgia:
a. Is a associated with ipsilateral facial weakness.
b. Is usually bilateral.
c. Is a severe, stabbing, paroxysmal pain.
d. Is usually familial.
e. Is associated treated with steroids.

79. A 57-year-old man is referred to a local neurologist. He has developed profound dizzy spells as soon as he stands up, prominent bouts of sweating after a heavy meal and increasing constipation. Causes of autonomic dysfunction include:
a. Hypothyroidsm.
b. Early idiopathic Parkinson's disease.
c. Multiple Sclerosis.
d. Guillain–Barré syndrome.
e. Myasthenia gravis.

80. Post-lumbar puncture headache:
a. Is related to the length of the needle used.
b. Often resolves spontaneously within one month.

c. Can be accompanied by neck stiffness and nausea.
d. Improves dramatically on standing.
e. Is related to draining greater than 10 mL of CSF.

81. A 39-year-old man complains of a throbbing unilateral about once a month and a headache after eating chocolate or drinking red wine. His mother and sister are known to have classical migraine. A diagnosis of migraine headache is also supported by:
a. Continuous daily headache.
b. Episodes of loss of consciousness.
c. Improved by standing.
d. Associated nausea, vertigo and photophobia.
e. Tight, band-like pain around the whole of the head.

82. The following are associated with anterior circulation (carotid territory) transient ischaemic attacks (TIAs):
a. Diplopia.
b. Weakness in all four limbs.
c. Loss of vision in one eye (amaurosis fugax).
d. Dysphagia.
e. Vertigo.

83. In myasthenia gravis the weakness:
a. Is associated with antibodies to the terminal axon.
b. May worsen transiently during treatment with steroids.
c. Often improves after removal of a thymoma.
d. Improves with exercise.
e. Is usually in the distal upper limbs.

84. The CSF glucose is usually 60 – 80% that of the plasma glucose. A low CSF glucose may be seen in:
a. Alzheimer's disease.
b. Ischaemic stroke.
c. Multiple sclerosis.
d. Guillain–Barré syndrome.
e. Tuberculous meningitis.

85. When considering stroke:
a. Hemiparesis is caused by a lacunar infarct in the anterior limb of the internal capsule.
b. Infarcts in the frontal lobes lobes are often silent.
c. A right incongruous hemianopia is caused by a left occipital infarct.
d. Seizures are uncommon in the acute phase if a stroke is haemorrhagic.
e. Gerstmann's syndrome is associated with constructional and geographical apraxia.

86. In myotonic dystrophy:
a. Myotonia may be transiently worse after a hot shower.
b. Is complicated by hypothyroidism.
c. Is complicated by cardiac conduction defects.
d. Only men demonstrate early frontal balding.
e. Anaesthetic complications are rare.

87. In Duchenne muscular dystrophy:
a. Is fatal in most patients before the age of 30.
b. Is associated with a normal CK.

c. Gower's sign is usually negative.

d. Is autosomal dominant.

e. Is associated with ocular, facial and bulbar weakness.

88. A 58-year-old man is brought to the A&E department by ambulance having been found unconscious on the pavement outside the chemist. He was carrying his medication and prescription which included Amlodipine, Metformin and Simvastatin. A CT brain identified a large intracerebral bleed. Primary intracerebral haemorrhage:

a. Can be differentiated clinically from ischaemic stroke.

b. Usually causes meningism.

c. Is often less clinically dangerous if in the posterior fossa.

d. Is usually within the internal capsule and basal ganglia in hypertensive patients.

e. Is best treated with emergency surgical evacuation.

89. A 29-year-old man is brought to casualty by his girlfriend who was concerned about his behaviour and change in personality over the preceeding week. He had become paranoid and was convinced that their home was under threat of burglary. He also described a dull headache that had been present for at least three days that woke him from his sleep. Within an hour of arriving in the department he had a generalised tonic clinic seizure. Herpes meningoencephalitis:

a. Is never associated with a low CSF glucose.

b. The CSF is often normal.

c. Imaging may show secondary haemorrhage in the temporal lobes.

d. The EEG shows slowing over one or both frontal lobes.

e. The ESR and CRP are usually normal.

90. A 68-year-old lady was accompanied by her husband to a neurology outpatient appointment. The husband described how his wife had changed considerably over the past 4 months with significant memory loss, unsteadiness on walking, a change in personality and some difficulty with her ability to speak. Prion diseases:

a. Are caused by slow viruses.

b. The infectious particles are easily destroyed by conventional sterilization techniques.

c. Can be genetically inherited.

d. Have a quicker clinical progression in the new variant than the sporadic form.

e. The MRI is usually normal.

Extended-matching questions (EMQs)

In each of the following questions, select the condition listed that is most likely to fit the given description.

1. Options:

a. Tension-type headache

b. Migraine with aura

c. Migraine without aura

d. Stroke

e. Subarachnoid haemorrhage

f. Bacterial meningitis

g. Tuberculous meningitis

h. Viral meningitis

i. Low-pressure headache

j. Raised intracranial pressure headache

For each of the following patients with headache, select the most likely answer from the list of options.

1. A 22-year-old man presents to casualty with a severe headache that came on 12 hours ago and is increasingly severe. He has vomited twice. On examination, he is confused, photophobic, and has a stiff neck. Kernig's sign is positive but the rest of the neurological examination is normal. His lumbar puncture shows an opening pressure of 23 cmH$_2$0, 160 polymorphs, 10 red cells, a protein of 1.2 g/L and a CSF glucose of 2 mmol/L (serum 5.4 mmol/L).

2. A 68-year-old smoker presents to clinic with a 3-week history of a progressive headache, which is increasing in severity. It is worse in the morning and after his afternoon nap. Over the past few days, he has been feeling increasingly nauseated and his right hand is becoming slow and clumsy. His wife feels that he is 'not himself' and that 'he cannot get his words out'. On examination, he has pyramidal weakness in the right arm and an expressive dysphasia. His optic disc margins are slightly indistinct.

3. A 24-year-old woman has recently started the contraceptive pill, and has noticed that three or four times per month she gets a numbness in her face which resolves in 20 minutes and is followed by numbness in her arm, which also resolves in 20 minutes. She then develops a bilateral retro-orbital and throbbing headache that makes her feel sick, although she does not usually vomit. She has to come home from work and rest in her bedroom with her curtains drawn but it is usually better by the next day. Her mother says that she had a few similar attacks in her teens but 'never as severe as her daughter's'.

4. A 40-year-old man comes to casualty with a 3-hour history of severe headache, which is now improving slightly. He normally gets headaches when he is stressed but he has never had anything as bad as this headache. On examination, he has slight neck stiffness, a right-sided ptosis, double vision on looking to the left and up as well as a slightly bigger pupil on the right compared to the left, but he is otherwise well now. His CT head is normal and his lumbar puncture shows an opening pressure of 25 cmH$_2$O, with 500 red cells and 3 lymphocytes. The protein is 0.8 g/L and the glucose is normal. He is kept in for observation overnight and during the night he alerts the nurses because his severe headache has returned. He subsequently becomes drowsy and has a tonic clonic seizure.

5. A 72-year-old man with diabetes presents to casualty with a 12-hour history of dull right-sided headache associated with acute onset of left-sided weakness. On examination, he is moderately drowsy but has a GCS of 15. He also has a left hemiparesis and a left homonomous hemianopia. His headache seems to be dull and nagging but he has no neck stiffness or photophobia. He is pyrexial to 37.4 °C. His wife tells you that 2 weeks ago the left side of his body went numb but it went away within a few hours.

2. Options:

a. Vasovagal syncope

b. Cardiogenic syncope

c. Complex partial seizure

d. Tonic-clonic seizure

e. Non-epileptic seizure

f. Narcolepsy

g. Hypoglycaemia

h. Absence seizure

i. Postural hypotension

j. Subarachnoid haemorrhage

For each of the following patients with impairment of consciousness, select the most likely answer from the list of options.

1. A 13-year-old girl is noticed by her teacher at school to be 'not concentrating on her work'. The teacher describes episodes where she stares into space for approximately a minute and returns to normal rapidly. The girl is otherwise very well and has a normal neurological examination. She had one febrile convulsion as a child.

2. An 18-year-old man complains of episodes where he suddenly collapses to the ground and starts to shake both upper limbs. He feels slightly 'distant' while the

shaking occurs but remembers people around him being concerned. The attacks last 30 seconds to 5 minutes and have occurred up to 10 times in a day. When the shaking stops, he complains of feeling slightly tired but can resume his activities. He is due to sit his A-levels in 4 months. There is a family history of epilepsy in his younger sister after she had meningitis as a baby.

3. A 24-year-old woman presents with episodes of loss of consciousness for a few minutes and recently one of the attacks was followed by some mild stiffening in all her limbs and urinary incontinence. The episodes tend to happen at the end of the day when she is standing on the train coming home. She is aware that she feels slightly nauseated before the attacks and feels as if a curtain is coming over her vision before she loses consciousness. Normally, she recovers fully in a few minutes after being given a seat by another passenger.

4. A 25-year-old woman has lapses of consciousness that occur anytime of the day. There are no associated movements or incontinence. She has also found that she has been feeling extremely tired throughout the day, despite having a good night's sleep. The attacks last from seconds to minutes and she does not get any warning they are going to occur. She also describes vivid 'dream-like' images on going to sleep and feels she cannot move her body on waking up for several minutes.

5. A 35-year-old man complains of episodes of confusion. His wife tells you that he will suddenly 'go blank and stare into space' for several minutes. He often wanders around the room and picks up and puts down objects repeatedly. His wife tells you he does not respond appropriately to her concerns during the attack, and he often feels extremely tired once they have finished. He sometimes gets a 'strange, horrible taste' in his mouth prior to the attacks.

3. Options:

a. Alzheimer's disease
b. Frontotemporal dementia
c. Normal pressure hydrocephalus
d. Acute confusional state
e. Non-convulsive status epilepticus
f. Multi-infarct dementia
g. Subcortical ischaemic leucoencephalopathy
h. New variant Creuztfeldt–Jakob disease (CJD)
i. Vitamin B_{12} deficiency
j. Pseudodementia

For each of the following patients with impairment of memory, select the most likely answer from the list of options.

1. A 60-year-old man lives in a nursing home after suffering a severe subarachnoid haemorrhage 5 years ago. Recently, his carers have noticed that his walking is becoming much slower and he is becoming slightly confused and forgetful. They have also noticed that, despite regular toileting, he has become incontinent of urine. On examination, he has old left-sided pyramidal signs, but coordination in his right side and sensory examination are normal. When he tries to stand up he slips backwards into his chair. His mini-mental test score is 21 out of 30, whereas 2 years ago it was noted to be 28. He informs you that he is simply unaware of needing to pass urine.

2. A young woman aged 20 dropped out of university recently because of a depressive illness. She has noticed that in retrospect she has also had strange sensations in her arms and legs over the past 2 months. In spite of treatment for her depression, her parents have noticed that she is becoming forgetful, disorientated, and clumsy.

3. A 75-year-old hypertensive patient had a small stroke 1 year ago, from which he made a good recovery although he was left with mild weakness on the left side and mild confusion. Since then, he has had two further acute episodes of slurred speech and then dysphasia, which have partially resolved but have left him functionally disabled. He is now very forgetful and shuffles when he walks. His wife suggests to you in confidence that he is 'not the man I used to know'. On examination, he has a pseudobulbar palsy, brisk but symmetrical reflexes, and extensor plantar responses with mild left-sided pyramidal weakness.

4. A 70-year-old woman comes to clinic with her daughter. The patient admits to having problems with her memory, which is frustrating for her, but she is mostly unaware of her difficulties. Her daughter then suggests that actually her mother has been becoming increasingly 'muddled and forgetful'. Two weeks previously, her mother was found wandering lost in her local shops. Two months before that the patient decided to stop attending her social meetings because she found it difficult to keep up with the conversation. She had also forgotten recent family events. Neurological examination was normal apart from a mini-mental test score of 22 out of 30.

5. A 82-year-old man presents to clinic with a 5-month history of 'apathy, loss of interest, and forgetfulness'. He has withdrawn from all his social engagements following the death of his wife 6 months previously. He recently had a small house fire because he left a chip pan on, but he was able to call the fire brigade. He has lost a significant amount of weight recently because he claims he is never hungry. He is often seen wandering around his local shops alone but his daughter claims his cupboards are empty and his house is in a bad condition. Neurological examination is normal and his mini-mental test score is 28 out of 30, but he was very slow in giving his answers.

4. Options:

a. Idiopathic Parkinson's disease
b. Multisystem atrophy
c. Huntington's disease
d. Wilson's disease
e. Benign essential tremor

f.   Spasmodic torticollis

g.   Physiological tremor

h.   Levodopa-induced dyskinesias

i.   Hemiballismus

j.   Pseudoathetosis

For each of the following patients with abnormal movements, select the most likely answer from the list of options.

1.   A 30-year-old woman presents to clinic with difficulty drinking a cup of tea because of a tremor. It is absent at rest but she also notices it as she is writing. She has noticed that it rarely affects her when she goes out at the weekend for a few drinks. On examination, she has a postural tremor of the upper limbs.

2.   A 21-year-old man presents with a 1-year history of slurring of his speech and difficulty swallowing. More recently, he has noticed that his legs and arms can go into 'spasms' and have become tremulous.

3.   A patient with Parkinson's disease has been managed successfully by his GP for the past 6 years but recently he has been experiencing writhing movements of his tongue, face, neck, trunk, and limbs that is worst 2 hours after he takes his dose of levodopa but resolves by the time he goes 'off'. It is now difficult for him to do anything during these episodes.

4.   A 70-year-old hypertensive woman has a sudden onset of wild flailing movements of her right arm and leg. She is otherwise well.

5.   A 42-year-old man, who has recently lost contact with his family because of 'differences', has noticed that he has become very fidgety. He functionally copes with constant fidgety movements but finds it frustrating and he has noticed that he loses his temper more frequently. He did not know his father very well because he had an unknown neurological illness that led to his father's early death.

5. Options:

a.   Multiple sclerosis

b.   Parkinson's disease

c.   Spinal cord compression

d.   Peripheral neuropathy

e.   Normal pressure hydrocephalus

f.   Subcortical ischaemic leucoencephalopathy

g.   Progressive supranuclear palsy

h.   Polymyositis

i.   Acute confusional state

j.   Motor neuron disease

For each of the following patients with imbalance, select the most likely answer from the list of options.

1.   A 74-year-old man presents with a 1-year history of feeling as if he is 'walking on stones'. He now has numbness and weakness, which involve both legs and recently he has had some numbness in the tips of his fingers. He recently fell over when he tried to get up during the night. On examination, he has weakness and sensory loss to the knees and he has lost all his tendon reflexes in his lower limbs. Plantars are flexor. His random glucose is 7 and his serum electrophoresis demonstrates an IgM paraprotein.

2.   A 65-year-old woman has noticed that over the last 3 months she has had increasing difficulty climbing stairs and standing from her chair. Over the past 2 weeks, her swallowing has also deteriorated. On examination, she has weakness around the shoulder and hip girdle and her swallow is slow. Her reflexes are slightly brisk but symmetrical. She has no sensory loss. Her creatine kinase is 3000.

3.   A 24-year-old woman presents acutely with slurred speech, double vision, vertigo, and imbalance on walking. On examination, her right optic disc is pale and she has a right relative afferent pupillary defect. She also has horizontal gaze-evoked nystagmus, which is worse on looking to the left, with a left internuclear ophthalmoplegia. On examination of her limbs, she has left-sided dysmetria, brisk but symmetrical reflexes and extensor plantar responses. Her gait is slightly broad and unstable. Five years previously she had an episode of blurred vision in her right eye and pain behind the eye for a few days but it has since returned to normal.

4.   A 75-year-old hypertensive woman presents to casualty with a 1-week history of difficulty walking. She has not passed urine or opened her bowels for the past 48 hours and she puts this down to the fact that she has not been eating much lately. On examination, she has reduced tone in her legs with only slight movement with gravity at the hip. Her reflexes are brisk in the legs and her abdominal reflexes are absent. She has lost pin-prick and vibration sensation to her upper chest. Her anal tone is reduced and her bladder is palpable. Her cranial nerves and arms are normal. She also informs you that she had a mastectomy over 10 years ago for breast cancer, but a recent check-up was 'all clear'.

5.   A 52-year-old man is referred to you from the ENT doctors because of imbalance, which was initially thought to be due to inner ear disease. He gives a 1-year history of falling over. His wife suggests that he is also becoming slower in everything he does and that he often cries or laughs at things he never used to feel emotional about. On examination, he has reduced down gaze, a brisk gag reflex, a starring face, prominent grasp reflexes, and symmetrical mild bradykinesia. As soon as you try and stand him up, he falls back into his chair.

6. Options:

a.   Multiple sclerosis

b.   Posterior interosseous nerve palsy

c.   Motor neuron disease

d.   Carpal tunnel syndrome

e. Brachial neuritis (neuralgic amyotrophy)

f. Ulnar nerve palsy at the elbow

g. Radial nerve palsy in the spiral groove.

h. Lower brachial plexus lesion

i. Ulnar nerve palsy at the wrist

j. Cervical myelo-radiculopathy

For each of the following patients with symptoms in their arms, select the most likely answer from the list of options.

1. A 74-year-old male smoker has developed severe pain and weakness in his right hand; he also describes some numbness over his right arm. On examination, he has wasting and power loss in his hand involving both thenar and hypothenar eminences as well as sensory loss over the C8 and T1 dermatomes. Closer inspection suggests that his right eyelid is drooping and he has a small right pupil. He has also lost a stone in weight over the past month.

2. A 25-year-old woman has noticed that, over the last 3 months, she has had increasing pain in her left arm and occasionally in her right. The pain wakes her up at night-time and she shakes her hands to relieve her symptoms. She has not noticed any weakness in her hands although she has recently been commenced on thyroxine replacement for hypothyroidism. Neurological examination is normal apart from a positive Phalen's test on the left.

3. A 46-year-old man had an acute onset of severe right shoulder pain which prevented him from working 6 weeks ago. Since then, he has noticed that his right shoulder has become weak. On examination, he has severe wasting and weakness of his deltoid, supraspinatus, rhomboids, and biceps. His reflexes in the right arm are all diminished. He has some slight numbness over his shoulder but it is relatively minor.

4. A 59-year-old secretary has noticed that her typing was not as good as it used to be 5 months ago and took early retirement. Recently, she has noticed that she has difficulty with getting dressed because her hands feel weak. Her swallowing has also become a problem, especially when drinking tea. She suffers from cramps at night-time in her legs and sometimes her arms. On examination, her tongue is small and possibly has some fasciculations in it. She has a brisk gag reflex and jaw jerk. She has fasciculations in her hands, biceps, quadriceps, and calves associated with wasting in her hands and forearms. Her reflexes are all brisk and her plantars are extensor.

5. A 62-year-old woman has recently been developing severe pain, especially at night, in her neck. She has also noticed that she gets shooting pains down her right arm, especially when she flexes her neck. On examination, she has weakness of her right elbow flexion and some numbness over the lateral surface of the arm. Her right biceps jerk is absent. You incidentally notice that her walking is slow and that her triceps, knee, and ankle jerks are brisk and her plantars are extensor.

7. Options:

a. Lacunar infarction of the internal capsule

b. Total right middle cerebral infarction

c. Total left middle cerebral infarction

d. Basilar artery thrombosis

e. Lateral medullary syndrome

f. Cerebellar haemorrhage

g. Partial left middle cerebral artery infarction

h. Transient ischaemic attack

i. Posterior cerebral artery infarction

j. Internal carotid artery occlusion

For each of the following patients with stroke, select the most likely answer from the list of options.

1. A 74-year-old hypertensive man developed an acute onset of severe weakness in his right side involving his lower face, arm and leg. On examination, he has a right hemiplegia with no sensory loss.

2. A 25-year-old woman was involved in a car accident and suffered a severe 'whiplash injury and shock' but was otherwise well. The following day she presents to casualty with weakness on her right side, confusion, and incomprehensible speech. On examination, she has a left-sided Horner's syndrome, a dense right hemiplegia, dysphasia, and probably a right homonomous hemianopia. Unfortunately she becomes very drowsy and obtunded over the next 24 hours and dies on ITU.

3. A 66-year-old man had an acute onset of right lower facial weakness and his wife tells you that he had severe difficulties 'in stringing his words together'. It has slowly improved over the past 4 days and, when you see him, he is only complaining of slight difficulties in expressing himself fully but he knows what he wants to say. On examination, he has a left carotid bruit and a mild expressive dysphasia.

4. A 59-year-old type 2 diabetic presents to casualty with acute onset of vertigo and imbalance. He also has problems swallowing and his right side of his face 'feels strange'. On examination, he has a right-sided Horner's syndrome, right-sided loss of pain and temperature sensation, his uvula moves to the left and he has pooling of his secretions in his pharynx. He has mild left-sided weakness and right-sided dysmetria. Over the next 2 weeks he almost makes a full recovery.

5. A 62-year-old hypertensive woman presents to casualty with a 4-hour history of rapidly progressive drowsiness. Her husband informs you that, prior to her becoming drowsy, she complained of a severe pain in the back of her head and she vomited twice. She tried to walk but was too unsteady. On examination, she has a Glasgow Coma Scale of 6 out of 15 and has a grossly dilated left pupil. There are no other obvious cranial nerve signs. She is too confused and drowsy to properly examine her but she appears to be moving all her limbs. Her reflexes are brisk but symmetrical and her plantars are extensor.

8. Options:

a.   An isolated third nerve palsy
b.   An isolated fourth nerve palsy
c.   An isolated sixth nerve palsy
d.   Myasthenia gravis
e.   Ocular myopathy
f.   Third and fourth nerve palsy
g.   A lesion in the cavernous sinus
h.   Pontine lesion
i.   A frontal lesion
j.   An occipital lesion

For each of the following patients with difficulties in moving their eyes, select the most likely answer from the list of options.

1.   A 64-year-old diabetic man developed an acute onset of double vision. On examination, his right eye is looking down and out and he has a ptosis of the right eyelid. The outer image is lost when he covers his right eye. The pupils are normal. The rest of the examination is normal.
2.   A 26-year-old woman has slowly developed worsening double vision over the past 4 weeks associated with a headache and nausea. On examination, she has gross papilloedema and failure of abduction of the right eye.
3.   A 30-year-old woman presents with worsening intermittent double vision over the past 2 weeks. She has noticed that it usually comes on when she is tired at the end of the day. On examination, she has limitation of movements in most directions except on looking down with the right eye and abducting the left eye. Her pupils are normal but she has bilateral ptosis, which gets worse on sustained upgaze. She is otherwise well and is a well-controlled type 1 diabetic for 16 years.
4.   A 59-year-old man presents with a 1-month history of progressive double vision and a 2-week history of deteriorating vision in the right eye and numbness over his right upper face. On examination, he has visual acuities of 6/6 on the left and 6/36 on the right. He has a partial right ptosis, slight movement of upgaze in his right eye but otherwise complete restriction of movement and loss of sensation in the ophthalmic and maxillary branches of the fifth nerve.
5.   A 62-year-old diabetic, hypertensive woman presents to casualty with sudden onset of left-sided weakness. On examination, she has a dense left hemiplegia and both her eyes deviate laterally to the right. She is drowsy and moderately confused.

9. Options:

a.   Optic neuritis
b.   Giant cell arteritis
c.   Parietal lobe lesion
d.   Occipital lobe lesion
e.   Pituitary macroadenoma
f.   Temporal lobe lesion
g.   Orbital tumour
h.   Craniopharyngioma
i.   Leber's optic neuropathy
j.   Idiopathic intracranial hypertension

For each of the following patients with loss of vision, select the most likely answer from the list of options.

1.   A 64-year-old man presents acutely with left-sided weakness and sensory loss. On examination, he has a left hemiplegia and hemisensory loss but also a left inferior homonymous quadrantinopia.
2.   A 24-year-old man develops worsening vision in his right eye over several days associated with pain on moving the eye. On examination of the affected eye, his visual acuity is 6/18 and he has lost perception of colour in the centre of his vision. His pupil is sluggish to react to a direct but not a consensual light stimulus and his fundi are normal. Over the next 4 weeks, his vision returns to normal.
3.   A 30-year-old woman presents with tiredness and lethargy and is found to have diabetes. You notice that her facial features are coarse and enlarged. The size of her hands and feet has increased over the past 5 years and colleagues at work have commented that she has a deep voice. She has also recently been developing tingling of her hands at night. On neurological examination, she has a bitemporal upper quadrantinopia and carpal tunnel syndrome.
4.   A 79-year-old woman has been feeling lethargic for 6 months and recently has developed severe right-sided headaches, which last most of the day and night. She finds it difficult to touch the right side of her face because of pain. Last night, she noticed that the vision in her right eye suddenly deteriorated and she has been left with a 'black area' at the bottom of her vision in the right eye. On examination, she has an altitudinal defect affecting the inferior portion of her right visual field.
5.   A 25-year-old man presents with episodes of brief loss of vision in both eyes. He is markedly overweight. On examination, he has peripheral restriction in his visual fields and swollen optic discs with a few peripapillary haemorrhages.

10. Options:

a.   Idiopathic Parkinson's disease
b.   Huntington's chorea
c.   Peripheral neuropathy
d.   Cerebellar syndrome
e.   Spastic paraparesis
f.   Spastic hemiparesis
g.   Subcortical ischaemic leucoencephalopathy
h.   Functional disorder

i.   Common peroneal nerve lesion

j.   Myopathy

For each of the following patients with abnormal gaits, select the most likely answer from the list of options.

1. A 35-year-old man has had progressive weakness in his shoulder and pelvic girdle for 10 years. When he walks he has a 'waddling' gait.
2. A 25-year-old man has had difficulties walking all his life. When he walks, his legs 'scissor' across one another. On examination, he has very stiff legs and clonus at the ankles. His reflexes are brisk and his plantars are extensor.
3. A 30-year-old alcoholic presents with difficulty walking. On examination, he has a broad-based gait and is severely imbalanced.

4. A 79-year-old hypertensive woman has recently had difficulty walking. Her gait is slow and shuffling and she takes very little steps. Even when she starts walking, she cannot speed up and easily comes to rest. On examination, she has a pseudobulbar palsy, brisk tendon reflexes and extensor plantars.
5. A 27-year-old man presents with episodes of sudden inability to walk. The attacks occur up to 10 times per day and are associated with twitching of his shoulder. He has fallen many times but not hurt himself. When you ask him to walk, he collapses to the floor, even though his bedside examination was normal. When he starts to walk, his gait is slow, intermittently clumsy and he has an asymmetrical posture with hunching of his right shoulder. He describes his feet as being 'stuck to the floor'.

1. A. Oculomotor. Cranial nerves III, VII and X and S3–5 spinal nerves carry parasympathetic fibres.
2. B. Acute subdural hematoma. The question outlines typical features of an acute subdural haematoma secondary to head trauma.
3. D. Reduction in power after repeated shoulder abduction and adduction. Fatigable weakness is a characteristic of myasthenia gravis. Brisk reflexes and a hemiparesis are signs of an upper motor neuron lesion. Muscle wasting is a sign of a lower motor neuron lesion. A glove and stocking loss of sensation is seen in a peripheral neuropathy.
4. C. Multiple sclerosis. This is a typical history of a relapsing-remitting illness with lesions separated in time and place, suggestive of multiple sclerosis.
5. D. Motor neuron disease. Guillain–Barré is a polyneuropathy and therefore a purely lower motor neuron syndrome. MS is a disease of the central nervous system and therefore is only associated with upper motor neuron signs. MND is associated with degeneration of the anterior horn and upper motor neuron cell bodies and so causes lower and upper motor neuron signs in the same patient.
6. A. Bell's palsy. Motor neuron disease does not tend to cause unilateral lower motor neuron weakness, but can cause wasting in the facial muscles (lower motor neuron) as well as slow movements of the face and brisk facial reflexes (upper motor neuron). Stroke causes an upper motor neuron facial weakness with sparing of the upper part of the face (due to bilateral cerebral representation of the upper part of the face). Trigeminal neuralgia is a purely sensory condition involving severe, short-lived episodes of pain on one side of the face. It is 'syringobulbia' not 'syringomyelia' that is associated with cranial nerve palsies, although syringobulbia is very rare.
7. B. Guillain–Barré syndrome. Guillain-Barré syndrome can cause bilateral facial weakness. Stroke causes a unilateral upper motor neuron weakness. Trigeminal neuralgia is a purely sensory condition involving severe, short-lived episodes of pain on one side of the face. Parkinson's disease causes a 'masklike' face with paucity and slowness of movement, but there is no facial weakness. A parasagittal meningioma causes damage to the leg area of both primary motor cortices and therefore causes upper motor neuron weakness of the legs.

8. E. A right sided throbbing headache which develops gradually. A headache worse in the morning suggests raised intracranial pressure. With a sudden and severe headache, it is important to rule out a bleed such as a subarachnoid hemorrhage. A tight band is indicative of a tension-type headache. Recurrent loss of consciousness should always warrant further investigations for an alternative diagnosis.
9. C. Shuffling gait. Spasticity is a feature of hypertonia associated with upper motor neuron lesions and is not a feature of PD. Rigidity, either lead-pipe or cogwheel, is the form of hypertonia associated with PD. Supranuclear vertical gaze palsies in the context of parkinsonism tend to occur with progressive supranuclear palsy. The tremor is a pill-rolling rest tremor, not a postural tremor. Incontinence is not a feature of Parkinson's disease.
10. A. Chlorpromazine. Chlorpromazine is a neuroleptic used in the treatment of psychosis and is a dopamine antagonist, so can cause parkinsonism. Trihexyphenydyl (Benzhexol) is used to treat tremor. Bromocriptine is a dopamine agonist and was used to treat PD until other agonists were developed. Sinemet contains L-dopa and is used to treat Parkinson's. Propranolol is a beta blocker used to treat postural tremor, among other conditions.
11. A. Tone is increased equally in flexor and extensor muscles. Rigidity is increased tone caused by extrapyramidal disease such as PD. Tone is increased throughout all movement whereas in spasticity, tone tends to be higher in the flexors in the upper limbs and extensors in the lower limbs. Extensor plantar responses are an upper motor neuron and not extra-pyramidal sign. A pill rolling rest tremor is typical of PD which is an extra-pyramidal disease, not a postural tremor. Patients with Parkinson's disease are often slow but should not exhibit any limb weakness. Deafness is not a feature of Parkinson's disease.
12. B. Huntington's chorea. Huntington's disease often starts with subtle cognitive changes which often do not present to doctors. This is followed by chorea and dementia in middle age. Myoclonus is seen in many diseases including Subacute Sclerosing Pan-Encephalitis (SSPE) and sporadic Creutzfeld–Jacob disease (CJD). Sporadic CJD typically presents with a rapidly progressive dementia and myoclonus, not chorea. Chorea is not a feature of Alzheimer's disease, normal pressure hydrocephalus (triad of

cognitive deficit, gait apraxia and incontinence) or schizophrenia.

13. E. Horner's syndrome. Horner's syndrome consists of meiosis, ptosis and anhydrosis and is seen in lesions of the sympathetic supply to the eye. A Holmes–Adie pupil is usually larger than normal in standard light. A third nerve palsy causes a ptosis but with associated dilated pupil and ophthalmoplegia (eye pointing down and out). Optic neuritis can lead to a relative afferent pupillary defect with a sluggish reacting pupil, not small pupils.

14. B. An enlarged blind spot. Papilloedema is caused by raised intracranial pressure which can prevent the retinal veins near the disc from pulsating. It is associated with an enlarged blind spot due to swelling of the optic disc. The optic disc may be swollen due to causes other than raised CSF pressure, e.g. inflammation of the anterior part of the optic nerve or 'papillitis'. Loss of colour vision, a central scotoma and a relative afferent pupillar defect are found in optic neuritis. A small pupil is found due to a number of causes, e.g. Horner's syndrome, secondary to certain drugs such as opiates.

15. C. A central scotoma with loss of colour vision. Optic neuritis is often painful especially on eye movement. Vision usually recovers with some residual loss of red–green colour perception and sometimes a reduction in visual acuity. Enlarged blind spot suggests papilloedema which is found with raised intracranial pressure. Tunnel vision usually develops due to retinal or ophthalmic disease.

16. D. Myotonic dystrophy. Bilateral ptosis is common in myotonic dystrophy, secondary to the associated myopathy. Horner's syndrome is associated with anhydrosis, meiosis and ptosis due to damage of the sympathetic supply to levator palpebrae superioris and is usually unilateral. The abducent nerve has no role in innervating the eyelid. The oculomotor nerve carries fibres which innervate levator palpebrae superioris and control voluntary eye closure. A third nerve palsy does cause a ptosis but is usually unilateral. Graves disease usually causes eyelid retraction.

17. D. Herniation of the uncus of the temporal lobe. Herniation of the uncus through the tentorial hiatus commonly causes third nerve compression due to raised supratentorial pressure and is an emergency. Idiopathic intracranial hypertension often causes papilledema. Myasthenia gravis may cause fatiguable ptosis and ophthalmoplegia but the pupil is normal. Multiple sclerosis can cause an optic neuritis. A Pancoast tumour often infiltrates the lower part of the brachial plexus and causes weakness and wasting of the hand in association with a Horner's syndrome.

18. C. An MRI of the cervical spinal cord. Brown–Séquard syndrome is associated with damage to half the spinal cord. In this case it involves the arms, so would need an MRI of the cervical spine. (If it had only affected the legs the lesion could be in the cervical or thoracic spine so both would need to be scanned.) N.B. If there are upper motor neurone signs, e.g. spastic paraparesis, the lesion has to be above L1 (the end of the spinal cord) and will not be in the lumbo-sacral spine (which is made up of nerve roots and therefore causes lower motor neurone signs only). None of the other investigations would help to make this diagnosis.

19. E. Sensory level on the trunk. In a thoracic myelopathy there will be no wasting or fasciculalations. A spastic paraparesis (increased tone) will develop pyramidal distribution weakness in the legs (but not the arms, as the arms are innervated by the cervical spine) and brisk reflexes in the lower limbs with extensor plantars. A sensory level may extend onto the trunk.

20. D. There should be no signs of sensory loss. Motor neuron disease can present with purely upper motor neuron signs and lower motor neuron signs may be present even in the absence of fasciculation's, e.g. severe wasting. Eye movements are not affected. Fatigueable weakness is found in myasthenia gravis. Patients often complain of sensory symptoms and cramps but do not have objective sensory loss. Sphincter dysfunction is not a feature.

21. A. In brachial neuritis, severe pain around the shoulder precedes rapid wasting. Severe pain preceding wasting is typical of brachial neuritis. Klumpke's paralysis affects mainly the distal upper limb, especially the hand and is caused by lesions to the lower brachial plexus. Erb's paralysis affects the upper part of the plexus (C5, 6) and causes the classical 'waiter's tip' posture of the arm with sparing of the hand and forearm. The brachial plexus lies in close proximity to the apex of the lung and the first rib and therefore Pancoast tumours (not pancreatic) can spread to involve the lower roots, including T1 which contains sympathetic fibres to the pupil. Brachial neuritis may occur after a viral infection or vaccination but not due to B12 deficiency which may be found with a vegan diet.

22. C. Polyarteritis nodosa. Polyarteritis nodasa is a vasculitis and can cause infarction of individual nerves. Other causes of a mononeuropathy include other vasculitides, diabetes, entrapment and pressure palsies. Diabetes causes microvascular infarcts in individual nerves, e.g. abducent nerve. Vincritine chemotherapy, HMSN, and Guillain–Barré syndrome are polyneuropathies. Multiple

sclerosis is a disease of the central nervous system and does not affect the peripheral nerves.

23. B. a glove and stocking sensory loss. Sensory polyneuropathy is a disorder of the peripheral nervous system. There may be a glove and stocking sensory loss and the patient may have absent or reduced reflexes (due to reduced afferent input). In a pure sensory polyneuropathy there should be no motor signs.

24. D. Weakness of dorsiflexion of the foot. The common peroneal nerve innervates the anterior tibialis (not quadriceps femoris) and dorsiflexes the ankle and the peronei which evert the foot and supplies sensation to the lateral aspect of the leg and dorsum of the foot, excluding the lateral border of the foot. Plantar flexion is mediated by soleus and gatrocnemius which are innervated by the tibial nerve. Abductor pollicis brevis is in the hand and innervated by the median nerve. The ankle reflex involves the tendon of soleus and gatrocnemius and is therefore not involved in common peroneal lesions. Tibial nerve lesions would cause a reduced, not brisk, ankle reflex.

25. D. A frontal meningioma. Any expanding frontal lesion can affect the first nerve – a frontal meningioma is the most common lesion in this area. Migrainous aura may be associated with olfactory hallucinations but not hyposmia. Temporal lobe epilepsy may be associated with olfactory hallucinations but not hyposmia. Alcohol use does not affect olfactory function – although head injuries may be more common. Hyposmia often follows head injuries as the delicate nerve fibres in the first nerve are sheared as they pass through the cribriform plate.

26. E. Absent 'doll's eye' reflexes. Extensor plantar responses reflect upper motor neuron damage and are not involved in the brainstem reflexes. They are often extensor, however, because lesions that cause brainstem death often involve the upper motor neurons as they pass through the brainstem. In order to examine the patient to assess the brainstem reflexes, the patient must be unsedated and off all respiratory support. Absent tendon reflexes represent a lower motor neuron disorder and are not involved in the brainstem reflexes. A flat EEG has many causes including diffuse cerebral cortical damage and deep anaesthesia but this is not a criterion for brainstem death. A patient's brainstem reflexes can be fully intact but the patient may be unconscious and unresponsive because of diffuse cortical damage. Doll's eye movements involve proprioceptive information from the neck muscles, visual input (second cranial nerve) and vestibular input (eighth) as well as output to the extraocular muscles (third, fourth and sixth).

27. B. Carotid embolism. Amaurosis fugax is transient visual loss caused by a blockage, from whatever cause, of the ophthalmic artery or its branches to the retina. This includes carotid embolism. Retinitis pigmentosa causes progressive visual loss which usually starts in the peripheral visual field and spreads to involve central vision. Papilloedema due to raised intracranial pressure can also cause progressive visual loss starting at the periphery but can also cause transient visual loss called 'visual obscurations' which is a warning of rising intracranial pressure. Migrainous aura is associated with both positive and negative visual phenomena which usually travels across the vision for up to 1 hour prior to the onset of the headache. Closed angle glaucoma can be associated with transient visual loss preceding chronic visual failure.

28. A. The optic chiasm. Homonymous hemianopia arises from lesions in the optic pathway posterior to the optic chiasm including optic tract, optic radiation and occipital lobe. Lesions in the optic chiasm cause bitemporal hemianopia, and lesions in the temporal and parietal lobes cause an upper and lower homonymous quadrantinopia respectively. Lesions in the optic nerve cause visual defects ranging from complete monocular blindness to a central scotoma to impairment of red–green perception only, but not homonymous field defects.

29. A. A grasp reflex. The frontal lobes represent 50% of the cerebral cortex but patients with frontal lobe disease often have few obvious clinical signs because the bulk of the frontal lobes deal with aspects that are difficult to quantify such as personality. The grasp reflex is one of the 'primitive reflexes' and is probably one of the most accurate primitive reflexes in localizing pathology to the frontal lobes. Constructional and dressing apraxia is due to dysfunction of the non-dominant parietal lobe. Receptive dysphasia occurs with damage to the posterosuperior part of the dominant temporal lobe or Wernicke's area. An expressive dysphasia is caused by a lesion in Broca's area in the posterior part of the dominant frontal lobe. Cortical blindess is caused by damage to the occipital cortex.

30. B. Broca's area. Dysphasia is a disorder of the production or understanding of speech and not failure of articulation, or dysarthria which is seen with hypoglossal nerve, cerebellar or basal ganglia pathology.

31. B. Motor neuron disease. Pseudobulbar palsy refers to a syndrome where both sets of upper motor neurons to cranial nerve nuclei are damaged, i.e. bilateral upper motor neuron lesions. Poliomyelitis only damages the lower motor neurons. Motor neuron disease is the commonest cause of a pseudobulbar palsy due to bilateral involvement of

the upper motor neurons. Huntington's disease is mostly associated with disease of the basal ganglia. Occlusion of the anterior cerebral artery causes weakness in the contralateral leg. Myasthenia gravis causes a bulbar palsy (affects the neuromuscular junction).

32. C. Dysarthria. Dysarthria is common with cerebellar disease and has a scanning, staccato form. Cerebellar disease causes intention tremor when approaching a target (seen when doing the finger nose test) and not a resting tremor. Spasticity is found in lesions of the pyramidal tracts or upper motor neuron and not in lesions of the cerebellum.

33. A. The cerebellopontine angle. The cerebellopontine angle lies in close proximity to the fifth, seventh and eighth cranial nerves. The facial nerve does supply a very small region of somatic sensation to the outer ear but not the face. The branches of the facial nerve run through the parotid gland. The cells bodies of the sensory nerves lie in the geniculate ganglion for the seventh nerve (Gasserian ganglion for the fifth nerve). The occipital lobe is not involved in the sensory pathway.

34. A. The patient was lying in bed at the onset. Syncope is often associated with patients standing whereas seizures can occur in any position. Jerks or convulsive movements can be seen during a syncopal episode but they are usually brief and not rhythmical. A bitten tongue (especially the side) or the inside cheek usually indicates a seizure but the tongue can be bitten (especially the tip) as a result of the fall which occurs in a true syncopal attack. Urinary incontinence is often not helpful diagnostically as it occurs in both seizures and less often in syncope (especially if the bladder is full). Malaise is often more prolonged after a seizure but can also occur after a syncopal attack.

35. E. Otosclerosis. Otosclerosis is associated with reduced compliance in the bony ossicles and is therefore a form of conductive deafness. All the others are forms of sensorineural deafness. Excess prolonged noise damages the cochlear hair cells. Gentamicin can damage both the auditory and vestibular components of the inner ear. Ménière's disease is associated with recurrent attacks of vertigo, tinnitus and nausea which eventually results in deafness due to damage within the cochlea. An acoustic neuroma develops on the vestibular portion of the eighth nerve and causes progressive unilateral deafness.

36. C. Brief, twitchy and jerky. Chorea is rapid, brief, twitchy movements. Slow and writhing movements with sustained postures is called dystonia. Shock-like jerks are myoclonic. Restlessness occurs with chronic neuroleptic usage and is called akathisia. Rhythmical oscillatory movements are usually associated with tremors.

37. D. Improved by beta-blockers. Both physiological and essential tremors can respond to beta-blockers. Parkinson disease is treated with L-dopa and deep brain stimulation. Neuroleptic medication may cause a tremor and a number of other movement disorders.

38. C. Hypertonia (spasticity). Hypertonia (spasticity) is an upper motor neuron sign (rigidity would be an extrapyramidal sign). The cutaneous reflexes, such as the abdominal reflexes, are reduced in an upper motor neuron syndrome. Wasting of muscles, especially individual muscles innervated by one nerve, is a lower motor neuron sign. Upper motor neuron weakness causes a pattern of weakness called 'pyramidal', which affects the extensors more than the flexors in the upper limbs and the flexors more than the extensors in the lower limbs. Focal weakness is typical of lower motor neuron syndromes. Fatigability is a sign of a problem at the neuromuscular junction, especially myasthenia gravis.

39. B. Horner's syndrome. Ipsilateral facial spinothalamic sensory loss not weakness. The facial nucleus and nerve are in the pons. Involvement of the sympathetic tract can give rise to a Horner's syndrome. The nucleus ambiguus, which is often involved in disorders of the lateral medulla, innervates the soft palate via the vagus nerve but affects the Ipsilateral palate. The hypoglossal nucleus is a paramedian structure in the medulla and is therefore not affected in a lateral lesion. The third nerve nucleus is mostly in the midbrain and is therefore not affected.

40. A. A lesion in the midbrain. A lesion in the midbrain can cause an enlarged pupil. The commonest cause of a small, poorly reactive pupil is old age. Horner's syndrome results from damage to the sympathetic fibres to the pupil and includes meiosis. Opiates cause meiosis. Pontine lesions cause small pin-point pupils.

41. D. Reduced abduction of the right eye. A right sixth-nerve palsy leads to reduced abduction of the right eye (lateral rectus palsy). The third nerve carries parasympathetic fibres to the constrictor pupillae which constrict the pupil so a lesion causes pupillary dilatation. The third nerve innervates levator palpebrae superioris which enable voluntary opening of the eye and a lesion causes ptosis. The third nerve innervates all the extraocular muscles except the lateral rectus (supplied by the sixth nerve) and superior oblique (supplied by the fourth cranial nerve) and is often associated with diplopia in all positions of gaze. In the context of a midbrain infarct, contralateral

hemiparesis or 'Weber's syndrome' can accompany a third nerve palsy.

42. C. A lesion of the medial longitudinal fasciculus. An internuclear ophthalmoplegia (INO) is caused by a lesion in the medial longitudinal fasciculus (MLF), most commonly by a plaque of multiple sclerosis or by an ischaemic lesion. None of the other answers listed will cause an INO.

43. C. Gower's sign may be present. Gower's sign is found in patients with proximal pelvic muscle weakness. Patients have to climb up their own legs with their hands in order to stand up. Sensation is unaffected. A scissoring gait is typical of a spastic paraparesis. Brisk reflexes and clonus are seen in lesions of the upper motor neuron.

44. B. Right sided cerebellar features. The deafness is sensorineural and not conductive. The ipsilateral cerebellar tracts can be involved which causes ipsilateral cerebellar signs. Lower facial weakness is an upper motor neuron deficit. Lesions at the CP angle affect the facial nerve and therefore cause lower motor neuron weakness, i.e. whole of the face. Pseudobulbardysarthria occurs in bilateral upper motor neuron deficits. A lower motor neuron bulbar dysarthria may occur due to involvement of the tenth cranial nerve. Vertigo tends to occur with acute rather than slowly progressive lesions of the vestibular system.

45. C. Hyperacusis. Ramsey–Hunt syndrome is caused by reactivation of herpes zoster within the geniculate ganglion of the seventh nerve. The upper motor neurons are not involved. A lower motor neuron seventh nerve lesion occurs. Diplopia does not tend to occur as the third, fourth and sixth nerves are spared. The nerve to stapedius, which if damaged causes hyperacusis, can be affected. The chorda tympani, which provides taste sensation to the anterior two-thirds of the tongue, can be affected. A small sensory branch from the seventh nerve supplies a portion of the auditory meatus and painful vesicles can occur.

46. E. Are spared following occlusion of the anterior spinal artery. The dorsal columns carry information regarding joint position and vibration sense. The dorsal columns decussate in the lower, not the upper brainstem. B_{12} and not B_1 deficiency can cause subacute combined degeneration of the spinal cord involving the dorsal columns and the corticospinal pathways. Romberg's test looks for a sensory ataxia associated with dorsal column damage. The spinal cord is mostly supplied by one anterior spinal artery which has poor anastomoses and is vulnerable to occlusion. The posterior cord, including the dorsal columns, is richly supplied by a posterior network of vessels and is therefore rarely involved following anterior spinal artery occlusion.

47. B. Anterior spinal artery occlusion. Dissociated sensory loss is a pattern of neurological damage caused by a lesion to a single tract in the spinal cord which involves selective loss of vibration and proprioception without loss of pain and temperature, or vice-versa. In an anterior spinal artery occlusion there is a dissociated loss of pain and temperature sensation but the dorsal columns (vibration and proprioception) are spared. Radiculopathy results in a dermatomal loss of sensation to all modalities. Middle cerebral artery infarcts usually cause cortical sensory loss and often involve all modalities, although if only the cortex and not the thalamus is involved, there is often relative sparing of pain and temperature sensation. A prolapsed intervertebral disc compressing the spinal cord will cause a myelopathy and affect all modalities.

48. E. May be associated with painless foot ulcers. Many patients are asymptomatic and only recognize something is wrong when they are examined. The most common finding is absent ankle jerks and some distal sensory loss, especially to vibration sense without gross wasting or weakness. There is evidence from trials that good blood glucose control slows or even slightly improves diabetic polyneuropathy. Diabetic polyneuropathy is common in both type I and II diabetics. Small pain-carrying fibres are often affected and therefore trophic ulcers can easily occur especially because microvascular and macrovascular arterial disease leads to ischemia in the feet.

49. B. Alcohol overuse. Painful neuropathies are caused by damage to the small unmyelinated 'slow' fibres in peripheral nerves that carry pain and temperature sensation. Conventional electrophysiology is often normal when patients have an isolated small fibre neuropathy. Patients often cannot tolerate even bed sheets touching their legs and may have spontaneous 'dysaesthetic' pain or pain only on touching the affected region. Diabetes is a common cause of small fibre neuropathy and so is alcohol. Charcot–Marie–Tooth disease is usually insidious and painless in onset as is a paraproteinemic neuropathy. Acute intermittent porphyria can cause a motor predominant polyneuropathy that can be mistaken for Guillain-Barré syndrome.

50. A. Guillain–Barré syndrome. It is important to recognize demyelinating neuropathies as some of them are potentially treatable. Guillain–Barré is the most common cause of an acute demyelinating neuropathy. Prolonged and/or severe demyelination may eventually cause axonal loss and therefore the patterns are often mixed. The remainder cause axonal neuropathies.

51. C. Pinprick testing may be abnormal over the medial aspect of the middle finger. Patients with carpal tunnel have parasthaesia confined to the hand but pain often extends right up the arm. There is sensory abnormality in the thumb, index and middle fingers (medial and lateral aspects) and the lateral aspect of the ring finger. Most patients have only sensory symptoms, but when wasting occurs it predominantly affects the abductor pollicis brevis and the thenar eminence, not the whole hand. The median nerve is affected which primarily supplies the thenar eminence including abductor pollicis brevis. The first dorsal interossei is supplied by the ulnar nerve.

52. B. Presents with sensory symptoms. Patients presenting with a spastic paraparesis have a poorer prognosis. Patients who present with sensory symptoms are more likely to have a relatively benign course. Patients who present before the age of 45 are more likely to have a relatively benign course. Patients presenting with sphincter disturbance, brainstem or cerebellar signs have a poorer prognosis.

53. A. Beta-interferon. Beta-interferon reduces relapses by approximately 30%. Steroids may speed up the recovery of a single episode but do not change the overall prognosis. There is no convincing evidence that methotrexate, cyclosporine or mycophenylate help in MS.

54. B. Urinary 24-hour copper is raised. Total serum copper is reduced in Wilson's disease because of a deficiency in the serum copper binding protein, caeruloplasmin. The reduction in caeruloplasmin leads to an increase in free, unbound copper, which is filtered at the glomerulus and therefore urinary copper levels are raised. Penicillamine treatment relies on its binding to accumulated copper and eliminating it through urine. Zinc, not magnesium, competes for copper absorption in the gut and therefore raises stool levels to help reduce dietary copper intake.

55. A. The creatinine kinase (CK) is usually raised. The CK is usually elevated in inflammatory muscle disease and swallowing is usually affected to some degree. Patients are often hyperreflexic and not hyporeflexic possibly due to the inflammatory changes in the muscle leading to hyperexcitability. Proximal muscles are more severely impaired in the upper and lower limbs. The heliotrope rash is assosciated with dermatomyositis.

56. A. Diplopia or ptosis in over 90% of patients at some time in their illness. Ocular involvement in myasthenia gravis occurs in the majority of patients at some time in their disease. Symptoms are often worse towards the end of the day and after exercise and are associated with fatigable weakness of the proximal muscles of the upper limbs and cranial nerves. Muscle cramps and myoblobinuria are not associated. Patients can develop type II respiratory failure due to neuromuscular weakness surprisingly quickly and measurement of the vital capacity is an absolute requirement in any new patient presenting with bulbar myasthenia. Tendon reflexes should be present unlike Lambert–Eaton myasthenic syndrome where they are often absent at rest.

57. D. A right middle cerebral artery ischaemic stroke. Amyotrophic lateral sclerosis is associated with bilateral degeneration of both upper and lower motor neurons. Any cause of myelopathy will usually cause bilateral extensor plantar responses. Multiple sclerosis is associated with diffuse white matter involvement which often involves both corticospinal tracts at some point in their long pathway. B_{12} deficiency can cause demyelination in both corticospinal tracts as well as the dorsal columns.

58. B. Temporal lobe pathology. Visual hallucinations can occur in ocular blindness but they tend not to be well-formed. Visual hallucinations can occur with lesions anywhere within the visual system but formed visual hallucinations of people, animals and objects often occur with diseases affecting the temporal lobes.or in diffuse Lewy body disease. Occipital lobe epilepsy tends to cause unformed images that are usually patterns. Migrainous aura is associated with fortification spectra and lights that move across the visual field. Psychosis rather than bipolar disorder, especially depressive psychosis, can be associated with morbid formed visual hallucinations.

59. A. Motor neuron disease. Fasciculations are spontaneous contractions of a group of muscle fibres innervated by one axon or a 'motor unit'. Fasciculations tend to occur when the axons are damaged or the muscle becomes hyperexcitable, e.g. thyrotoxicosis. Processes that affect the central nervous system (unless it involves the anterior horn cell) or muscle do not tend to cause fasciculations. Parkinson's disease affects the basal ganglia in the central nervous system.

60. B. Tuberculous meningitis. Any process that causes a blockage in the passage of CSF between the choroid plexus and arachnoid granulations can cause hydrocephalus. Basal meningitis caused by *Mycobacterium tuberculosis* and some fungi and bacteria can block the passage of CSF around the fourth ventricle and basal cisterns. Viral meningitis does not tend to block the passage of CSF. Idiopathic or 'benign' intracranial hypertension causes an increase in total brain water which increases intracranial pressure but does not cause

hydrocephalus. Subarachnoid rather than a subdural haemorrhage can cause blockage of the arachnoid granulations or basal cisterns to cause hydrocephalus.

61. C. Post-traumatic epilepsy. Typical absence seizures (previously termed 'Petit mal') is a form of generalized epilepsy that occurs in children and often resolves spontaneously with age. Children of normal intelligence can underperform at school when the absence episodes become frequent and they are missing what is being said in class. The absence attack usually lasts seconds and are not usually accompanied by any post-ictal confusion.The seizures tend to be relatively easily treatable. There is a distinctive 3-per-second spike and wave discharge on EEG during an attack. There is no association with an underlying structural lesion.

62. A. Multiple in 15% of cases. Berry aneurysms are often multiple in 15% of cases. Aneurysms of the posterior communicating artery can cause pain in the eye and an associated third (and not a sixth) nerve palsy. Intracerebral and intraventricular haemorrhage are relatively common with MCA aneurysms. Aneurysms are less common in the posterior circulation than the anterior circulation but are more likely to rupture. Blood can block the passage of CSF through the arachnoid granulations and basal cisterns causing hydrocephalus and is not uncommon.

63. E. Is usually the drug of choice in primary generalized epilepsy. Sodium valproate has a high incidence of teratogenicity and should be avoided in women of child-bearing age. A screen of both the white cell count and LFTs are requiste. Weight gain is a common problem. Phenytoin and carbamazepine can cause hirsuitism but valproate causes hair loss. It is usually the drug of choice in primary generalized epilepsy.

64. A. Can be associated with Coeliac's disease. Coeliac's disease can be associated with an ataxia. B_{12} rather than B_1 deficiency causes an cerebellar syndrome. A cerebellar syndrome may be the presenting feature of coeliac disease. Alzheimer's disease does not tend to affect the cerebellum but other neurodegenerative diseases such as multiple system atrophy can cause a severe cerebellar syndrome. Anticonvulsants, especially toxic levels of phenytoin can very rarely cause irreversible damage to the cerebellum but most cases are reversible. Small cell lung cancer as well as gynaecological malignancies can cause a severe cerebellar syndrome often in association with anti-Yo antibodies.

65. A. Causes pain over the anterior thigh and medial leg. Compression of the L4 nerve root causes pain into the thigh and medial leg rather than L5 and S1 lesions where the pain can extend into the foot. The knee jerk is supplied by L3 and L4 can therefore be reduced. The ankle jerk is innervated by S1 and should be spared. Foot drop is associated with lesions of the common peroneal nerve which is innervated by L4 and partly L5 and therefore L4 root lesions can mimic the motor signs of a common peroneal nerve palsy but the sensory deficit is very different. Degenerative disc disease is a common cause of lumbar radiculopathies but the level should be L4/5. The hamstrings are supplied by the sciatic nerve from L5/S1 roots. Tibialis anterior may be wasted with L4 root lesions.

66. A. There may be upper motor neuron signs in the upper limbs. Cervical spondylosis can cause compression either of the cervical spinal cord causing a cervical myelopathy with upper motor neuron signs in the arms and legs and/or the cervical roots causing lower motor neuron signs in the arms. Pain is often worse at night. Secondary headaches are common. Most patients do not have neurological signs but have neck pain. Neck traction is contraindicated as it can lead to destabilization of the neck and subsequent cord compression.

67. E. Steroid treatment should be initiated as soon as the diagnosis is strongly suspected. Temporal arteritis is five times more common in women and rarely affects patients below 50. It can be associated with a systemic inflammatory disease called *polymyalgia rheumatica* in up to 20% of cases and not optic neuritis. Ischaemiaa of the scalp and muscles of mastication can cause jaw claudication and scalp tenderness but not neck pain Up to 30% of biopsy-proven temporal arteritis have a normal ESR. If the history is highly compatible with the diagnosis, steroids should be commenced and an ESR and temporal artery biopsy then commenced.

68. B. May be affected as a 'false localizing' sign. The third nerve carries parasympathetic fibres to the pupil. Raised intracranial pressure may cause downward displacement of the brain and pressure on the fragile sixth nerve leading to a sixth nerve palsy. This is said to be a 'false localizing sign' because the anatomical site of the sign is distant to the site of the initial lesion. A sixth nerve palsy arises from the pons and travels from the brainstem through the cavernous sinus and superior orbital fissure into the orbit. The facial nerve (seventh nerve) travels through the stylomastoid foramen. The sixth nerve supplies the lateral rectus muscle which abducts the eye.

69. B. Dressing apraxia. The dominant cerebral cortex is on the left in the majority of right-handed people

and is specifically involved in reading, maths (dyscalculia), writing and language. Apraxias involving visuospatial tasks, e.g. dressing and drawing shapes, is a symptom of dysfunction in the non-dominant right hemisphere. More subtle functions of the dominant parietal lobe include naming fingers (if abnormal this is called a finger agnosia) and left–right discrimination.

70. D. If damaged usually causes numbess over the ring and little finger of the hand. The radial nerve is the main branch of the posterior cord of the brachial plexus and supplies most of the muscles on the extensor surface of the arm and forearm including brachioradialis. The radial nerve can be easily damaged as it runs in the bony spiral groove of the humerus especially by pressure from misplaced crutches and by leaning an arm over a chair. Most of the sensation to the hand is supplied by the ulnar and median nerves.

71. A. May produce 'tunnel-vision'. Chronic papilloedema can cause damage to the optic nerve which usually involves the fibres that supply peripheral vision initially, but can extend to involve all fibres. Papilloedema also causes an enlarged blind spot. The disc in temporal arteritis may appear pale but not swollen. Papillitis caused by optic nerve inflammation can resemble the swollen disc but is not papilloedema. Papillitis is often associated with pain on eye movement, a reduction in visual acuity and impaired red–green colour vision. A high CSF protein, as seen in Guillain–Barré, can cause papilloedema probably through a local effect on the flow of CSF. It can also be associated with transient blurring or loss of vision or 'visual obscurations'.

72. A. Monocular visual loss associated with pain on eye movement. Loss of vision in one eye associated with pain on moving the eye is typical of optic neuritis and is a common initial presentation. Typically there is initially a normal looking disc that later turns pale. Hemianopias are surprisingly uncommon in MS. Focal weakness described is that of a peripheral ulnar nerve lesion. Seizures are relatively uncommon in MS but do occur.

73. A. Worsening with coughing, sneezing or bending over. Coughing, sneezing and bending overall increase intracranial pressure and worsen the headache. Fortification spectra are typical of aura associated with migraine headache. Patients with raised pressure often have a dull, progressive headache. The headache is worse on waking in the morning and on prolonged lying flat and better with standing in contrast to low-pressure headaches seen after LP. Nausea and subsequent vomiting are common symptoms of increasing intracranial pressure.

74. B. The ulnar nerve supplies most of the intrinsic muscles of the hand. The median nerve supplies most of the muscles in the forearm. The ulnar nerve supplies all the intrinsic hand muscles, including all the interossei, except the lateral two lumbricals, abductor pollicis brevis, opponens pollicis and flexor pollicis brevis which are supplied by the median nerve. The hypothenar eminence is supplied by the ulnar nerve – the median nerve supplies most of the thenar eminence. The radial does not supply any of the intrinsic hand muscles. The intrinsic hand muscles are mostly supplied by T1 and to a lesser extent C8.

75. B. Lip-smacking and chewing automatisms. Temporal lobe epilepsy can be associated with epigastric rising sensations (panic-like feelings), and *deja vu* (simple partial seizures), various automatisms such as lip smacking, chewing, hand wringing (complex partial seizures) and can secondarily generalise. Much more rarely temporal seizures may present with formed visual, olfactory and gustatory hallucinations. Adopting a 'fencing posture' is a feature of frontal lobe epilepsy. Patients who shake only the upper limbs and have repetitive conjugate eye movements often have pseudoseizures but these can reflect seizures in the frontal lobes and be difficult to diagnose.

76. E. There is a 20% chance of rebleed within the first two weeks. The raised pressure in subarachnoid haemorrhage (SAH) is usually communicating and it is therefore safe and sometimes necessary to perform a LP to aid diagnosis. Patients often become hypertensive and only when it becomes malignant with signs of end-organ damage or greater than 240 mmHg systolic should hypertension be treated. Berry aneurysms are more common in the anterior circulation but are at a greater risk of rupturing in the posterior circulation. Approximately 90% of SAH can be detected on CT within the first 24 hours. The highest incidence of rebleeding is within the first two weeks and therefore many surgeons and radiologists advocate early treatment of aneurysms.

77. D. Geographical apraxia and language deficits are often early features. Patients who are acutely confused present with disorientation, but patients are often initially quite well-orientated in Alzheimer's disease. Later in the disease, patients become disorientated. Patients are often unaware of the degree of memory loss but can retain some insight into their illness in the initial stages of the disease. Alzheimer's disease typically involves the parietal (including apraxias and aphasias) and temporal lobes initially and therefore spares the frontal lobes at presentation. Alzheimer's disease typically involves the parietal lobes – causing

dyspraxia and dysphasia – as well as the temporal lobes in the initial stages. The disease becomes more global as it progresses. Capgras syndrome is more in keeping with dementia with Lewy bodies.

78. C. Is a severe, stabbing, paroxysmal pain. By definition, idiopathic trigeminal neuralgia should not be associated with neurological signs. It is not usually familial. It is usually unilateral – if bilateral then other conditions which affect the trigeminal nuclei and exit zone of the nerve need to be considered, e.g. Multiple sclerosis. The pain is often paroxysmal and is triggered by touching particular parts of the face and mouth, e.g. during chewing and shaving. It is often very sensitive to the anti-epileptics carbamazepine and lamotrigine. Steroids do not help in this condition.

79. D. Guillain–Barré syndrome. Autonomic dysfunction causes include postural hypotension, cardiac arrhythmias, gastric stasis, paralytic ileus, anhydrosis and pupillary abnormalities. Thyroid dysfunction, MS and myasthenia gravis are not a cause of this type of neuropathy. If patients present with parkinsonism and severe autonomic failure then the diagnosis of idiopathic Parkinson's disease is highly unlikely and multi system atrophy is more probable. Autonomic neuropathy can be life-threatening and is a major cause of mortality in Guillain–Barré syndrome. Lambert–Eaton myasthenic syndrome, not myasthenia gravis, is associated with an autonomic neuropathy.

80. C. Can be accompanied by neck stiffness and nausea. The post-LP low-pressure headache is probably related to ongoing CSF leakage after the needle has been removed and therefore larger gauge needles (rather than length) which make a bigger hole in the dura, and repeated unsuccessful attempts are the primary cause. The headache usually resolves within 48 hours although it may continue for several weeks. Patients may develop slight neck stiffness, dizziness and nausea, especially on standing, and some patients vomit. A low pressure headache is worse on standing and is mostly relieved on lying flat. Up to 500 mL of CSF are produced by the choroid plexus daily and therefore draining 10 mL of CSF will not cause the headache.

81. D. Associated nausea, vertigo and photophobia. Chronic form of tension-type headache occurs most days in the month unlike migraine which tends to occur periodically. There should be no loss of consciousness. Further investigation for a structural lesion is warranted. Standing helps headaches associated with raised intracranial pressure. A tight band-like pain around the head is the typical character of tension type headache.

82. C. Loss of vision in one eye (amaurosis fugax). Diplopia can be caused by TIAs involving the pons and midbrain supplied by the posterior circulation. Weakness of all four limbs or 'tetraparesis' is usually caused by TIAs involving the basilar artery, which supplies both corticospinal tracts in the brainstem. Amaurosis fugax is due to blockage in the ophthalmic artery or its branches. It is especially common in the elderly and may be associated with temporal arteritis. Dysphasia (rather than dysphagia) results from lesions to the dominant frontal, parietal or temporal lobes which are supplied by the middle cerebral artery. Vertigo can be caused by lesions to the pons or cerebellum supplied by the posterior circulation.

83. B. May worsen transiently during treatment with steroids. Myasthenia gravis (MG) is associated with antibodies to the acetylcholine receptor. Steroids may temporarily worsen the symptoms but are often necessary to control the disease. The removal of thymomas is to remove the potential risk of malignant transformation and not to improve the underlying disease. Weakness usually is fatigable, worsens with exercise and affects the proximal upper limbs as well as the extraocular muscles, neck flexion, swallowing and speech.

84. E. Tuberculous meningitis. A low CSF glucose occurs in conditions where there are cells or organisms in CSF that consume large quantities of glucose as part of their metabolism – such as bacteria, fungi, tuberculosis, and neoplastic cells but not viruses or inflammation, although very high white cell counts and viral loads in the CSF can reduce the CSF glucose. Alzheimer's disease is a neurodegenerative disorder and does not cause a low CSF glucose. Ischaemic stroke can be associated with a mildly raised CSF protein but not a low glucose. During acute attacks of multiple sclerosis the lymphocyte count and protein can be raised but this is not associated with a low glucose. Guillain–Barré is typically associated with a high CSF protein in isolation due to inflammation of the proximal nerve roots.

85. B. Infarcts in the frontal lobes lobes are often silent. Hemiparesis is the commonest syndrome resulting from a lacunar infarct of the posterior limb of the internal capsule (not anterior). The frontal lobes can often be affected by strokes that are clinically silent. Incongruous (i.e. not the same amount of visual field affected) hemianopias typically occur following damage to the optic tract. Seizures are relatively common in the acute phase of haemorrhagic stroke whereas they are not common in the acute phase of ischaemic stroke. Gerstmann's syndrome is often caused by a stroke involving the

dominant parietal lobe and results in finger agnosia, left/right discrimination difficulties, dysgraphia and dyscalculia.

86. C. Is complicated by cardiac conduction defects. Myotonia typically is worse in the cold. Myotonia is a failure or slowing of relaxation following contraction of a muscle and patients not only have a myopathy with myotonia but also dysfunction of other organ systems, e.g. cardiac conduction defects and diabetes but not hypothyroidism. Myotonic dystrophy (MD) is one a several neurodegenerative conditions that has been found to be associated with an expanded trinucleotide repeat sequence which demonstrate 'anticipation'. Frontal balding is especially common in male patients but also present in female patients. Patients with myotonia are often difficult to anaesthetise due to affects on the respiratory muscles.

87. A. Is fatal in most patients before the age of 30. It usually causes a severe and progressive myopathy resulting in death by the third decade. The creatine kinase (CK) is often in the 1000s due to death of muscle fibres. It causes a severe proximal symmetrical myopathy resulting in the patient having to use their arms to push on their thighs in order to stand from sitting on the ground. This is called 'Gower's sign'. Duchenne muscular dystrophy is an X-linked disorder that affects a protein called dystrophin. It tends to spare the muscles in the head and neck as well as the hands.

88. D. Is usually within the internal capsule and basal ganglia in hypertensive patients. There may be distinguishing features such as headache and altered level of consciousness in a large intracerebral haemorrhage. However, usually the presentation of a haemorrhgic and ischaemic stroke are identical and can only be distinguished on imaging. Meningism only occurs if the haemorrhage extends into the subarachnoid space. A cerebellar haemorrhage in the posterior fossa is a neurological emergency and if suspected clinically a CT head should be performed as the patient can rapidly deteriorate because of the proximity of the brainstem. Patients who are hypertensive tend to have subcortical haemorrhages in the basal ganglia, internal capsule or thalamus. Surgical evacuation is only really indicated if the haemorrhage is in the posterior fossa or is on the convexity of the brain and is having a pressure effect.

89. C. Imaging may show secondary haemorrhage in the temporal lobes. Herpes meningitis is associated with a low CSF glucose in only 20% of patients. The CSF is very rarely normal. The virus has a predilection for the temporal lobes and may be associated with haemorrhagic changes within the temporal lobes. There may be slow waves or epileptiform discharges over the temporal rather than frontal regions on the EEG. In an infective meningoencephalitis the inflammatory markers are usually raised.

90. C. Can be genetically inherited. Prion diseases are caused by a novel infectious agent called a 'prion'; prions are abnormally conformed proteins that do not contain RNA or DNA. The infectious particle is highly resistant to all usual methods of sterilisation and requires special techniques to inactivate it. Surgical instruments used on an infected patient should therefore not be used again. There are several rare forms of inherited prion disease but most are sporadic with no known cause. Recently, there has been a link between a prion disease that affects cows or 'bovine spongiform encephalopathy' and a new variant of a human form of prion disease called 'new variant Creutzfeldt–Jakob disease' or 'nvCJD'. This form is slower in onset than the sporadic form and often presents with psychiatric features and myoclonus. MRI may show characteristic changes in both new variant and sporadic CJD.

EMQ answers

1

1. F The CSF confirms that the patient has a bacterial meningitis, although he should have been given broad-spectrum antibiotics based on the history alone without waiting for the CSF results.
2. J The features of raised intracranial pressure combined with a progressive course suggest a space-occupying lesion such as a neoplasm and, since he is a smoker, it is likely to be lung metastases.
3. B The recent onset of the contraceptive pill can precipitate migraine in a susceptible individual.
4. E The patient has had a partial third nerve palsy with a sentinel bleed from a Berry aneurysm of the posterior communicating artery.
5. D Patients who have had a stroke can complain of a headache.It is much more common with haemorrhagic strokes but a headache should not rule out an ischaemic stroke, especilly if it is a large ischaemic stroke accompanied by oedema and mass effect or if there is haemorrhagic transformation.

2

1. H Absence attacks are rare in adulthood and often patient's attacks will disappear as they get older. Poor performance at school is one possible presentation, although relatives and patients often recognize that there is a problem before this occurs.
2. E Non-epileptic seizures are common even in patients with epilepsy. The awareness during what is apparently a generalised event and the shaking of only the upper limbs with rapid return to normality are suggestive but occasionally strange episodes can occur as part of frontal lobe seizures.
3. A Vasovagal syncope often has a prodrome of impending loss of consciousness and patients can even have some myoclonic jerking of the limbs and urinary incontinence especially if they are kept upright which delays the return of normal cerebral blood flow.
4. F Narcolepsy often presents with excessive daytime sleepiness and hallucinations on going to sleep (hypnagogic hallucinations).
5. C This is a typical complex partial seizure of temporal lobe origin.

3

1. C The triad of dementia, gait apraxia, and urinary incontinence, especially when there is a previous history of subarachnoid haemorrhage, suggests normal pressure hydrocephalus.
2. H New variant CJD has a slower onset than sporadic CJD and often starts non-specifically with psychiatric features and non-specific sensory symptoms.
3. F A stepwise progressive deterioration in neurological function in an elderly patient with vascular risk factors suggests multi-infarct dementia, although there is considerable cross-over with ischaemic leucoencephalopathy.
4. A This is atypical presentation of Alzheimer's disease.
5. J The patient has an excellent MMSE score and is actually able to walk to the shops and call the fire brigade but is too depressed to take an active part in life.

4

1. E Essential tremor may be responsive to alcohol.
2. D Any progressive abnormal movements in young patients especially with bulbar dysfunction suggests Wilson's disease.
3. H Most patients with idiopathic Parkinson's disease who are treated with levodopa develop peak-dose dyskinesias within 5–10 years of commencing treatment.
4. I This is usually caused by a lacunar infarct in the contralateral subthalamic nucleus.
5. C Huntington's disease typically starts with cognitive and psychiatric features and progresses to a movement disorder (usually chorea which presents with fidgety movements). Patients often have no family history even though it is autosomal dominant because their affected parent was becoming symptomatic when they were conceived.

5

1. D A 'glove and sock' loss of sensation and power in a patient with a paraprotein suggests a peripheral neuropathy.
2. H The proximal weakness with a raised CK is suggestive of an inflammatory myopathy such as polymyositis.
3. A The previous episode of optic neuritis and currently the brainstem and cerebellum are affected making MS most probable.

4. C She has a thoracic myelopathy probably secondary to metastatic breast disease. The reduced tone and sometimes loss of reflexes in her legs is common initially in acute myelopathy.

5. G The early loss of postural reflexes, the supranuclear gaze palsy and the frontal signs (grasp reflexes and emotional lability) is characteristic of progressive supranuclear palsy.

6

1. H This story is typical of a Pancoast tumour, which is usually caused by squamous cell carcinoma of the lung invading the lower brachial plexus and roots.

2. D Young patients may have pain throughout the arm and no neurological signs whereas older patients may have severe signs of median nerve damage with relatively few symptoms.

3. E There is often little sensory involvement and recovery occurs over months and may not be complete.

4. C A mixture of upper and lower motor neuron signs above and below the neck is highly suggestive of motor neuron disease.

5. J She has signs and symptoms consistent with a right C6 radiculopathy as well as a cervical myelopathy.

7

1. A Pure motor loss is usually due to a lacunar infarct.

2. J Complete carotid occlusion can be fatal due to post-infarction oedema. In this example, it is probably due to left carotid artery dissection following a deceleration car accident and the sympathetic fibres are involved.

3. G His symptoms have not fully resolved after 24 hours, therefore he has not had a TIA. His stroke did not involve all the territory supplied by the middle cerebral artery.

4. E The posterior inferior cerebellar artery is usually involved but patients often make a good recovery.

5. F This woman is starting to develop 'transtentorial herniation' with a false localizing early third nerve palsy and tonsillar herniation causing drowsiness. She needs an urgent CT head and referral to neurosurgery.

8

1. A Diabetic patients are at risk of acute mononeuropathies. Diabetes tends to cause a pupil-sparing third nerve palsy as it is caused by a vasculitic event inside the third nerve. The parasympathetic supply, which controls the pupil,

travels along the outside of the third nerve and is only affected with external compressive lesions.

2. C A sixth nerve palsy is a common finding in idiopathic intracranial hypertension and can be bilateral.

3. D Ocular symptoms are very common in myasthenia gravis and are often fatigable.

4. G This is a classic presentation of a cavernous sinus syndrome and is probably due to a benign tumour such asa meningioma, but because of their location they are very difficult to treat.

5. I This woman has had a large right middle cerebral stroke and it involves the frontal gaze centre causing weakness of gaze to the left and hence deviation of her eyes to the right.

9

1. C A quadrantanopia usually occurs when one half of the optic radiation is affected – in this case the upper half in the parietal lobe.

2. A Pain on moving the eye is typical of optic neuritis.

3. E A pituitary macroadenoma is often associated with a bitemporal hemianopia that starts from the upper quadrants and progresses down.

4. B The new onset of severe headache should be taken seriously in the elderly and giant cell arteritis can cause infarction of the optic nerve which may cause an altitudinal defector complete visual loss.

5. J Episodes of visual loss and constriction of the visual fields or 'tunnel vision' are concerning signs of impending further visual loss in patients with chronic progressive intracranial hypertension.

10

1. J A waddling gait can occur with orthopaedic problems, but when it is symmetrical and associated with muscle weakness and wasting it is usually caused by a long-standing myopathy.

2. E This is the history of someone with a spastic paraparesis often associated with cerebral palsy.

3. D Cerebellar disease causes a broad-based gait and it may be the only feature, especially with lesions of the cerebellar vermis.

4. G Small, slow, shuffling steps in the context of frontal lobe disease is sometimes called 'marche à petit pas'. In contrast to Parkinson's disease, there is no festination and patients have no problem stopping, having started to walk.

5. H The inconsistency of his disorder and the normal bedside examination are suggestive of an underlying functional disorder.

1. This 33 year old lady has developed clumsiness and has difficulty walking. Please conduct a physical examination of her cerebellar system. Describe to the examiner what you are doing as you go along

Checklist

- Introduce yourself to the patient and obtain consent.
- General inspection – does the patient have any axial instability when sitting?
- Assess for dysarthria – ask the patient to repeat after you 'West Register Street' and/or 'baby hippopotamus' and/or 'British Constitution'.
- Assess for nystagmus:
  - Firstly look at the pursuit eye movements by slowly moving a target (usually finger or a pen) from a position of about 30 cm from the patient's nose in a cross shape, looking to see if the eyes follow smoothly and looking for nystagmus. Note in which direction nystagmus is most pronounced and whether it is horizontal or vertical.
  - Then assess saccadic movements. Hold a finger of one hand 30 cm in front of the nose and the fist of the other hand about 30 cm lateral to the finger. Ask the patient to move his or her gaze rapidly back and forth between finger and fist without moving their head. This is repeated in the four positions of the cross, the finger staying at the level of the nose and the fist moved for each testing. Look for nystagmus, slowed saccades and evidence of inter-nuclear opthalmoplegia.
- Assess for dysdiadochokinesis (difficulty carrying out rapid alternating movements) – ask the patient to alternately pronate and supinate his or her arm and tap the palm and then the dorsum of the hand on his or her other hand.
- Finger–nose test:
  - The examiner holds a finger about 50 cm for the patient's nose and asks the patient to move his or her index finger between the patient's nose and the examiner's finger. Look for an intention tremor (coarse oscillations as the target is approached).

- Heel–shin test:
  - From a lying position on the couch, ask the patient to place one heel on the other knee and slowly slide the heel down the shin, then lift the heel off the shin and place it accurately back on the knee and repeat.
- Assess stance with eyes open and then closed (Rhomberg's test) – ensure that it is safe to do so and that you are close enough to support the patient if they are unsteady (NB: Rhomberg's test is a test of proprioceptive loss but it is often included at this stage to assess whether unsteadiness is cerebellar or due to a sensory ataxia).
- Assess gait and heel-to-toe, but first ensure the patient is sufficiently safe and able to walk. Stand close to them throughout, ready to support as needed. First ask for normal walking and then ask the patient to walk heel-to-toe 'as if walking on a tightrope'.

2. This 48 year old man has had progressive difficulty in walking over the last 2 months. He has also experienced some urgency of micturition. Examine the motor system in his legs. Describe to the examiner what you are doing as you go along

Checklist

- Introduce yourself to the patient and obtain consent.
- Ensure patient is comfortable on the couch in a semi-reclined or sitting position, with legs stretched out in front.
- General inspection – ensure the legs are exposed but the patient is sufficiently covered to avoid embarrassment.
- General inspection – inspect for any obvious abnormalities (e.g. deformity, pes cavus, clawing of the toes and involuntary movements).
- Comment on the absence (or presence) of wasting and fasciculations

- Tone – assess legs for tone at the hip (rolling each leg from side to side), at the knee (by rapidly jerking up each knee) and for clonus at the ankle.
- Test power by assessing the following on each side and scoring out of 5 according to the MRC score:
  - Hip flexion
  - Hip extension
  - Knee flexion
  - Knee extension
  - Ankle dorsi flexion
  - Ankle plantar flexion
- Assess knee and ankle reflexes on each side (use reinforcement if necessary).
- Assess plantar response using an orange stick.
- Assess stance and gait – ensuring that it is sufficiently safe to do so and that you are close enough to support the patient if they are unsteady.
- Identify major abnormalities and suggest a likely cause (e.g. spastic paraparesis, which may be caused most commonly in a gentleman of this age by a prolapsed disc in the cervical or thoracic region or an area of inflammation such as is found in 'demyelination')

---

3. This 60-year-old man is complaining of numbness and pins and needles in his feet. Examine the sensory system in his legs. Describe to the examiner what you are doing as you go along

Checklist

- Introduce yourself to the patient and obtain consent.
- Ensure patient is comfortable on the couch in a semi-reclined or sitting position, with legs stretched out in front.
- General inspection – ensure the legs are exposed but the patient is sufficiently covered to avoid embarrassment.
- Inspect for any obvious abnormalities (e.g. hair loss, ulcers, skin changes, joint swelling, pes cavus, toe clawing).
- Ask patient to describe or indicate area of abnormal sensation.
- Demonstrate sensory testing first, with eyes open, in an area of normal sensation. Then test sensation with eyes closed.
- Test light touch (using cotton wool – touching briefly, not stroking) and then pin prick (using a Neurotip™) in all dermatomes and in small steps from distal to proximal to assess for a 'stocking' distribution.
- Map out any deficit with light touch and pinprick.

- Test vibration sense at hallux on each side with a 128Hz tuning fork. Move proximally, if there is a deficit (ankle, knee, anterior superior iliac spine).
- Test joint position sense at hallux on each side. Move proximally if there is a deficit (ankle, knee, hip).
- For extra marks – suggest carrying out an ankle reflex to assess for the afferent limb of the reflex which will be absent in a large fibre peripheral neuropathy.
- Identify major abnormalities and suggest a likely cause (e.g. stocking distribution of sensory loss suggestive of a peripheral sensory neuropathy. In a gentleman on this age common causes include diabetes, renal disease, alcohol, vitamin B12 deficiency, and a number of medications).

---

4. Please examine the 3rd, 4th, 5th, 6th and 7th cranial nerves of this patient. Describe to the examiner what you are doing as you go along

Checklist

- Introduce yourself to the patient and obtain consent.
- Ensure patient is comfortable on the couch or chair.
- General inspection of patient (e.g. facial asymmetry, obvious ophthalmoplegia, ptosis)
- Ensure patient has adequate visual acuity to be able to follow a target – explain what you are doing to the examiner as you have not been asked to test visual acuity ("can you see my finger?" test each eye in turn).
- If obvious ptosis – comment if unilateral or bilateral, partial or complete, and check for fatiguability.
- Test pupillary reaction to light.
- Test pupillary reaction to accommodation.
- Test eye movements horizontally and vertically, asking the patient to report any double vision (ask the patient repeatedly throughout the examination if they see double).
  - Firstly look at the pursuit eye movements by slowly moving a target (usually finger or a pen) from a position of about 30 cm from the patient's nose, looking to see if the eyes follow smoothly and looking for opthalmoplegia and nystagmus. (H shape or 6-gear stick pattern).
  - Then assess saccadic movements. Hold a finger of one hand 30 cm in front of the nose and the fist of the other hand about 30 cm lateral to the finger. Ask the patient to move his or her gaze rapidly back and forth between finger and fist without moving their head. This is repeated in the four positions of the cross, the finger staying at the level of the nose and the fist moved for each testing. Look for nystagmus,

ophthalmoplegia, slowed saccades and evidence of inter-nuclear opthalmoplegia.

- Check skin sensation in all three trigeminal areas (light touch with cotton wool) and map out sensory deficit. Offer to repeat with a pin prick.
- Offer to carry out a corneal reflex.
- Test motor functions of the trigeminal (look for wasted temporalis, ask patient to clench their teeth and palpate masseter. Offer to test pterygoids by resisting patient's attempts to keep their mouth open (risk of dental injuries so often not carried out).
- Check muscles of facial expression – elevate eyebrows, screw up the eyes and resist attempts to open them, blow out cheeks with air, purse lips tightly and resist attempts to open them, show teeth.
- Mention that the facial nerve delivers taste to the anterior 2/3 of the tongue and offer to test.
- Offer to test the jaw jerk (use reinforcement if necessary).
- Describe abnormal findings and make an attempt to make a diagnosis, e.g:
  - Lower motor neurone facial weakness, likely to be a Bell's palsy.
  - Complete ptosis, eye deviated down and out, with a large, unreactive pupil likely to be a third nerve palsy.
  - Failure of abduction of the right eye, likely to be a right sixth nerve palsy.
  - Unilateral loss of facial sensation and lower motor neurone facial weakness may represent an lesion in the cerebello–pontine angle such as an acoustic neuroma.

5. Paul, who is a 36-year-old gentleman, needs to have an elective lumbar puncture. Can you explain the procedure to him?

Checklist

- Introduce yourself and obtain consent.
- Enquire as to what Paul understands about the procedure and why it is needed.
- Describe the procedure and its purpose:
  - A lumbar puncture (sometimes called a spinal tap) is a routine procedure where a sample of cerebrospinal fluid (CSF) is taken for testing.
  - CSF is the fluid that surrounds the brain (cerebrum) and the spine and by examining its contents, we can help make certain neurological diagnoses or rule out certain conditions.

- It is usually done in a clinic room or hospital bed. If you are not an inpatient, it can often be done as a day case.
- It is important that you are not taking any blood thinners such as warfarin or heparin at the time of the test. You will need to let us know if you take these medications.
- There are no special preparations for the procedure. You can eat normally.
- You will be asked to change into a hospital gown, opening at the rear.
- You will be asked to lie on the couch or bed on your left hand side and asked to curl up in a fetal-like position. Your knees will be positioned up near your chest and your head will be positioned on your chest. This position flexes the back and widens up the spaces between your vertebrae making it easier to insert a needle. It is very important to maintain this position and not move during the procedure.
- The doctor will expose your back and may initially feel with his or her finger to find the best space. The doctor will then scrub up and put on sterile gloves.
- Your back will be washed with antiseptic soap or iodine. This will feel cold. And then you will be covered with a sterile sheet.
- Next a local anaesthetic will be injected into your lower back. The needle will sting briefly as it is injected but then the area will begin to feel numb.
- Once your back feels numb (you will be able to feel pressure, but not sharpness, or actual pain), a thin hollow needle is inserted between two lower lumbar vertebrae in the midline. It will pass through the spinal membrane (dura) and into the spinal canal.
- Once in the spinal canal, CSF will flow through the hollow part of the needle. A manometer may be attached and a pressure measurement may be taken first. Then a few drops of fluid are collected into, usually, three containers. The needle is only usually in the back for about 1 to 2 minutes. (but the whole procedure may take 30 minutes or longer with all the preparations).
- The needle is then removed and a bandage is used to cover the puncture site.

After the procedure

- You will asked to remain lying down for a number of hours (no longer in the fetal position) and subsequently asked not to participate in any strenuous activity or heavy carrying on the day of your procedure.
- You may be given simple painkillers for any slight headache or ache around the lumbar puncture site.

- All the results will not be available on the day of the procedure and you may have to return to an outpatient clinic to get the results.

Risks

Often there are no side effects at all after a lumbar puncture. But the following should be mentioned.

- Post lumbar puncture headache – a low-pressure headache (worse on getting up) due to a delay in healing of the puncture site and a slight leak of CSF. The treatment would be bed-rest and painkillers. Very rarely, further in-patient treatment is required if it is severe and resistant.
- Rare other risks include infection or bleeding at the site of the needle entry.
- The procedure is carried out below the level of the spinal cord so no damage to the spinal cord is possible.
- Check with the patient: does that make sense? Any questions? Any concerns?

---

6. This 22-year-old lady presents with headaches. Please take a focused headache history

Checklist

- Introduce yourself and obtain consent.
- Establish the age when the symptoms first started.
  - Was there a hormonal link (with the onset of menstruation or the oral contraceptive pill)?

- Establish the frequency of the attacks.
- Establish the onset of the headaches – acute, subacute, gradual or preceded by an aura.
- Establish duration of each headache.
- Establish characteristics of the headaches:
  - Site
  - Radiation
  - Nature and severity
  - Relieving factors
  - Precipitating factors
  - Exacerbating factors
- Establish associated symptoms
  - Warning aura, e.g. visual disturbances
  - Nausea and vomiting
  - Meningism
  - Rash
  - Watering or reddening of the eye
  - Ptosis
- Exclude family history of headaches e.g. migraine, subarachnoid haemorrhage.
- Relevant past medical history including head injury.
- Drug history (any medications that cause headaches eg nitrates).
- Elicit patient's concerns.
- Respond appropriately to concerns.
- Summarise history back to patient and ask if there is anything more they wish to add or ask.
- Make a reasonable attempt at the diagnosis. e.g. In a young woman, with recurrent unilateral headaches since her teenage years, preceded by flashing lights, with associated nausea and vomiting, which were made worse by starting the oral contraceptive pill, the most likely diagnosis is migraine headaches.

Glossary

A

acalculia difficulty in performing simple mental arithmetic.

ageusia loss of taste sensation.

agnosia deficit of higher sensory processing caused by impaired recognition.

agraphaesthesia loss of the ability to recognize numbers or letters traced on the skin.

akathisia feeling of inner restlessness associated with repetitive movements of a purposeless nature.

akinesia inability to initiate a voluntary movement.

amyotrophy wasting of muscle.

anarthria inability to articulate.

anisocoria unequal pupil size.

anosognosia patients unawareness of their illness.

apraxia inability to perform a motor sequence with preserved motor, sensory and coordination functions.

astereognosis inability to recognize an object placed in the hand with eyes closed and intact peripheral sensation.

athetosis involuntary movements characterized by slow writhing purposeless movements.

aura a neurological phenomenon occurring seconds to minutes before a migraine headache or epileptic seizure.

B

ballismus wild flailing movements of the limbs.

Broca's aphasia non-fluent, slow, laboured effortful speech, but patient can recognize errors in own speech. Comprehension often preserved for simple material. Repetition, reading, writing and naming impaired, but naming may be helped by contextual cues.

C

cataplexy sudden loss of lower limb tone leading to falls without loss of consciousness.

chorea involuntary hyperkinetic movement disorder associated with jerky, restlessness, purposeless movements, which move from one part of the body to another in an unpredictable way.

coma a state of unresponsiveness to verbal or mechanical stimuli.

conjugate gaze palsy a disorder affecting the ability to move both eyes in the same direction. These palsies can affect gaze in a horizontal, upward or downward direction.

D

déjà vu an inappropriate feeling of overfamiliarization with the environment.

delirium a neurobehavioural syndrome associated with problems with attention.

dementia loss of intellectual functions leading to impaired function or behaviour.

dissociated sensory loss impairment of some, but not all, sensory modalities.

dysdiadochokinesia difficulty in performing rapid alternating movements.

dysgeusia a distortion of the sense of taste.

dyskinesia excessive involuntary movements, e.g. chorea, athetosis.

dysmetria abnormal control of range of movement.

dysphagia difficulty swallowing.

dysphonia disorder of volume, pitch or quality of voice due to dysfunction of the larynx.

dystonia sustained involuntary muscle contraction.

E

encephalopathy general term for diffuse disturbance of brain function.

F

fasciculation rapid, flickering movements within a muscle associated with spontaneous activity of a motor unit. Sometimes described as 'worms under the skin'.

fibrillation spontaneous contraction of single muscle fibres. These cannot be seen by eye and are detected electrophysiologically.

frontal release signs a group of reflexes that are usually absent in healthy adults but may be found following a wide range of disorders of the CNS. Their anatomical localization is vague, even though they are still referred to as the 'frontal release signs', and 'primitive reflexes' may be a more appropriate term as it suggests that these are reflexes which are inhibited as the brain develops.

G

gait apraxia the inability/impairment to walk in spite of preserved motor sensory and coordination functions. It usually occurs with lesions of the frontal lobes and its white matter connections.

glabellar tap reflex tap on the forehead produces blinking, which habituates in most people. If this fails to habituate, then it used to be felt that it was a useful diagnostic sign of idiopathic Parkinson's disease. Unfortunately, it is often positive in normal aged individuals and in other extrapyramidal disorders and is, therefore, usually not clinically useful.

'glove and sock' sensory/motor loss the loss of sensation and power in a polyneuropathy is typically worse distally than proximally. This is often referred to as 'glove and stocking' but the loss rarely extends up to the mid-thigh and usually stops mid-calf.

Gower's sign a typical movement made by a patient with proximal lower limb weakness where the arms are used to climb up the legs in order to stand from lying on the floor.

H

hemianopia a defect of one-half of the visual field.

Horner's syndrome partial ptosis, meiosis and anhydrosis associated with dysfunction in the sympathetic supply to the eye.

hypomimia reduction of voluntary facial expression.

hypoosmia a decreased sense of smell.

I

internuclear ophthalmoplegia failure or slowing of adduction during horizontal conjugate gaze with or without gaze-evoked nystagmus in the abducting eye secondary to a lesion in the medial longitudinal fasciculus.

J

Jacksonian march sequential spread of a simple partial usually motor seizure, e.g. hand, elbow then shoulder, which may terminate spontaneously or with a secondary generalized seizure.

K

Kayser–Fleischer rings green/brown deposits of copper in Descemet's membrane, which can usually only be seen with slit-lamp examination and is highly suggestive of Wilson's disease.

Kernig's sign pain in the lower back and neck and resistance to passive extension of the knee when the thigh is flexed secondary to meningitis.

L

Lhermitte's sign electric shock-like sensation down the arms and legs following flexion of the neck due to a lesion within the cervical cord.

locked-in syndrome severe damage to the ventral pons causing loss of the ascending and descending tracts to the spinal cord, pons and medulla so that the patient can only move the eyes, often vertically, and blink. It is usually caused by basilar artery thrombosis.

M

marche à petit pas small-stepped, often wide-based, shuffling gait without a flexed posture or festination

of idiopathic Parkinson's disease caused by bilateral frontal cortical or white matter damage usually secondary to small vessel disease.

Marcus Gunn pupil delay or failure of constriction of a pupil to direct light due to a lesion in the optic nerve.

micrographia small handwriting. This is often seen in idiopathic Parkinson's disease and starts normally, but fatigues and becomes small.

myelopathy a disorder of the spinal cord which is usually associated with a sensory level near the level of the lesion, upper motor neuron weakness below the lesion, sometimes lower motor neuron signs at the level of the lesion and sphincter disturbance.

myoclonus involuntary 'shock-like' contraction resulting in a jerking movement, usually of the limbs, trunk or neck.

myotonia inability to relax a muscle following contraction.

N

neglect inability to respond to or attend to a sensory stimulus.

nystagmus involuntary oscillation of the eyes that can be pathological or physiological.

O

oculocephalic response (doll's eye movements) the eyes remain fixated on an object when the head is passively moved, which is a sign of an intact pontine brainstem reflex.

optokinetic nystagmus a physiological involuntary conjugate pursuit eye movement in response to a moving object with a return saccade when the object disappears out of vision, e.g. looking out of a moving train.

P

papilloedema swelling of the optic disc head secondary to raised intracranial pressure.

paraplegia severe/total weakness of both legs.

parkinsonism a constellation of signs associated with some or all of the features of bradykinesia, rigidity, tremor and postural instability.

pes cavus high arched feet due to imbalance in the muscular contractions acting on the feet usually associated with genetic neuropathies, e.g. Charcot–Marie–Tooth, or due to an early neurological insult, e.g. cerebral palsy.

Phalen's sign tingling in the distribution of the median nerve when the wrist is forced flexed at 90°; it is associated with carpal tunnel syndrome.

phonophobia dislike or fear of loud noises.

photophobia dislike or fear of bright lights.

pseudobulbar palsy impairment of bilateral corticobulbar fibres associated with dysphagia, dysarthria, brisk jaw jerk, slow and spastic tongue and exaggerated gag reflex.

pseudodementia global impairment of cognitive functions due to affective disorders (anxiety/depression) which mimics dementia caused by organic pathology, e.g. Alzheimer's disease.

ptosis drooping of the eylid.

pyramidal synonymous with corticospinal and upper motor neuron.

Q

quadrantanopia loss of a quarter of the visual field.

quadriplegia total or severe loss of power in all four limbs.

R

radiculopathy disorder of the nerve roots causing sensory loss in the corresponding dermatome, motor loss in the corresponding myotome, reflex loss and pain in a radicular distribution.

rigidity increased resistance to passive movement that is equal throughout the range of movement and is associated with extrapyramidal disease.

Romberg's sign increase in unsteadiness when a standing patient closes their eyes; it is associated with proprioceptive loss to the feet.

S

saccades rapid movements of the eyes, which move the focus from one point to another.

scotoma a localized area of impaired vision.

spasticity increased resistance to passive movement at a joint that varies with amplitude and velocity and is associated with a lesion in the upper motor neuron.

supranuclear gaze palsy impairment of the supranuclear connections to the nuclei of the nerves supplying the extraocular muscles leading to preservation of reflex, but loss of voluntary, eye movements.

syncope loss of consciousness.

T

tandem gait the ability to walk in a straight line with one foot in front of the other. This is impaired in midline cerebellar disorders.

Tinel's sign paraesthaesia following tapping of a trapped or regenerating peripheral nerve.

Todd's paresis transient localized weakness following a seizure usually lasting seconds or minutes.

U

Uhthoff's phenomenon worsening of visual acuity with exercise or other causes of increased body temperature in optic neuritis related to temperature sensitivity of demyelinated axons.

upper motor neuron the cell in the primary motor cortex which projects its axon down through the internal capsule and spinal cord to synapse with the lower motor neuron.

V

vegetative state clinical syndrome associated with extensive loss of cognitive function but preserved vegetative function, e.g. respiration and autonomic. It has a very poor prognosis.

W

Wernicke's aphasia fluent aphasia with phonemic and semantic paraphasias, impaired comprehension, impaired repetition, and severely impaired naming, reading and writing.

Index

Notes: *vs.* indicates a comparison or differential diagnosis
To save in the index, the following abbreviations have been used:
LMN - lower motor neuron
TIA - transient ischaemic attack
UMN - upper motor neuron

Page numbers followed by *f* indicate figures.

A

ABC approach, coma 44
Abducens nerve (cranial nerve VI)
  anatomy 73*f*
  assessment 12–15
  cavernous sinus 77*f*
  lesions 74*f*, 154–155, 154*f*
    binocular diplopia 70
Abscesses
  cerebellar dysfunction 95*f*
  cerebral 228–229
  intracranial 51*f*
Absence seizures 134
ACA *see* Anterior cerebral artery (ACA)
Accessory nerve (cranial nerve XI)
  assessment 17
  lesions 154*f*, 158
Accommodation, pupil assessment 13
Accommodation reflex 64
Acetylcholine receptor, myasthenia gravis 190
Acetylcholinesterases 191
Acoustic neuromas (schwannomas) 157, 216, 217*f*
Acquired myopathies 195*f*
  electrolyte myopathies 195*f*, 198
  endocrine myopathies 195*f*, 198
Activated partial thromboplastin time (APT) 26*f*
Acute brachial neuropathy 175–176
Acute disseminated encephalomyelitis (ADEM) 241
Acute dystonic reaction 150
Acute glaucoma, subacute-onset headache 51*f*
Acute hydrocephalus, subacute-onset headache 51*f*
Acute intermittent porphyria 253–254
Acute-onset headaches 51
  causes 52*f*

Acute toxicity, antiepileptic drugs 136
Acute transient visual impairment 61
Acute vestibular failure 158
Acute visual impairment 61–62
  differential diagnosis 61–62
Acyclovir
  Bell's palsy 157
  encephalitis treatment 227
ADEM (acute disseminated encephalomyelitis) 241
Adson's sign 176
Affect, neurological examination 7
Ageusia 53–54
  definition 54
Agnosia
  auditory 36
  visual 38
Akathisia 150
Akinesia, Parkinson's disease 146
Akinetic mutism, coma *vs.* 42
Akinetic-rigid syndromes 145–150
Alcohol, cerebellar dysfunction 95*f*
Alcoholic neuropathy 184
Alertness, consciousness evaluation 7
Alpha-synuclein, Parkinson's disease 145
ALS *see* Amyotrophic lateral sclerosis (ALS)
Alzheimer's disease 128
Amaurosis fugax 61
4-Aminopyridine (4-AP), Lambert–Eaton myasthenic syndrome 192
Amoxycillin 234
Ampulla 82*f*
Amyloidosis, paraneoplastic polyneuropathy 184
Amyloid precursor protein (APP) gene 128
β-Amyloid protein 128
Amyotrophic lateral sclerosis (ALS) 169, 170*f*
  differential diagnosis 171
ANA (antinuclear factor antibodies) 27*f*
Anaemia 244
Anaesthesia, saddle 106*f*, 107
Analgesic overdose headache 139
  causes 50*f*
ANCA (antineutrophil cytoplasmic antibodies) 27*f*
Angiography 30

cerebral 208
  subarachnoid haemorrhage 210
ANI (asymptomatic neurocognitive impairment) 231
Anisocoria 64–65
  physiological 65
Anosmia 10, 53
  definition 54
  frontal lobe lesions 35
  olfactory nerve lesions 153
Antalgic gait 121
Anterior cerebral artery (ACA) 58, 58*f*, 203*f*
  distribution 204*f*
  frontal lobes 33
  occlusion 204–205
Anterior choroidal artery 58, 58*f*
Anterior communicating artery 58, 58*f*, 203*f*
Anterior horn cell disease 109
  LMN limb weakness 108
Anterior semicircular canal 82*f*
Anterior spinal artery occlusion 164
Anterior spinal artery syndrome 212–213
Anterior spinal nerve roots 173
Anterior superior vermis (spinocerebellum) 93
Anti-acetylcholine receptor (AChR) antibodies, tests 27*f*
Antibiotics, cerebral abscesses 228
Anticholinergic drugs, Parkinson's disease treatment 148
Anticonvulsant side effects 95*f*
Anti-double-stranded DNA (dsDNA) antibodies 27*f*
Anti-epileptic drugs 135–137
  adverse effects 136
  dose increases 136
  pharmacokinetics 136
  start of 135
  types 135–136
  withdrawal of 136–137
Anti-GM1 antibodies 27*f*
Anti-Hu antibodies
  paraneoplastic polyneuropathy 183
  tests 27*f*
Anti-La antibodies 27*f*
Anti-MUSK antibodies 190
Antineutrophil cytoplasmic antibodies (ANCA) 27*f*

Antinuclear factor antibodies
    (ANA) 27*f*
Antiphospholipid antibodies 27*f*
Antiphospholipid syndrome 244
Antiplatelet medication, stroke
    management 208
Antiretroviral toxic neuropathy 232
Anti-Ri antibodies 27*f*
Anti-ribonucleoprotein (RNP)
    antibodies 27*f*
Anti-Ro (SSA) antibodies 27*f*
Anti-voltage-gated potassium channel,
    tests 27*f*
Anti-Yo antibodies 27*f*
Aortic disease 246*f*
Apneustic respiration, coma 45
Apomorphine 148
Appearance, neurological
    examination 7
APP (amyloid precursor protein) gene
    128
Apraxia
    bilateral ideational 36
    bilateral ideomotor 36
    constructional 36
    dressing 36
Apraxic gait 121
APT (activated partial thromboplastin
    time) 26*f*
Aqueduct, anatomy 146*f*
Aqueduct of Sylvius 94*f*
Argyll Robertson pupil 12, 65
Arms
    coordination 23
    motor system assessment 18–19,
        20*f*, 21*f*
Arnold–Chiari malformation 95*f*
Arrhythmias 246*f*
Arterial dissection 211
    acute-onset headache 52*f*
    stroke 202
Arteriovenous malformations,
    intramedullary spinal 165
Articulation 89
    neural pathways 90*f*
    speech assessment 9
Associated symptoms, history taking 3
Astrocytomas 215
Asymmetrical nystagmus 73
Asymptomatic neurocognitive
    impairment (ANI) 231
Asymptomatic neurosyphilis 230
Ataxias
    cerebellar 120
    hereditary conditions 253
    multiple sclerosis 241*f*
    sensory *see* Sensory ataxia
    spinocerebellar 253
    spinocerebellar degeneration 253
Ataxia telangiectasia 253
Ataxic dysarthric speech 93

Ataxic gait 93
Atherosclerosis, stroke 202
Athetosis, dysarthria 91
Atonic seizures 134
Atrial myxoma 246*f*
Atrophic skin changes, motor system
    assessment 18
Attention, Mini-Mental State
    Examination 8, 8*f*
Auditory agnosia 36
Auditory cortex 34*f*
    temporal lobes 36
Auditory information, parietal lobes 35
Auditory ossicles 82*f*
Auditory system 81
    anatomy 82*f*
Auditory (eustachian) tube 82*f*
Auras 131
Autoantibodies
    myasthenia gravis 191
    polymyositis/dermatomyositis 198
    tests 27*f*
    see also specific antibodies
Autosomal dominant myopathies,
    194
Autosomal recessive myopathies 194
Axial dystonia 100–101
Axonal neuropathy 29*f*
Axons 178*f*
    unmyelinated 57
Azathioprine 191

B

Bacterial infections
    cerebral abscesses 228
    see also specific infections
Bacterial meningitis 223, 224*f*
Ballism 98*f*, 101
Basal ganglia
    anatomy 97
    lesions, dysarthria 9, 90–91
Basilar artery 58*f*, 203*f*, 204*f*
    occlusion 206–207
Basilar migraine 140
Becker's muscular dystrophy 195
Behaviour
    frontal lobe lesions 34
    neurological examination 7
Behçet's disease 245–246
Bell's palsy 156–157
Benign coital headache 50*f*
Benign paroxysmal positional vertigo
    (BPPV) 84, 85*f*, 158
Benserazide 147
Benzatropine 148
Benzhexol (trihexyphenidyl) 148
Beri-beri 247
Beta-interferon 240
Bilateral fixed eye position, coma 45

Bilateral fixed pupils, coma 45
Bilateral ideational apraxia 36
Bilateral ideomotor apraxia 36
Bilirubin 27*f*
Binocular diplopia 68–70
    abducens nerve lesions 70
    brainstem lesions 70
    cranial nerve dysfunction 69–70
    extraocular muscle dysfunction 68
    neuromuscular junction
        dysfunction 68
    oculomotor nerve lesions 69
    trochlear nerve lesions 69
Binocular visual field defects 59
Binocular visual impairment 61
Biochemical tests 27*f*
Biopsies
    dementia 127
    muscle 198
    myopathies 194
    peripheral neuropathies 179
    stereotactic brain biopsy 219
Bladder dysfunction, multiple sclerosis
    241*f*
Blepharospasm 100
Blindness
    cortical 38
    see also Visual impairment
Blind spot assessment 12
Blood supply
    anatomy 203, 203*f*
    frontal lobes 33
    occipital lobes 37
    parietal lobes 35
    temporal lobes 36
    see also specific vessels
Blood tests
    dementia 126
    peripheral neuropathies 179
    see also specific tests
Borderzone ischaemia 207
Borrelia burgdorferi infection *see* Lyme
    disease
Botulinum toxin 192
Bovine spongiform encephalopathy
    (BSE) 234
BPPV (benign paroxysmal positional
    vertigo) 84, 85*f*, 158
Brachial neuritis 175–176
Brachial neuropathy, episodic painful
    175–176
Brachial plexus
    anatomy 109–110, 109*f*, 173
    plexopathies 109, 175–176
Bradykinesia 145
    Parkinson's disease 146
Brain injury 101
Brainstem
    anatomy 94*f*
    auditory evoked potentials 240
    lesions *see below*

multiple sclerosis 239
sensorineural deafness 83
stroke 206–207, 206f
trauma, deafness/tinnitus 83f
Brainstem death 47
Brainstem lesions
binocular diplopia 70
dizziness/vertigo 86
facial sensory loss 76–77
limb sensory symptoms 117–118, 117f
Broca's area 34f
frontal lobes 33
lesion 9–10
Bromocriptine 148
Brown–Séquard syndrome 116–117, 160, 161, 162f
BSE (bovine spongiform encephalopathy) 234
Bulbar palsy 171
progressive 170

C

Cabergoline 148
Caeruloplasmin 150
Café-au-lait spots 251
Calcium 27f
Calculation, Mini-Mental State Examination 8, 8f
Caloric test 86–87
Canal paresis, Caloric test 86
Carbidopa 147
Cardiac disease 245
stroke 202
see also specific diseases/disorders
Cardiac embolism, stroke 202
Cardiac surgery 246f
Cardiolipin tests, syphilis diagnosis 230
Cardiomyopathies, primary 246f
Cardiomyopathy, Becker's muscular dystrophy 195
Cardiovascular disease 246f
Carotid artery occlusion 206
Carotid Doppler ultrasound 208
Carotid embolism, stroke 202
Carotid sinus disease 41
Carpal tunnel syndrome 180, 180f
hypothyroidism 243
Cataplexy 41
Catatonia, coma vs. 43
Catheter angiography 30
Cauda equina 160f
Cavernous haemangiomas 165
Cavernous sinus lesions 77, 77f
Cavernous sinus thrombosis 211
Ceftriaxone 234
Cefuroxime 234
Central field assessment 12
Central (Rolandic) fissure 34f

Central lumbar disc protrusion 175
Central nervous system lymphoma, primary see Primary central nervous system lymphoma
Central nervous system toxoplasmosis 231
Central neurogenic hyperventilation, coma 45
Central nystagmus 73
Central pontine myelinolysis (CPM) 242
Cerebellar dysfunction 93–96
causes 95f
clinical features 93–95
abnormal eye movements 93
ataxic dysarthric speech 93
ataxic gait 93, 120
hypotonia 94–95
movement incoordination 93
postural changes 94, 94f
titubation 94
lesions 95
Cerebellar syndrome, toxins 248f
Cerebellar tremor see Intention tremor (cerebellar tremor)
Cerebellar vermis lesions 95
Cerebellopontine angle lesions
dizziness/vertigo 86
facial sensory loss 77
Cerebellum
anatomy 93, 94f
multiple sclerosis 239
Cerebellum lesions
dizziness/vertigo 86
dysarthria 9, 91
Cerebral abscesses 228–229
Cerebral angiography, stroke/TIAs 208
Cerebral cortex 34f
Cerebral hemispheres
anatomy 33, 34f
focal damage 33
lesions 95
paraparesis 106–107
trauma, deafness/tinnitus 83f
Cerebral infarction (ischaemic stroke) 201
Cerebral oedema treatment 219
Cerebral venous thrombosis 211
Cerebropontine angle lesions 83, 157
Cerebrospinal fluid (CSF)
culture 225
low volume in headache 141–142
staining 225, 225f
Cerebrospinal fluid examination 227
multiple sclerosis 239–240
peripheral neuropathies 179
Cerebrovascular disease 201–209
definitions 201
diabetes mellitus 243
parkinsonism 150
vasculitis 211
see also specific diseases/disorders

Cervical discs, lateral protrusion 174
Cervical dystonia 100
Cervical rib syndrome 176
Cervical spinal cord 160f
Charcot joint 113
Charcot–Marie–Tooth (CMT) disease 186
Chemotherapy
intracranial tumour treatment 219
neurotoxicity 221
Cheyne–Stokes respiration 45
Chorea 98f, 101
dysarthria 90
toxins 248f
Chronic cluster headache 50f
Chronic daily headache 49
causes 50f
Chronic inflammatory demyelinating polyradiculoneuropathy (CIDP) 185
HIV infection 232
Chronic migraine 50f
Churg Strauss syndrome 246f
CIDP see Chronic inflammatory demyelinating polyradiculoneuropathy (CIDP)
Circle of Willis 203, 203f, 204f
CK see Creatine kinase (CK)
Classical migraine see Migraine with aura (classical migraine)
Clotting disorders 244
Cluster headache 140–141
causes 50f
CMT (Charcot–Marie–Tooth) disease 186
Coagulation tests 26f
Cochlea 82f
disorders 83
trauma, deafness/tinnitus 83f
Cochlear nerve disorders 83
Cognition
definition 33
history taking 3
multiple sclerosis 239
neurological examination 7–8
Parkinson's disease 147
Coital headache 52f
Colour vision assessment 11
Coma 42–47
causes 43, 44f
clinical approach 43
consciousness evaluation 7
differential diagnosis 42–43
examination 45–46
investigations 46–47
prognosis 47
Combined ocular palsies 155, 155f
Common carotid artery 204f
Common migraine 140
Common peroneal nerve palsy 181, 182f

Community-acquired meningitis 226
Complex partial seizures 133–134
Comprehension, dysphasia assessment 9
Compression, brachial plexopathies 176
Compression mononeuropathies, diabetes mellitus 243
Computed tomographic angiography (CTA), stroke/TIAs 207–208
Computed tomography (CT) 29
  Alzheimer's disease 128
  cerebral abscesses 228
  dementia 127
  epilepsy diagnosis 135
  extradural haematoma 210, 210f
  intracranial tumours 218, 219f
  lateral cervical disc protrusion 174
  meningitis 224, 224f
  stroke/TIAs 207
  subarachnoid haemorrhage 209–210
  transient loss of consciousness 42
COMT (catechol-O-methyltransferase) inhibitors 148
Conduction dysphasia 10f, 37
  causes 10
Conductive deafness 81, 82–83
Cones 57
Confusion
  consciousness evaluation 7
  Parkinson's disease treatment 148
Congenital aqueduct stenosis 95f
Congenital myasthenia gravis 192
Congenital nystagmus 72
Conjugate eye movements 14
  frontal lobe lesions 33
Conjugate gaze 66–68
  definition 66
Connective tissue diseases/disorders 245, 246f
  peripheral neuropathies 183–184, 187f
  transverse myelitis 165
  see also specific diseases/disorders
Consciousness disturbances 39–48
  driving implications 42
  transient loss of consciousness 39–42, 40f
  see also specific diseases/disorders
Consciousness, neurological examination 7
Constructional ability, Mini-Mental State Examination 8, 8f
Constructional apraxia, parietal lobe lesions 36
Contraceptives, stroke 203
Contralateral homonymous field defect, occipital lobe lesions 38
Contralateral nasal fibres, light stimulation path 57

Contralateral sensory weakness, parietal lobe lesions 36
Contralateral weakness, frontal lobe lesions 33
Conus medullaris 159, 160f
Coordination, motor system assessment 19–23
Copper deficiency
  myelopathy 166
  spinal cord diseases 166
  see also Wilson's disease (hepatolenticular degeneration)
Corneal reflex 16
  coma 46
Cortical blindness, occipital lobe lesions 38
Cortical contralateral sensory loss, parietal lobe lesions 35
Cortical deafness, temporal lobe lesions 36
Cortical micturition centre, frontal lobes 33
Corticobasal degeneration 149
Corticospinal tracts 146f
Corticosteroids
  Bell's palsy 157
  cluster headache therapy 141
  giant-cell arteritis therapy 143
  multiple sclerosis management 240
  myasthenia gravis management 191
  polymyositis/dermatomyositis 198
Cough headache 50f
Cough syncope 40
Counselling, dementia management 127
CPK (creatine phosphokinase) 194
CPM (central pontine myelinolysis) 242
Cranial nerve(s)
  binocular diplopia 69–70
  cranial nerve I see Olfactory nerve (cranial nerve I)
  cranial nerve II see Optic nerve (cranial nerve II)
  cranial nerve III see Oculomotor nerve (cranial nerve III)
  cranial nerve IV see Trochlear nerve (cranial nerve IV)
  cranial nerve V see Trigeminal nerve (cranial nerve V)
  cranial nerve VI see Abducens nerve (cranial nerve VI)
  cranial nerve VII see Facial nerve (cranial nerve VII)
  cranial nerve VIII see Vestibulocochlear nerve (cranial nerve VIII)
  cranial nerve IX see Glossopharyngeal nerve (cranial nerve IX)
  cranial nerve X see Vagus nerve (cranial nerve X)

  cranial nerve XI see Accessory nerve (cranial nerve XI)
  cranial nerve XII see Hypoglossal nerve (cranial nerve XII)
  lesions 153–158, 154f
  see also specific nerves
  neurological examination 10
Craniofacial pain 139–144
Creatine kinase (CK)
  myopathies 194
  tests 27f
Creatine phosphokinase (CPK) 194
Creatinine 27f
Creutzfeldt–Jakob disease 234
Critical illness myopathies 199
Critical illness polyneuropathy 186
CSF see Cerebrospinal fluid (CSF)
CTA (computed tomographic angiography) see computed tomography (CT)
CTA (computed tomographic angiography), stroke/TIAs 207–208
Cushing's syndrome 198
Cyclosporin adverse effects 245

D

Dandy–Walker syndrome, cerebellar dysfunction 95f
Deafness 81
  causes 83f
  conductive 81, 82–83
  cortical 36
  differential diagnosis 81–83
  investigations 83
  sensorineural 81, 82–83
  see also specific types
Decerebrate positioning, coma 46, 46f
Decorticate positioning, coma 46, 46f
Degenerative diseases/disorders
  epilepsy causes 132
  spastic paraparesis 107f
  spinal cord compression 163, 163f
  see also specific diseases/disorders
Delirium, intracranial tumours 220
Dementia 123–130
  clinical features 125, 126f
  definition 125
  differential diagnosis 125
    depression vs. 126f
  epidemiology 125
  examination 126
  history taking 126
  HIV infection 231–232
  investigations 126–127
  management 127
  other degenerative diseases 130
  prevalence 125
  primary neurodegenerative 128–130
  toxins 248f

Dementia with Lewy bodies (DLB) 128–129
Demyelination
  nerve conduction studies 29f
  peripheral nerves 177
Denervation, electromyography 29f
Depression
  dementia vs. 126f
  history taking 3
  multiple sclerosis 241f
Dermatomyositis 197–198
Developmental disorders
  cerebellar dysfunction 95f
  see also specific diseases/disorders
Dexamethasone 226
Diabetes mellitus 243
  stroke 202
Diabetic amyotrophy 243
  lumbosacral plexopathy 176
Diabetic neuropathy 183
Diaphragm, enervation 161
Diet, stroke 203
Diffusion-weighted imaging (DWI), intracranial tumours 219
Dilated pupils, coma 45
Dilator pupillae muscle 63
Diplopia
  binocular see Binocular diplopia
  monocular 68
Directional preponderance, Caloric test 87
Discitis 164
Disease-modifying treatment, multiple sclerosis 240–241
Distal symmetrical polyneuropathy
  diabetes mellitus 243
  HIV infection 232
Distal weakness 104
Dizziness 84–86
DLB (dementia with Lewy bodies) 128–129
Doll's eye movements see Oculocephalic reflex (doll's eye movements)
Donald Duck voice (spastic dysarthria) 170
Donepezil 128
Dopamine agonists 148
Dopa-responsive dystonia 100
Dorsal (posterior) column pathway, limb sensory symptoms 113
Dorsal spinal nerve roots 173
  lesions 115, 115f
Doxycycline 234
Dressing apraxia 36
Driving
  consciousness disturbances 42
  epilepsy 138
Drug(s)
  induced myopathies 199
  peripheral neuropathies 184
  see also specific drugs

Drug history, history taking 4
Drug-induced confusional state, toxins 248f
Duchenne muscular dystrophy 195
Duplex ultrasonography 30
Dural arteriovenous fistulas, vascular spinal cord lesions 165
Dura mater 159
DWI (diffusion-weighted imaging), intracranial tumours 219
Dysarthria 89–91
  assessment 9
  basal ganglia lesions 90–91
  causes 92f
  cerebellar lesions 91
  definition 89
  LMN lesions 90
  myopathies 91
  neuromuscular junction disorders 91
  oropharyngeal lesions 91
  spastic 170
  UMN lesions 89–90
Dysdiadochokinesia 23
  cerebellar dysfunction 93
Dysgeusia 53–54
  definition 54
Dyskinesia, tardive 150–151
Dysmetria 93
Dysphagia 91
  causes 92f
  definition 89
  lesion sites 91
Dysphasia 37
  assessment 9–10
  classification 10f
  conduction see Conduction dysphasia
  expressive see Expressive dysphasia
  fluent see Wernicke's receptive (fluent) dysphasia
  global see Global dysphasia
  mixed 10
  nominal see Nominal dysphasia
  receptive see Receptive dysphasia
  see also specific types
Dysphonia 91–92
  assessment 8–9
  causes 92f
  definition 89
Dystonia 98f, 99–101
  cervical 100
  classification 99–100
  dopa-responsive 100
  early-onset generalized 100
  focal 99–100
  generalized 99–100
  multifocal 99–100
  oromandibular 100
  paroxysmal 101
  primary 100
  primary focal 98f
  primary generalized 98f

  secondary 98f, 100–101
  segmental 99–100
  tardive 100–101
  toxins 248f
  tremor 99
Dystonia-plus syndromes 98f, 100
Dystrophia myotonica 111
Dystrophia myotonica (myotonic dystrophy) 196–197, 196f

E

Early-onset generalized dystonia 100
ECG see Electrocardiogram (ECG)
Echocardiography, stroke/TIAs 208
EEG see Electroencephalography (EEG)
EIA (enzyme immunosorbent assay), syphilis diagnosis 230
Eighth cranial nerve. see Vestibulocochlear nerve (cranial nerve VIII)
Electrocardiogram (ECG)
  primary cardiac dysfunction 40–41
  transient loss of consciousness 42
Electroencephalography (EEG) 25
  abnormal rhythms 28f
  dementia 127
  encephalitis 227
  epilepsy diagnosis 134–135
  normal rhythms 28f
  transient loss of consciousness 42
Electrolyte myopathies, acquired 195f, 198
Electrolytes
  imbalances of 244
  tests 27f
Electromyography (EMG) 25–29
  abnormalities 29f
  Lambert–Eaton myasthenic syndrome 191–192
  motor neuron disease diagnosis 171
  myasthenia gravis 191
  myopathies 194
  peripheral neuropathies 179
Electrophysiology, ulnar nerve compression 181
Eleventh cranial nerve see Accessory nerve (cranial nerve XI)
EMG see Electromyography (EMG)
Emotional disturbances
  affect evaluation 7
  temporal lobe lesions 36
Encephalitis 226–228
  aetiology 226, 227, 227f
  clinical features 227
  definition 226
  diagnosis 227
  incidence 226
  prognosis 228
  subacute-onset headache 51f
  treatment 227

Encephalopathy
  definition 226
  toxins 248f
Endocrine disorders 243–244
  see also specific diseases/disorders
Endocrine myopathies, acquired 195f,
  198
Endolymphatic duct 82f
Endolymphatic sac 82f
Endoneurium 178f
Entacapone 148
Enteroviruses, viral meningitis 224
Entrapment neuropathies 180–181
Environment, Parkinson's disease 145
Enzyme immunosorbent assay (EIA),
  syphilis diagnosis 230
Eosinophils 26f
Ependymoma 215
Epidural haemorrhage, spinal cord
  compression 164
Epilepsy 131–138
  aetiology 131–133
    degenerative diseases 132
    family history 131–132
    hypoxia 132
    infections 132
    inflammation 132
    intracranial tumours 132
    metabolic causes 132
    perinatal factors 132
    photosensitivity 132
    prenatal factors 132
    sleep deprivation 133
    surgery 132
    toxic causes 132
    trauma 132
    vascular causes 132
  clinical features 133–134, 133f
  definitions 131
  differential diagnosis 135
  driving 138
  drug treatments 135–137
    see also Anti-epileptic drugs
  epidemiology 131
  history taking 134–135
  investigations 134–135
  mortality 137–138
  myoclonic 102
  neurosurgery 137
  progressive myoclonic 102
Epileptic seizures 131
Epineurium 178f
Episodic headache, recurrent see Recurrent
  episodic headache
Episodic painful brachial neuropathy
  175–176
EPs see Evoked potentials (EPs)
Erythrocyte sedimentation rate (ESR)
  26f
  giant-cell arteritis (temporal arteritis)
  142

ESR see Erythrocyte sedimentation rate
  (ESR)
Essential tremor 99
Euphoria, affect evaluation 7
Eustachian tube 82f
Evoked potentials (EPs) 29
  multiple sclerosis 240
  somatosensory 240
Exertional headache 50f, 52f
Expressive dysphasia 10f
  Broca's area lesion 9–10
  frontal lobe lesions 34
Extensor plantar responses, UMN limb
  weakness 105
External auditory canal 82f
External carotid artery 204f
Extradural haematoma 210
Extradural haemorrhage 210–211
Extradural tumours, spinal cord
  compression 164
Extraocular muscle dysfunction,
  binocular diplopia 68
Extrapyramidal rigidity 19
Eyelids, assessment 12, 14f
Eye movements 63–74
  assessment 13–15
  coma 45–46
  conjugate see Conjugate eye
    movements
  disorders 66–74
    supranuclear lesions 71–72
    see also specific diseases/disorders
  muscles 67, 68f
  pursuit 13, 14
  saccadic see Saccadic eye movements
Eye position
  bilateral fixed, coma 45
  coma 45
  resting 45

F

Facial nerve (cranial nerve VII) 78–79
  anatomy 78, 78f
  assessment 16
  headache 49
  lesions 154f, 156–157, 156f
  LMN facial weakness 78
  UMN facial weakness 78
Facial sensory loss 75–80
  brainstem lesions 76–77
  cavernous sinus lesions 77, 77f
  cerebellopontine angle lesions 77
  differential diagnosis 75–77
  supranuclear lesions 76
Facial weakness
  differential diagnosis 79, 79f
  LMN 78
  UMN 78
Factor 5 Leiden 26f

Fainting (vasovagal syncope) 39
Familiar object naming, dysphasia
  assessment 9
Family history
  epilepsy 131–132
  history taking 4
  stroke 203
Fasciculation potentials,
  electromyography 28–29
Fasciculations
  LMN limb weakness 108
  motor system assessment 18
Fatigue, multiple sclerosis 241f
FBC (full blood count) 26f
FIA-abs (fluorescent treponema
  antibody absorbed), syphilis
  diagnosis 230
Fibrillation potentials,
  electromyography 28
Fifth cranial nerve see Trigeminal nerve
  (cranial nerve V)
Finger–nose test 23
Fingolimod 240–241
First cranial nerve see Olfactory nerve
  (cranial nerve I)
Flaccid paraparesis 107
Flexor plantar response, LMN limb
  weakness 108
Flocculonodular lobe
  cerebellum 93
  lesions 95
Fluent dysphasia see Wernicke's
  receptive (fluent) dysphasia
Fluorescent treponema antibody
  absorbed (FIA-abs), syphilis
  diagnosis 230
Focal damage, cerebral hemispheres 33
Focal dystonia 99–100
  primary 98f
Focal neurological signs
  intracranial tumours 218
  LMN limb weakness 108
Focal seizures 34
Focal syndromes 98f
Folate 26f
Foramen magnum 160f
Fourth cranial nerve see Trochlear nerve
  (cranial nerve IV)
Friedreich's ataxia 253
Frontal eye field, frontal lobes 33
Frontal lobes 33–35, 34f
  blood supply 33
  lesions 33–35, 37f
  normal function 33
Frontal lobe, seizures 133f
Frontotemporal dementia (FTD) 169
Frontotemporal lobar dementia (FTLD)
  129
FTD (frontotemporal dementia) 169
FTLD (frontotemporal lobar dementia)
  129

Full blood count (FBC) 26f
Functional gait 121
Functional seizures, epilepsy vs. 135
Fundoscopy
    coma 46
    optic nerve assessment 12, 13f
Fungal meningitis 224

G

'Gag' reflex 17
Gait 119–122
    antalgic 121
    apraxic 121
        frontal lobe lesions 33
    assessment 119
    ataxic 93
    causes 120–121
    coordination 23
    functional 121
    hemiparetic 120
    myopathic 121
    neurological examination 10
    Parkinsonian 120
    spastic 120
    steppage 120–121
    vestibular nerve lesions 85
    vestibular system disorders 84
        see also specific types of gait
Galantamine 128
Ganglion cells 57
Gastrointestinal disorders 244–245
        see also specific diseases/disorders
Gaze
    horizontal 67, 67f
    pursuit 66
GCS (Glasgow Coma Scale) 42, 43f
Gene mutations, Parkinson's disease
        145
Generalized dystonia 99–100
    primary 98f
Generalized seizures 134
    investigations 134
    secondary 134
Generalized tonic-clonic seizures 134
General paralysis of the insane 230
Genetic counselling
    Duchenne muscular dystrophy 195
    hereditary conditions 251
Genetic testing
    dementia 127
    myopathies 195
Gerstmann's syndrome 36
Giant-cell arteritis (temporal arteritis)
        142–143, 246f
    subacute-onset headache 51f
Gilles de la Tourette syndrome 102
Glasgow Coma Scale (GCS) 42, 43f
Glatiramir acetate 240
Glaucoma, acute 51f

Glioblastoma multiforme 215
Gliomas 215
Global dysphasia 10f, 37
    causes 10
Global weakness 104
Glossopharyngeal nerve (cranial
        nerve IX)
    assessment 17
    headache 49
    lesions 154f, 158
Glove-and-stocking distribution,
        polyneuropathies 179
Glucose 27f
Gower's sign 195, 196f
Gram stain, CSF in meningitis 225
Grave's disease 243
Guanethidine hydrochloride 192
Guillain–Barré syndrome
        (postinfectious polyneuropathy)
        184–185
    HIV infection 232

H

HAD (HIV-associated dementia) 231
Haemangioblastomas 216
Haematological disorders 244
        see also specific diseases/disorders
Haematological tests 26f
Haematoma
    extradural 210
    spinal cord compression 164
    subdural see Subdural haematoma
Haemoglobin testing 26f
Haemorrhage(s)
    cerebellar dysfunction 95f
    epidural, spinal cord compression
        164
    extradural 210–211
    intracerebral see Intracerebral
        haemorrhage
    intracranial see Intracranial
        haemorrhage (haemorrhagic
        stroke)
    subarachnoid see Subarachnoid
        haemorrhage
    subdural 210–211
Haemorrhagic stroke see Intracranial
        haemorrhage (haemorrhagic
        stroke)
Hallpike manoeuvre 85f, 86
Hallucinations
    olfactory see Olfactory hallucinations
    Parkinson's disease treatment 148
Handedness, dysphasia assessment 9
Handwriting, Parkinson's disease,
        146
Harlequin syndrome 117
Headaches 49–52, 139–144
    acute-onset see Acute-onset headaches

analgesic overdose see Analgesic
        overdose headache
    assessment 49
    benign coital 50f
    chronic cluster 50f
    chronic daily see Chronic daily
        headache
    classification 49
    cluster see Cluster headache
    cough 50f
    examination 52
    exertional 50f, 52f
    history-taking 51–52
    hypnic 50f
    low CSF volume 141–142
    new daily persistent 49
    non-neurological causes 142–143
    post-traumatic 51f
    progressive 50
    raised intracranial pressure 141
    recurrent episodic see Recurrent
        episodic headache
    referred pain 49, 50f
    secondary 50f
    subacute-onset see Subacute-onset
        headache
    tension-type see Tension-type
        headache
        see also specific headaches;
        specific types of headache
Head trauma
    cochlea 83
    coma 45
Hearing
    loss see Deafness
    vestibular nerve lesions 85
    vestibular system disorders 84
    vestibulocochlear nerve assessment
        17
Heel–shin test 17
Hemianopia 59
Hemidystonia 99–100
Hemiparesis 105, 106f
Hemiparetic gait 120
Hemiplegic migraine 140
Hepatic encephalopathy 245
Hepatolenticular degeneration
        (Wilson's disease) 150, 254
Hereditary conditions 251–254
    ataxias 253
    genetic counselling 251
    neurocutaneous syndromes 251–252
    peripheral neuropathies 186, 187f
        see also specific diseases/disorders
Hereditary myopathies 195–197, 195f
Hereditary neuropathy with liability to
        pressure palsies (HNPP)
        175–176
Herniation
    intracranial tumours 217, 218f
    raised intracranial pressure 141, 142f

Herpes simplex virus (HSV), viral
    meningitis 224
Herpes zoster, trigeminal nerve lesions
    77
Higher cerebral functions
    disorders 31–38
        see also specific diseases/disorders
    neurological examination 7–8
History taking 1–6
    drug history 4
    family history 4
    past medical history 4
    presenting complaint 3–5
    presenting complaint history 3–4
    review of systems 4
    social history 4–5
HIV-associated dementia (HAD) 231
HIV-associated mild neurocognitive
    disorder 231
HIV infection 231–232, 231*f*
    dementia 231–232
    encephalopathy 231
    myopathy 232
    peripheral neuropathies 185–186,
        232
    spinal cord inflammation 164
    viral meningitis 224
HNPP (hereditary neuropathy with
    liability to pressure palsies)
    175–176
Hodgkin lymphoma 244
Holmes–Adie pupil 66
Holter monitoring, stroke/TIAs 208
Homonymous hemianopia 62
Horizontal gaze 67, 67*f*
Horizontal gaze palsy 71
Horner's syndrome 14*f*
    causes 65*f*
    small constricted (miotic) pupil 65
HSV (herpes simplex virus), viral
    meningitis 224
HTLV-1 (human T-cell lymphocytic
    virus type 1) infection 164
Human T-cell lymphocytic virus type 1
    (HTLV-1) infection 164
Huntington's disease (Huntington's
    chorea) 101
Hydrocephalus, acute 51*f*
5-Hydroxytryptamine (5-HT), migraine
    139
Hyperglycaemia, diabetes mellitus 243
Hyperkalaemic periodic paralyses 197
Hyperkinetic disorders 97
Hyperlipidaemia, stroke 202
Hyperosmia 54
    definition 54
Hypertension
    idiopathic intracranial 51*f*
    management 208
    stroke 202
Hyperthyroidism 243

Hypertropia 67
Hyperventilation 41
Hypnic headache 50*f*
Hypoglossal nerve (cranial nerve XII)
    assessment 17–18
    lesions 154*f*, 158
Hypoglycaemia 41
    diabetes mellitus 243
    epilepsy *vs.* 135
Hypokalaemia, myopathies 198
Hypokalaemic periodic paralyses 197
Hypokinesia 145
    Parkinson's disease 146
Hypopituitarism 244
Hyposmia 53
    definition 54
    olfactory nerve lesions 153
Hypotension, postural 40, 86
Hypothyroidism 243
Hypotonia, cerebellar dysfunction
    94–95
Hypotropia 67
Hypoxia, epilepsy causes 132

Iatrogenic Creutzfeldt–Jakob disease
    234–235
Iatrogenic mydriasis 66
IBD (inflammatory bowel disease)
    244–245
ICES (International Classification of
    Epileptic Seizures) 131, 132*f*
Ictus 131
Ideational apraxia, bilateral 36
Ideomotor apraxia, bilateral 36
Idiopathic intracranial hypertension
    51*f*
Idiosyncratic toxicity, antiepileptic
    drugs 136
Imaging 29–30
    dementia 127
    meningitis 225
    stroke/TIAs 207–208
        see also specific methods
Immunocompromised patients,
    cerebral abscesses 228
Immunological tests 27*f*
Immunomodulation, multiple sclerosis
    management 240–241
Immunosuppressive drugs
    myasthenia gravis management 191
    polymyositis/dermatomyositis 198
Inborn errors of metabolism,
    253–254
Inclusion body myositis 198
Incontinence, frontal lobe lesions 35
Incus 82*f*
Indian-ink stain, CSF in meningitis 225
Infarction, cerebellar dysfunction 95*f*
Infections 223–236

cerebellar dysfunction 95*f*
cochlea 83
dementia *vs.* 125
epilepsy causes 132
intracranial tumours 220
peripheral neuropathies 185–186,
    187*f*
spinal column 164
    see also specific diseases/disorders
Inferior oblique muscles 67
Inferior recti muscle 67
Inflammation
    epilepsy causes 132
    optic neuropathy 60*f*
Inflammatory bowel disease (IBD)
    244–245
Inflammatory disorders
    dementia *vs.* 125
    myopathies 197–198
    peripheral neuropathies 187*f*
    spastic paraparesis 107*f*
Inflammatory lesions, spinal cord
    compression 164
Inner ear anatomy 82*f*
INO *see* Internuclear ophthalmoplegia
    (INO)
Inspection, motor system assessment 18
Intention tremor (cerebellar tremor) 99
    cerebellar dysfunction 93
Interferon-β 240
Internal carotid artery 58, 58*f*, 203*f*,
    204*f*
    cavernous sinus 77*f*
International Classification of Epileptic
    Seizures (ICES) 131, 132*f*
Internuclear ophthalmoplegia (INO)
    67*f*
    causes 70
Intracerebral haemorrhage
    primary 207
    stroke 202
Intracranial abscess, subacute-onset
    headache 51*f*
Intracranial haemorrhage
    (haemorrhagic stroke) 52*f*, 201,
    209–211
    subarachnoid haemorrhage
        209–210
Intracranial hypertension, idiopathic
    51*f*
Intracranial tumours 215–222
    clinical features 216–218
        focal neurological signs 218
        herniation 217, 218*f*
        raised intracranial tumours
            217–218
        seizures 218
    epilepsy causes 132
    investigations 218–219
    neurological complications
        220–221, 220*f*

prognosis 219
relative frequencies 216f
subacute-onset headache 51f
treatment 219
types 215–216
Intradural tumours, spinal cord
compression 164
Intramedullary spinal arteriovenous
malformations 165
Intramedullary tumours, spinal cord
compression 163
Intravenous immunoglobulin (IvIg)
191
Intrinsic lesions, spinal cord diseases
166–167, 166f
Investigations 25–30
biochemical tests 27f
coma 46–47
immunological tests 27f
microbiology 28f
neurophysiological 25–29
transient loss of consciousness 42
see also specific investigations
Involuntary movements 18
Ipsilateral temporal fibres, light
stimulation path 57
Iris disorders 66
Ischaemic stroke (cerebral infarction)
201
IvIg (intravenous immunoglobulin)
191

J

Jarisch–Herxheimer reactions 231
Jaw jerk 76
trigeminal nerve assessment 15
Jerky nystagmus 72
Jerky pursuit 93
Jo-1 antibodies 27f
Joint-position sense assessment 24
Jugular foramen syndrome 158

K

Kennedy's disease, motor neuron
disease vs. 171
Kinetic tremor 97, 98f, 99

L

Lacunar stroke 206
Lambert–Eaton myasthenic syndrome
(LEMS) 191–192
Language
Mini-Mental State Examination 8, 8f
parietal lobes 35
production 9–10
Large dilated (mydriatic) pupils 66
Large posterior lobe, cerebellum 93

Lateral cervical disc protrusion 174
Lateral cutaneous nerve of the thigh
(Meralgia paraesthetica) 181,
183f
Lateral geniculate nucleus (LGN)
blood supply 58f
light stimulation path 57, 58
Lateral lumbar disc protrusion
174–175, 174f
Lateral medullary syndrome 206–207,
206f
Lateral recti muscle 67
Lateral semicircular canal 82f
L-dopa 147–148
Legs
coordination 23
motor system assessment 19, 21f
LEMS (Lambert–Eaton myasthenic
syndrome) 191–192
Lens opacities, toxins 248f
Leptomeningeal metastases, intracranial
tumours 220
Leucodystrophies 241
Leukaemia 244
meningeal 244
Levator palpebrae superioris muscle 189
Levodopa (L-dopa) 147–148
Lewy bodies, Parkinson's disease 145
LFTs (liver function tests) 27f
LGN see Lateral geniculate nucleus
(LGN)
Lhermite's syndrome, multiple sclerosis
239
Light responses, pupil assessment 12–13
Light touch, assessment 24
Limb(s)
LMN pathway 103
movement in coma 46
muscle pathway 103–104
neuroanatomy 103–104
neuromuscular junction pathway
103–104
position in coma 46
sensory symptoms see Limb sensory
symptoms
UMN pathway 103, 104f
weakness see Limb weakness
see also Arms; Legs
Limbic system, temporal lobes 36
Limb sensory symptoms 113–118
dorsal (posterior) column pathway
113
dorsal root lesions 115, 115f
peripheral nerve lesions 114–115
spinal cord lesions 115–117, 116f
spinal nerve root lesions 115, 115f
spinothalamic pathway 113, 114f
syndromes 114–118
see also specific diseases/disorders
trophic skin changes 113–114
ulcers 113–114

Limb weakness 103–112
anatomical sites 104f
LMN syndrome 108–110
LMN weakness 107–108, 111f
myopathy 110–111
neuromuscular junction disorders
110
terminology 104
UMN syndrome 105–107
UMN weakness 104–105
see also specific diseases/disorders
Lipohyalinosis, stroke 202
Liver enzyme tests 27f
Liver function tests (LFTs) 27f
Locked-in syndrome 207
coma vs. 43
Loss of interest, affect evaluation 7
Loss of sight see Visual impairment
Lower-limb parkinsonism 150
Lower motor neuron (LMN) lesions
170f
dysarthria 9, 90
limb weakness 21f
Lower motor neuron (LMN) pathway
103
lesions see above
limb weakness 107–108
Lumbar disc protrusion
central 175
lateral 174–175, 174f
Lumbar plexus 173
Lumbar puncture, dementia 127
Lumbosacral plexopathy 110, 110f,
176
Lumbosacral plexus 110f, 173
Lyme disease 233–234
peripheral neuropathies 185–186
Lymphocyte counts 26f
Lymphoma, primary central nervous
system see Primary central
nervous system lymphoma

M

Macula 57
Magnetic resonance angiography
(MRA), stroke/TIAs 207–208
Magnetic resonance imaging (MRI)
29–30
dementia 127
encephalitis 227
epilepsy diagnosis 135
intracranial tumours 218–219
lateral cervical disc protrusion 174
lateral lumbar disc protrusion 175
multiple sclerosis 239
myopathies 195
perfusion techniques 219
stroke/TIAs 207
transient loss of consciousness 42

Magnetic resonance spectroscopy (MRS), intracranial tumours 219

Malignancies *see* Tumours

Malleus 82*f*

MAOIs (monoamine oxidase inhibitors) 148

Mastoid air cavities 82*f*

Maxillary nerve 77*f*

MCA *see* Middle cerebral artery (MCA)

McDonald criteria, multiple sclerosis diagnosis 240

MCV (mean cell volume) 26*f*

Mean cell volume (MCV) 26*f*

Medial recti muscle 67

Medical Research Council (MRC), power testing 19, 19*f*, 20*f*, 21*f*

Medication-induced parkinsonism 150

Medications
  cochlea 83
  small constricted (miotic) pupil 65

Medulla
  anatomy 94*f*
  lesions 117, 117*f*

Medulla oblongata 159

Memantine 128

Memory impairment, temporal lobe lesions 36

Ménière's disease 84, 157–158
  cochlea 83

Meningeal leukaemia 244

Meningiomas 215

Meningitis 223–226
  bacterial 223, 224*f*
  causative agents 223
  chemoprophylaxis 226
  clinical features 223–224
  community-acquired 226
  complications 225–226
  diagnosis 224–225
  infection control 226
  notification 226
  subacute-onset headache 51*f*
  treatment 226
    see also specific types

Meningoencephalitis 226

Meningovascular syphilis 230

Mental state, neurological examination 7–8

Meralgia paraesthetica 181, 183*f*

Metabolic disease
  dementia *vs.* 125
  epilepsy causes 132
  peripheral neuropathies 187*f*
  spastic paraparesis 107*f*
  spinal cord diseases 165–166
    see also specific diseases/disorders

Metabolic encephalopathies 254*f*

Metabolic myopathies 195*f*, 197

Metabolic storage diseases 254*f*
    see also specific diseases/disorders

Metastatic tumours 216
  intracranial tumours 220

Microbiological tests 28*f*

Micrographia, Parkinson's disease 146

Micturition syncope 40

Midbrain
  anatomy 94*f*
  cross-section 146*f*
  lesions 118

Middle cerebral artery (MCA) 58, 203*f*, 205*f*
  distribution 204*f*
  frontal lobes 33
  occlusion 203–204, 204*f*, 205*f*
  parietal lobes 35
  temporal lobes 36

Middle ear
  anatomy 82*f*
  trauma, deafness/tinnitus 83*f*

Midline vermis lesions 95

Migraine 139–140
  basilar 140
  causes 50*f*, 52*f*
  chronic 50*f*
  classical *see* Migraine with aura (classical migraine)
  common 140
  epilepsy *vs.* 135
  hemiplegic 140
  management 140
  prophylaxis 140
  without aura 139

Migraine with aura (classical migraine) 139, 140
  differential diagnosis 61

Miller–Fisher syndrome 184

Mini-mental State Examination 7–8, 8*f*

Miotic pupil 65

Mitochondrial myopathies 194, 197

Mitoxantrone 240

Mixed dysphasia 10

Mixed tremor 99

MND *see* Motor neuron disease (MND)

Monoamine oxidase inhibitors (MAOIs) 148

Monocular diplopia 68

Monocular visual field defects 59

Monocular visual impairment 61

Mononeuritis, HIV infection 232

Mononeuritis multiplex *see* Multifocal neuropathy (mononeuritis multiplex)

Mononeuropathies
  compression 243
  definition 177
  motor syndromes 110
  multiple *see* Multiple mononeuropathies
  peripheral neuropathies 180–182
  sensory syndromes 114–115, 115*f*

Monoparesis 106*f*, 107

Mood, history taking 3

Motor function
  facial nerve assessment 16
  glossopharyngeal nerve assessment 17
  trigeminal nerve 76
  trigeminal nerve assessment 15
  vagus nerve assessment 17

Motor neuron disease (MND) 169–172
  clinical features 169–170
  diagnosis 171
  differential diagnosis 171
  drug treatment 171
  pathogenesis 170
  symptomatic treatment 172
  treatment 171–172
  types 169–170
    see also specific diseases/disorders

Motor neuropathy
  multifocal 185
  painful proximal asymmetrical 243

Motor pathways, spinal cord 160

Motor system assessment 18–23
  arms 18–19, 20*f*, 21*f*
  coordination 19–23
  inspection 18
  legs 19, 21*f*
  power 19
  reflexes 19, 22*f*, 23*f*
  tone 18–19

Movement disorders 97–102, 98*f*
  classification 97
  hyperkinetic disorders 97–99, 101
  neuroleptic-induced 150–151
    see also specific diseases/disorders

Movement incoordination, cerebellar dysfunction 93

Movements, involuntary 18

MRA (magnetic resonance angiography), stroke/TIAs 207–208

MRI *see* Magnetic resonance imaging (MRI)

MRS (magnetic resonance spectroscopy), intracranial tumours 219

MSA *see* Multiple system atrophy (MSA)

Multifocal dystonia 99–100

Multifocal motor neuropathy 185

Multifocal neuropathies, diabetes mellitus 243

Multifocal neuropathy (mononeuritis multiplex) 181–182
  definition 177
  diabetes mellitus 243
  HIV infection 232

Multiple mononeuropathies
  motor syndromes 110
  sensory syndromes 115

Multiple sclerosis 165, 237–242
  clinical features 237–239, 238*f*

brainstem 239
cerebellum 95f, 239
cognitive defects 239
myelopathy 239
optic neuritis 238–239
retrobulbar neuritis 238–239
spinal cord lesions 239
diagnosis 240
differential diagnosis 239
motor neuron disease vs. 171
epidemiology 237
investigations 239–240
life expectancy 238
management 240–241
pathogenesis 237
pathology 237
primary progressive 238
relapsing and remitting 237
secondary progressive 237
symptomatic treatment 241f
Multiple system atrophy (MSA) 149
cerebellar dysfunction 95f
Muscle(s)
anatomy 193, 194f
eye movements 67, 68f
see also specific muscles
Muscle biopsy, polymyositis/
dermatomyositis 198
Muscle bulk, myopathies 193
Muscle lesions
dysarthria 9
limb weakness 21f
Muscle pathway, limbs 103–104
Muscle tone, myopathies 193
Muscle wasting, motor system
assessment 18
Muscular disorders see Myopathies
Muscular dystrophies 195–196
see also specific types
Myasthenia gravis 110, 189–191
causes 189
clinical features 189–190, 190f
congenital 192
electromyography 29f
epidemiology 189
investigations 190–191
management 191
neonatal 192
ptosis 14f
Myasthenia, penicillamine-induced 192
Mydriasis, iatrogenic 66
Mydriatic pupils 66
Myelitis, transverse 165
Myelography 30
lateral lumbar disc protrusion 175
Myelopathies
multiple sclerosis 239
toxins 248f
Myoclonic epilepsy 102
progressive 102
Myoclonic seizures 134

Myoclonus 98f, 102
Myopathic gait 121
Myopathies 193–200
acquired 195f
acquired electrolyte 195f, 198
acquired endocrine 195f, 198
autosomal dominant 194
autosomal recessive 194
clinical features 193–194
critical illness 199
definition 103
drug-induced 199
dysarthria 91
electromyography 29f
hereditary 195–197, 195f
HIV infection 232
inflammatory 197–198
investigations 194–195
limb weakness 110–111
LMN limb weakness 108
metabolic 195f, 197
mitochondrial 194, 197
paraneoplastic 199
periodic paralyses 197
ptosis 14f
toxins 248f
X-linked 194
see also specific diseases/disorders
Myotonia, myopathies 193–194
Myotonic dystrophy (dystrophia
myotonica) 196–197, 196f
Myxoedema, cerebellar dysfunction 95f

N

Narcolepsy 41
Natalizumab 240
Neck stiffness, coma 45
Neocerebellum 93
Neonatal myasthenia gravis 192
Neoplasms see Tumours
Nerve conduction studies 25, 29
abnormalities 29f
peripheral neuropathies 179
Nerve sheath tumours 216
Neuralgic amyotrophy 175–176
Neurodegenerative conditions
cerebellar dysfunction 95f
dementia vs. 125
secondary dystonia 101
see also specific diseases/disorders
Neurodegenerative dementia, primary
128–130
Neurofibrillary tangles, Alzheimer's
disease 128
Neurofibromas 216
Neurofibromatosis 251
type 1 (von Recklinghausen's disease)
251–252, 252f
type 2 252

Neurogenic claudication 175
Neuroleptic-induced movement
disorders 150–151
Neuroleptic malignant syndrome 151
Neuroleptic medication 127
Neurological examination 7–24
affect 7
appearance 7
behaviour 7
cognitive function 7–8
consciousness 7
cranial nerves see specific nerves
gait 10
general examination 24
higher cerebral functions 7–8
mental state 7–8
motor system see Motor system
assessment
sensory system 23–24
speech see Speech assessment
Neurological symptoms, history taking
3
Neurological syphilis 230–231
Neuromuscular blockade, toxins 248f
Neuromuscular junction 189, 190f
Neuromuscular junction disorders
189–192
binocular diplopia 68
dysarthria 91
lesions see below
limb weakness 110
LMN limb weakness 108
see also specific diseases/disorders
Neuromuscular junction lesions
dysarthria 9
limb weakness 21f
Neuromuscular junction pathway,
limbs 103–104
Neuro-oncology 215–222
see also Tumours; specific diseases/
disorders
Neuropathic tremor 99
Neuropathies
definition 177
demyelinating, nerve conduction
studies 29f
entrapment 180–181
episodic painful brachial 175–176
multifocal see Multifocal neuropathy
(mononeuritis multiplex)
peripheral see Peripheral
neuropathies
Neurophysiological investigations
25–29
Neuropsychology, dementia 127
Neurosurgery, epilepsy 137
Neurosyphilis, asymptomatic 230
Neutrophils, counts 26f
New daily persistent headache 49
Nicotinic acid (vitamin B$_3$) deficiency
248

Nimodipine 210
Ninth cranial nerve *see* Glossopharyngeal nerve (cranial nerve IX)
Nodes of Ranvier 177
Nominal dysphasia 10*f*, 37
  causes 10
Non-atherosclerotic diseases, stroke 202
Non-convulsive status epilepticus, coma *vs.* 42
Non-epileptic seizures 42
  epilepsy *vs.* 135
Non-Hodgkin's lymphoma 215–216, 244
Numeracy, parietal lobes 35
Nutritional deficiencies
  optic neuropathy 60*f*
  peripheral neuropathies 185–186, 187*f*
  spastic paraparesis 107*f*
  see also Vitamin deficiency
Nystagmoid jerks 72
Nystagmus 15, 72–74
  asymmetrical 73
  causes 15*f*
  central 73
  cerebellar dysfunction 93
  congenital 72
  differential diagnosis 85*f*
  jerky 72
  optokinetic 73
  pathological 73–74
  pendular 72
  peripheral 73–74
  physiological 72–73
  vertical 73
  vestibular nerve lesions 85
  vestibular system disorders 84

O

Obesity, stroke 203
Obtundation, consciousness evaluation 7
Occipital cortex
  lesions 60
  light stimulation path 58
Occipital lobes 34*f*, 37–38
  blood supply 37
  function 37
  lesions 37*f*, 38
Occipital lobe, seizures 133*f*
Ocular bobbing 73
Ocular nerve palsy 15
  combined 155, 155*f*
Oculocephalic reflex (doll's eye movements) 14–15
  coma 45, 45*f*
Oculomotor nerve (cranial nerve III)
  anatomy 69*f*

assessment 12–15
  cavernous sinus 77*f*
  lesions 66, 70*f*, 154–155, 154*f*
    binocular diplopia 69
  palsy 14*f*
Oculovestibular reflex, coma 45*f*, 46
Oedema, cerebral 219
Old age, small constricted (miotic) pupil 65
Olfactory hallucinations 54
  definition 54
Olfactory nerve (cranial nerve I)
  anatomy 54*f*
  assessment 10
  lesions 153, 154*f*
Oligodendrogliomas 215
One-and-a-half syndrome 71
Onset
  history taking 3
  myopathies 194
Ophthalmic artery 58, 58*f*, 204*f*
Ophthalmic nerve 77*f*
Optic atrophy 62
  optic nerve lesions 154
Optic chiasm 58*f*, 203*f*
  anatomy 59*f*
  blood supply 58*f*
  lesions 58*f*, 60
  light stimulation path 57
Optic disc, fundoscopy 13*f*
Optic nerve (cranial nerve II) 203*f*
  assessment 11–12
  blood supply 58*f*
  ischaemia 62
  lesions 58*f*, 59, 60*f*, 153–154, 154*f*
  light stimulation path 57, 58*f*
Optic neuritis 60*f*, 62
  multiple sclerosis 238–239
  optic nerve lesions 153, 154*f*
Optic neuropathy
  causes 60*f*
  toxins 248*f*
Optic tract
  blood supply 58*f*
  lesions 60
Optokinetic nystagmus 73
Oral acetylcholinesterases 191
Oral contraceptives, stroke 203
Organ of Corti 81
Orientation, Mini-Mental State Examination 7, 8*f*
Oromandibular dystonia 100
Oropharyngeal lesions 91
Osteomyelitis 164
Ototoxicity 248*f*
Outer ear, anatomy 82*f*
Oval window 82*f*
Oxygen therapy, cluster headache, 141

P

Pain
  assessment 23–24
  craniofacial 139–144
  LMN limb weakness 108
  multiple sclerosis 241*f*
  myopathies 194
  referred, headache 49, 50*f*
  spinal cord pathways 159
Painful proximal asymmetrical motor neuropathy, diabetes mellitus 243
Palatal movement assessment 17
Palsy
  progressive supranuclear 149
  pseudobulbar *see* Pseudobulbar palsy
  Saturday-night 180
Pancoast tumour 176
Papilloedema
  differential diagnosis 61
  optic nerve lesions 153, 154*f*
Paraesthesia (pins and needles) 178
Paralysis 104
Paralytic poliomyelitis 232
Paraneoplastic myopathies 199
Paraneoplastic polyneuropathy 183
Paraparesis 106–107, 107*f*, 160–161, 161*f*
  flaccid 107
  spastic *see* Spastic paraparesis
Paraplegia 160–161
Parapontine reticular formation (PPRF) 66–67
Parasagittal brain lesions 107*f*
Parasagittal meningioma 106–107
Parasympathetic pathway, pupillary reflexes 63, 64*f*
Parietal lobes 34*f*, 35–36
  blood supply 35
  functions 35
  lesions 37*f*
    limb sensory symptoms 117*f*, 118
  lesion symptoms 35
  syndromes 35–36
Parietal lobe, seizures 133*f*
Parkinsonian gait 120
Parkinsonian tremor 97
Parkinsonism
  differential diagnosis 148
  lower-limb 150
  medication-induced 150
  toxins 248*f*
Parkinson's disease 145–149
  aetiology 145
  atypical disorders 149
    see also specific diseases/disorders
  clinical features 146–147
    akinesia 146
    bradykinesia 146
    cognitive features 147

dysarthria 90
  handwriting 146
  hypokinesia 146
  micrographia 146
  non-motor features 147
  posture 147, 147f
  psychiatric features 147
  rigidity 146, 146f
  speech alterations 146
  tremor 146
 differential diagnosis 148–149
 investigations 147
 natural history 147
 pathology 145, 146f
 treatment 147–148
  confusion 148
  hallucinations 148
  psychosis 148
  surgery 148
Paroxysmal dystonia 101
Partial seizures 133, 133f
 simple 133
Past medical history, history taking 4
Pathological nystagmus 73–74
Pathological tremor 97
PCA see Posterior cerebral artery (PCA)
PCR see Polymerase chain reaction (PCR)
Pendular nystagmus 72
Penicillamine-induced myasthenia 192
Pergolide 148
Perilymph 82f
Perimetry, assessment 12
Perinatal factors, epilepsy 132
Perineurium 178f
Periodic paralyses, myopathies 197
Peripheral nerve(s)
 anatomy 177, 178f
 compression 180–181
 functions 177
 lesions in diabetes mellitus 243
Peripheral neuropathies 110, 177–188,
  187f
 autonomic symptoms 179
 definitions 177–188
 drugs 184
 hereditary diseases 186
 HIV infection 232
 infections 185–186
 inflammatory demyelinating
  184–185
 investigations 179
 LMN limb weakness 108
 mononeuropathies 180–182
 motor symptoms 179
 nutritional deficiencies 185–186
 polyneuropathies 183–186
 sensory symptoms 178–179
 skeletal symptoms 179
 symptoms 178–179
 toxins 184, 248f
 see also specific diseases/disorders

Peripheral nystagmus 73–74
Peripheral visual field assessment
  11–12
Persistent vegetative state, coma vs. 43
Personality changes, frontal lobe
  lesions 34
Pes cavus 186
PET (positron emission tomography),
  intracranial tumours 219
Phonation 91–92
 speech assessment 8–9
Photosensitivity, epilepsy causes 132
Physiological anisocoria 65
Physiological nystagmus 72–73
Physiological tremor 97, 99
Pinna 82f
Pin-point pupils, coma 45
Pins and needles (paraesthesia) 178
Pituitary gland disorders 244
 tumours 216, 244
Plain radiography 29
Plasma cell dyscrasias 244
Plasmapheresis 191
Platelet count 26f
Plexopathies 109, 175–176
 definition 103, 173
 LMN limb weakness 108
PLS (primary lateral sclerosis) 169,
  170
PMA see Progressive muscular atrophy
  (PMA)
PMA (primary muscular atrophy) 169
PML see Progressive multifocal
  leucoencephalopathy (PML)
Poliomyelitis 232–233
 paralytic 232
Polyarteritis nodosa 246f
Polymerase chain reaction (PCR)
 encephalitis 227
 meningitis 225
Polymyositis 197–198
 HIV infection 232
Polyneuropathies
 critical illness 186
 definition 177
 distal symmetrical see Distal
  symmetrical polyneuropathy
 glove-and-stocking distribution 179
 motor syndromes 110
 paraneoplastic 183
 peripheral neuropathies 183–186
 postinfectious see Guillain–Barré
  syndrome (postinfectious
  polyneuropathy)
 sensory syndromes 115
Pons
 anatomy 94f
 lesions 118
Porphyria
 acute intermittent 253–254
 paraneoplastic polyneuropathy 184

Positron emission tomography (PET),
  intracranial tumours 219
Posterior cerebral artery (PCA) 58, 58f,
  203f, 204f
 distribution 204f
 occlusion 205–206
 temporal lobes 36
 thromboembolism 62
Posterior communicating artery 58f,
  203f, 204f
Posterior inferior cerebellar artery
  syndrome 206–207, 206f
Posterior semicircular canal 82f
Postherpetic neuralgia 156
Postictal period 131
Postinfectious polyneuropathy
  see Guillain–Barré syndrome
  (postinfectious polyneuropathy)
Post-polio syndrome 233
 motor neuron disease vs. 171
Post-traumatic headache 51f
Postural hypotension 40, 86
Postural tremor 98f, 99
Posture
 cerebellar dysfunction 94
 motor system assessment 18
 Parkinson's disease 147, 147f
Potassium 27f
Pott's disease (spinal tuberculosis) 229
Power, motor system assessment 19
PPRF (parapontine reticular formation)
  66–67
Pramipexole 148
Prednisolone
 cluster headache therapy 141
 giant-cell arteritis therapy 143
Prefrontal cortex 34f
 frontal lobes 33
Pregnancy, antiepileptic drugs 136
Premotor cortex 34f
 frontal lobes 33
Prenatal factors, epilepsy 132
Presbycusis, cochlea 83
Presenting complaint, history taking
  3–5
Primary cardiac dysfunction, syncope
  40–41
Primary cardiomyopathies 246f
Primary central nervous system
  lymphoma 215–216
 HIV infection 231
Primary dystonia 100
Primary focal dystonia 98f
Primary generalized dystonia 98f
Primary intracerebral haemorrhage 207
Primary lateral sclerosis (PLS) 169, 170
Primary motor cortex 34f
 frontal lobes 33
Primary muscular atrophy (PMA) 169
Primary neurodegenerative dementia
  128–130

Primary neurodegenerative diseases, dementia *vs.* 125
Primary progressive multiple sclerosis 238
Primary somatosensory cortex 34*f*
  parietal lobes 35
Primary tics 98*f*
Primary visual cortex 34*f*
Primitive reflexes, frontal lobe lesions 35
Prion disease 234–235
  cerebellar dysfunction 95*f*
  see also specific diseases/disorders
Procaine penicillin 231
Procyclidine 148
Prodrome 131
Progressive bulbar palsy 170
Progressive headache 50
Progressive multifocal leucoencephalopathy (PML) 241
  HIV infection 231
Progressive muscular atrophy (PMA) 169
  differential diagnosis 171
Progressive myoclonic epilepsy 102
Progressive supranuclear palsy 149
Prolactinomas 216
Proprioception pathways, spinal cord 159
Protein C 26*f*
Protein S 26*f*
Proximal weakness 104
Pseudobulbar palsy 170
  differential diagnosis 171
  dysarthria 89
Pseudodementia 130
Psychiatric features, Parkinson's disease 147
Psychosis, Parkinson's disease treatment 148
Ptosis
  assessment 12, 14*f*
  senile 14*f*
Pupil(s)
  bilateral fixed 45
  coma 45
  dilated 45
  Holmes–Adie 66
  large dilated 66
  mydriatic 66
  small constricted 65
Pupil assessment 12–13
  accommodation 13
  light responses 12–13
  size and shape 12
Pupil disorders 63–74
  differential diagnosis 64–66
  relative afferent 66
  see also specific diseases/disorders
Pupil reflexes 63–64

accommodation reflex 64
parasympathetic pathway 63, 64*f*
sympathetic pathway 63–64, 64*f*
Pursuit eye movements 13, 14
Pursuit gaze 66
Pyramidal hypertonia assessment 18–19
Pyramidal-pattern weakness 105
Pyramidal weakness 104
Pyridostigmine 191

Q

Quadrantanopia 59, 62
Quadriparesis 161
Quadriplegia 161

R

Radial nerve compression 181, 182*f*
Radiculopathies 109, 173–175
  clinical features 174
  definition 173
  LMN limb weakness 108
  see also specific diseases/disorders
Radiography 29
Radiotherapy
  induced brachial plexopathies 176
  intracranial tumour treatment 219
  neurotoxicity 221
Raised intracranial pressure
  headache 141
  herniation 141, 142*f*
  intracranial tumours 217–218
  treatment 219
Ramsay–Hunt syndrome 156–157
Rasagiline 148
Rebound phenomenon 23
Recall tests, Mini-Mental State Examination 7, 8*f*
Receptive dysphasia 10*f*
  Wernicke's area lesion 10
Recurrent episodic headache 49
  causes 50*f*
Red nuclear 'rubral' tremor 99
Red nucleus 146*f*
Referred pain, headache 49, 50*f*
Reflexes
  motor system assessment 19, 22*f*, 23*f*
  myasthenia gravis 189–190
  myopathies 193
  primitive 35
  spinal cord transection 161
Registration, Mini-Mental State Examination 7, 8*f*
Rehabilitation, stroke management 208
Relapsing and remitting multiple sclerosis 237
Relative afferent pupillary defects 66

Renal disorders 245
  peripheral neuropathies 183
  see also specific diseases/disorders
Respiratory pattern, coma 45
Responsivity, history taking 3
Resting tremor 97–98, 98*f*
Restless legs syndrome 151
Retina
  fundoscopy 13*f*
  ischaemia 62
  lesions 59
  light stimulation path 57, 58*f*
Retinal arteries 13*f*
Retinal veins 13*f*
Retrobulbar neuritis, multiple sclerosis 238–239
Review of systems (ROS), history taking 4
Rheumatoid arthritis 246*f*
Rheumatoid factor 27*f*
Rhine's test 81
Rigidity
  Parkinson's disease 146, 146*f*
  spasticity *vs.* 146*f*
Riluzole 171
Risk factors, history taking 3
Rivastigmine 128
Rods 57
Rolandic (central) fissure 34*f*
Romberg's test 119, 179
Ropinirole 148
ROS (review of systems), history taking 4
Round window 82*f*

S

Saccadic eye movements 13, 14–15
  cerebellar dysfunction 93
Saccule 82*f*
Sacral plexus anatomy 173
Saddle anaesthesia 106*f*, 107
Sarcoidosis 245, 246*f*
Saturday-night palsy 180
Scars, motor system assessment 18
SCDC (subacute combined degeneration of the cord) 165–166
Schwann cells 177
Schwannomas (acoustic neuromas) 157, 216, 217*f*
  vestibular *see* Vestibular schwannoma
Sciatica, lateral lumbar disc protrusion 174–175
Sciatic nerve anatomy 173
Scleroderma 246*f*
Secondary dystonia 98*f*, 100–101
Secondary generalized seizures 134
Secondary headache 50*f*
Secondary progressive multiple sclerosis 237

Secondary tics 98f
Second cranial nerve see Optic nerve
    (cranial nerve II)
Segmental dystonia 99–100
Seizures 41
    absence 134
    atonic 134
    classification 131, 132f
    complex partial 133–134
    epileptic 131
    focal 34
    frontal lobe 133f
    functional, epilepsy vs. 135
    generalized see Generalized seizures
    generalized tonic-clonic 134
    intracranial tumours 218
    myoclonic 134
    non-epileptic see Non-epileptic
        seizures
    parietal lobe 133f
    partial see Partial seizures
    secondary generalized 134
    simple partial 133
    syncope vs. 40f
    tonic 134
    toxins 248f
    treatment 219
Selegiline 148
Senile ptosis 14f
Sensorineural deafness 81, 82–83
Sensory ataxia 179
    gait 120
Sensory loss, face see Facial sensory loss
Sensory system
    LMN limb weakness 108
    neurological examination 23–24
Sensory testing 23
    facial nerve assessment 16
    glossopharyngeal nerve assessment
        17
    trigeminal nerve assessment 16
    vagus nerve assessment 17
Septic arthritis 164
Serology
    encephalitis 227
    meningitis 225
    syphilis diagnosis 230
Serum acetylcholine receptor,
    myasthenia gravis 190
Seventh cranial nerve see Facial nerve
    (cranial nerve VII)
Shape, pupil assessment 12
Simple partial seizures 133
Single photon emission computed
    tomography (SPECT),
    Parkinson's disease 147
Situational syncope 40
Sixth cranial nerve see Abducens nerve
    (cranial nerve VI)
Size, pupil assessment 12
Sjogren's syndrome 246f

Skull
    fractures 77
    plain radiography 29
SLE (systemic lupus erythematosus)
    246f
Sleep deprivation, epilepsy causes 133
Small anterior lobe, cerebellum 93
Small constricted (miotic) pupil 65
Smell disorders 53–56
    differential diagnosis 53–54
    examination 54–55
    investigations 55
    see also specific diseases/disorders
Smoking, stroke 202
Snellen charts 11, 11f
Social disinhibition
    affect evaluation 7
    frontal lobe lesions 34
Social history, history taking 4–5
SOD-1 (superoxide dismutase-1 gene)
    170
Sodium 27f
Sodium valproate, teratogenicity 136
Somatosensory evoked potentials,
    multiple sclerosis 240
Somatosensory information, parietal
    lobes 35
Space occupying lesions, optic
    neuropathy 60f
Spastic dysarthria (Donald Duck voice)
    170
Spastic gait 120
Spasticity
    assessment 18–19
    multiple sclerosis 241f
    rigidity vs. 146f
    UMN limb weakness 105
Spastic paraparesis 106, 107f, 160–161
    causes 107f
Spastic tetraparesis 161
SPECT (single photon emission
    computed tomography),
    Parkinson's disease 147
Speech assessment 8–10
    articulation 9
    language production 9–10
    phonation 8–9
Speech, Parkinson's disease 146
Sphenoid sinus, cavernous sinus 77f
Sphincter pupillae muscle 63
Spinal arachnoiditis 229
Spinal canal stenosis 163
Spinal cord
    anatomy 159, 160f
    anterior lesions 116
    central lesions 117
    cervical 160f
    hemisection 116–117
    limb sensory symptoms 115f,
        116–117
    pathways 159–161

    motor 160
    pain 159
    proprioception 159
    temperature 159
    vibration 159
    posterior lesions 116
    tetraparesis 105
    transection see below
    vascular diseases 212–213, 212f
Spinal cord compression 162–164
    causes 163–164
        degenerative disease 163
        spastic paraparesis 107f
Spinal cord diseases 159–168
    causes 161–167
    clinical syndromes 160–161
    compression see above
    copper deficiency 166
    inflammation 162–164
    lesions see below
    metabolic/toxic disease 165–166
    see also specific diseases/disorders
Spinal cord lesions
    intrinsic lesions 166–167, 166f
    limb sensory symptoms 115–117,
        116f
    multiple sclerosis 239
Spinal cord transection 115f, 116,
    161–162
    differential diagnosis 162
    reflexes 161
    spinal shock 161
    treatment 162
Spinal nerve root(s)
    anatomy 173, 174f
    dorsal roots 173
    nomenclature 173, 174f
    ventral (anterior) 173
    ventral (anterior) roots 173
Spinal nerve root lesions
    limb sensory symptoms 115, 115f
    see also Radiculopathies
Spinal shock, spinal cord transection
    161
Spinal tuberculosis (Pott's disease) 229
Spine
    intramedullary arteriovenous
        malformations 165
    plain radiography 29
Spinocerebellar ataxia 253
Spinocerebellar degeneration, ataxias
    253
Spinocerebellum (anterior superior
    vermis) 93
Spinothalamic pathway, limb sensory
    symptoms 113, 114f
Spirometry, myasthenia gravis 191
Spondylotic disease 163
Sporadic Creutzfeldt–Jakob disease 234
SSPE (subacute sclerosing
    panencephalitis) 241

Stapes 82f
Statins, side effects 199
Status epilepticus 137
    definition 131
Steppage gait 120–121
Stereotactic brain biopsy, intracranial
    tumours 219
Storage disorders, dementia vs. 125
Strabismus 67
Stroke
    aetiology 202
    definition 201
    differential diagnosis 202f
    haemorrhagic see Intracranial
        haemorrhage (haemorrhagic
        stroke)
    incidence 201
    investigations 207–208
    ischaemic 201
    lacunar 206
    management 208
    monoparesis 107
    prognosis 209
    risk factors 202–203
    types of 201, 202f
Stupor, consciousness evaluation 7
Sturge–Weber syndrome 252, 253f
Subacute combined degeneration of the
    cord (SCDC) 165–166
Subacute-onset headache 50
    causes 51f
Subacute sclerosing panencephalitis
    (SSPE) 241
Subarachnoid haemorrhage 209–210
    acute-onset headache 52f
Subdural haematoma 210
    subacute-onset headache 51f
Subdural haemorrhage 210–211
Substantia nigra
    anatomy 146f
    Parkinson's disease 145
Sudden unexpected death in epilepsy
    (SUDEP) 137–138
SUDEP (sudden unexpected death in
    epilepsy) 137–138
Sumatriptan 141
Superior colliculus anatomy 146f
Superior medullary vellum anatomy
    94f
Superior oblique muscles 67
Superior recti muscle 67
Superoxide dismutase-1 gene (SOD-1)
    170
Supplementary motor cortex 34f
    frontal lobes 33
Supportive care, subarachnoid
    haemorrhage 210
Supranuclear lesions
    facial sensory loss 76
    sensorineural deafness 83
Supranuclear palsy, progressive 149

Surgery
    epilepsy causes 132
    intracranial tumour treatment 219
    Parkinson's disease treatment 148
Sylvian fissure 34f
Sympathetic pathway, pupillary reflexes
    63–64, 64f
Symptomatic myoclonus 102
Symptoms, history taking 3
Syncope 39–41
    carotid sinus disease 41
    cough 40
    differential diagnosis
        epilepsy vs. 135
        seizures vs. 40f
    micturition 40
    postural hypotension 40
    primary cardiac dysfunction 40–41
    situational 40
    vasovagal syncope (fainting) 39
Syphilis 229–231
    associated conditions 230
    diagnosis 230–231
    meningovascular 230
    neurological 230–231
    treatment 231
Syringobulbia 166–167, 166f
Syringomyelia 166–167, 166f
Systemic diseases 243–246
    see also specific diseases/disorders
Systemic lupus erythematosus (SLE)
    246f

T

Tabes dorsalis 230
Tacrine 128
Tapping test 17
Tardive dyskinesia 150–151
Tardive dystonia 100–101
Taste disorders 53–56
    differential diagnosis 53–54
    examination 54–55
    investigations 55
    see also specific diseases/disorders
Taste, facial nerve assessment 16
TBM see Tuberculous meningitis (TBM)
Temperature assessment 24
Temperature pathways, spinal cord
    159
Temporal arteritis see Giant-cell arteritis
    (temporal arteritis)
Temporal lobes 34f, 36
    blood supply 36
    function 36
    lesions 36, 37f
Temporal lobe, seizures 133f
Tendon reflexes
    LMN limb weakness 108
    UMN limb weakness 105
Tensilon test, myasthenia gravis 190

Tension-type headache 139
    causes 50f
Tenth cranial nerve see Vagus nerve
    (cranial nerve X)
Teratogenicity, antiepileptic drugs 136
Terminology, history taking 3
Tetraparesis 105–106, 160, 161
    spastic 161
Tetraplegia 161
Thalamus, lesions 117f, 118
Thiamine deficiency see Vitamin B_1
    (thiamine) deficiency
Third cranial nerve see Oculomotor
    nerve (cranial nerve III)
Thoracic outlet syndrome 176
Thoracic spinal cord 160f
Thromboembolism, posterior cerebral
    artery 62
Thrombolysis, stroke management 208
Thrombophilias 244
Thrombotic thrombocytopenic purpura
    (TTP) 244
Thymectomy, myasthenia gravis
    management 191
Thymus imaging, myasthenia gravis 191
Thyroid function tests 27f
Thyroid-stimulating hormone (TSH)
    27f
Thyrotoxicosis, myopathies 198
Thyroxine (T_4) 27f
TIAs see Transient ischaemic attacks
    (TIAs)
Tibial nerve anatomy 173
Tic douloureux (trigeminal neuralgia)
    155–156
Tics 98f, 101–102
    primary 98f
    secondary 98f
Tinnitus 81
    causes 83f
    differential diagnosis 83–84
Tolcapone 148
Tone
    LMN limb weakness 108
    motor system assessment 18–19
Tongue, weakness patterns 18f
Tonic-clonic seizures, generalized 134
Tonic seizures 134
Tonsillar herniation 217, 218f
Topographic disorientation, parietal
    lobe lesions 36
Toxicity, antiepileptic drugs 136
Toxins 248, 248f
    cerebellar dysfunction 95f
    epilepsy causes 132
    optic neuropathy 60f
    peripheral neuropathies 184, 187f
Toxoplasmosis, central nervous system
    231
T. pallidum haemagglutination assay
    (TPHA) 230

T. pallidum particle agglutination assay (TPPA) 230
Transient ischaemic attacks (TIAs) 202*f*
  causes 203, 205*f*
  clinical features 205*f*
  definition 201
  differential diagnosis 202*f*
    epilepsy *vs.* 135
  investigations 207–208
  management 208–209
Transient visual impairment, acute 61
Transverse myelitis 165
Trauma
  brachial plexopathies 175
  cerebellar dysfunction 95*f*
  epilepsy causes 132
  peripheral neuropathies 187*f*
  spastic paraparesis 107*f*
Tremor 97, 98*f*
  cerebellar *see* Intention tremor (cerebellar tremor)
  dystonic 99
  essential 99
  intention *see* Intention tremor (cerebellar tremor)
  kinetic 97, 98*f*, 99
  mixed 99
  multiple sclerosis 241*f*
  neuropathic 99
  parkinsonian 97
  Parkinson's disease 146
  pathological 97
  physiological 97, 99
  postural 98*f*, 99
  red nuclear 'rubral' 99
  resting 97–98, 98*f*
  toxins 248*f*
Trigeminal nerve (cranial nerve V) 75
  anatomy 76*f*
  assessment 15–16
  clinical syndromes 16*f*
  cutaneous distribution 76*f*
  headache 49
  lesions 77, 154*f*, 155–156, 155*f*
  mandibular branch (V₃) 75
  maxillary branch (V₂) 75
  ophthalmic branch (V₁) 75
Trigeminal neuralgia (tic douloureux) 155–156
Trochlear nerve (cranial nerve IV)
  anatomy 71*f*
  assessment 12–15
  cavernous sinus 77*f*
  lesions 72*f*, 154–155, 154*f*
    binocular diplopia 69
Trophic skin changes, limb sensory symptoms 113–114
TTP (thrombotic thrombocytopenic purpura) 244
Tuberculin testing 229
Tuberculomas 164, 229

Tuberculosis 229
Tuberculous meningitis (TBM) 224, 229
  treatment 226
Tuberous sclerosis 252, 252*f*
Tumours
  brachial plexopathies 176
  cerebellar dysfunction 95*f*
  dementia *vs.* 125
  extradural 164
  intracranial *see* Intracranial tumours
  intradural 164
  intramedullary 163
  nerve sheath 216
  peripheral neuropathies 187*f*
  spinal cord compression 163–164
Twelfth cranial nerve *see* Hypoglossal nerve (cranial nerve XII)
Two-point discrimination, assessment 24
Tympanic membrane 82*f*

U

Ulcers 113–114
Ulnar nerve compression 180–181, 181*f*
Ultrasonography, duplex 30
Uncal herniation 217, 218*f*
Unmyelinated axons 57
Upper motor neuron (UMN) lesions 170*f*
  dysarthria 9, 89–90
  limb weakness 21*f*
Upper motor neuron (UMN) pathway 103, 104*f*
  limb weakness 104–105
Urea 27*f*
Utricle 82*f*

V

Vaccination, poliomyelitis 233
Vagus nerve (cranial nerve X)
  assessment 17
  headache 49
  lesions 154*f*, 158
Variant Creutzfeldt–Jakob disease 234
Vasa nervorum 178*f*
Vascular dementia 129
Vascular diseases/disorders 201–214
  dementia *vs.* 125
  epilepsy 132
  intracranial tumours 220
  optic neuropathy 60*f*
  spastic paraparesis 107*f*
  spinal cord 212–213, 212*f*
  see also specific diseases/disorders
Vascular spinal cord lesions, 164–165

Vasculitides 245
  peripheral neuropathies 183–184
  see also specific diseases/disorders
Vasculitis 130
  cerebrovascular disease 211
  peripheral neuropathies 187*f*
Vasovagal syncope (fainting) 39
Venous sinus thrombosis, subacute-onset headache 51*f*
Ventral (anterior) spinal nerve roots 173
VEPs *see* Visual evoked potentials (VEPs)
Verapamil 141
Vertebral artery 203*f*, 204*f*
  occlusion 206–207
Vertebrobasilar ischaemia 41–42
Vertical gaze palsy 71–72
Vertical nystagmus 73
Vertigo
  differential diagnosis 84–86, 85*f*
  investigations 86–87
  vestibular nerve lesions 85
  vestibular system disorders 84
Vestibular cortex, temporal lobes 36
Vestibular failure, acute 158
Vestibular schwannoma 217*f*
  deafness/tinnitus 81
Vestibular system 84
  anatomy 82*f*
  vestibulocochlear nerve assessment 17
Vestibular system disorders
  clinical features 84
  examples 84–85
  nerve lesions 85–86
  neuronitis 85–86
  see also specific diseases/disorders
Vestibule 82*f*
Vestibulocochlear nerve (cranial nerve VIII)
  assessment 17
  deafness/tinnitus 81, 82*f*
  lesions 154*f*, 157–158, 157*f*
  trauma, deafness/tinnitus 83*f*
Vibration assessment 24
Vibration pathways, spinal cord 159
Viral encephalitis 95*f*
Viral infections
  transverse myelitis 165
  see also specific infections
Viral meningitis 224
  treatment 226
Visual acuity assessment 11, 11*f*
Visual agnosia 38
Visual cortex
  blood supply 58*f*
  primary 34*f*
Visual evoked potentials (VEPs) 29
  multiple sclerosis 240
Visual field(s)
  assessment 11
  peripheral assessment 11–12

Visual field defects 58–59, 58*f*
  binocular 59
  monocular 59
  optic nerve lesions 153
Visual illusions 38
Visual impairment 57–62
  acute 61–62
  acute transient 61
  binocular 61
  diabetes mellitus 243
  differential diagnosis 60–62
  giant-cell arteritis (temporal arteritis) 142
  lesion localization 59–60
  monocular 61
  parietal lobe lesions 35
  temporal lobe lesions 36
Visual information, parietal lobes 35
Visual pathways 57–58, 58*f*
  blood supply 58*f*
  parietal lobes 35
Vitamin deficiency 247–248
  cerebellar dysfunction 95*f*
Vitamin B$_1$ (thiamine) deficiency 247
  peripheral neuropathies 185

Vitamin B$_3$ (nicotinic acid) deficiency 248
Vitamin B$_6$ (pyridoxine) deficiency 247
  peripheral neuropathies 185
Vitamin B$_{12}$ deficiency 242, 247–248
  peripheral neuropathies 185
  subacute combined degeneration of the cord 165
Vitamin B$_{12}$, testing 26*f*
Vitamin D deficiency 248
  myopathies 198
Vitamin E deficiency 248
  peripheral neuropathies 185
Von Recklinghausen's disease (neurofibromatosis type 1) 251–252, 252*f*

W

Wallenberg's syndrome 206–207, 206*f*
Wallerian degeneration 177
Wasting, hereditary neuropathies 186, 186*f*
WBC (white cell count) 26*f*
Weakness, myopathies 193

Weber's syndrome 207
Weber's test 82
Wegener's granulomatosis 246*f*
Wernicke–Korsakoff syndrome 247
Wernicke's area 34*f*
  lesions, receptive dysphasia 10
  temporal lobes 36
Wernicke's receptive (fluent) dysphasia
  parietal lobe lesions 35
  temporal lobe lesions 36
White cell count (WBC) 26*f*
Wilson's disease (hepatolenticular degeneration) 150, 254
Writer's cramp 100

X

X-linked myopathies 194
X-rays 29

Z

Zidovudine (AZT), side effects 199
Ziehl–Neelsen stain 225